Dentistry: A Case-Based Approach

Dentistry: A Case-Based Approach

Editor: Preston Bailey

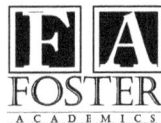

FA FOSTER
A C A D E M I C S

www.fosteracademics.com

www.fosteracademics.com

F A
FOSTER
ACADEMICS

Cataloging-in-Publication Data

Dentistry : a case-based approach / edited by Preston Bailey.
    p. cm.
Includes bibliographical references and index.
ISBN 978-1-63242-614-7
1. Dentistry. 2. Dentistry--Case studies. 3. Oral medicine. 4. Teeth.
I. Bailey, Preston.
RK51 .D46 2019
617.6--dc23

Foster Academics,
118-35 Queens Blvd., Suite 400,
Forest Hills, NY 11375, USA

ISBN 978-1-63242-614-7 (Hardback)

Contents

Preface

Over the recent decade, advancements and applications have progressed exponentially. This has led to the increased interest in this field and projects are being conducted to enhance knowledge. The main objective of this book is to present some of the critical challenges and provide insights into possible solutions. This book will answer the varied questions that arise in the field and also provide an increased scope for furthering studies.

The diagnosis and treatment of diseases and disorders of the oral cavity is under the scope of dentistry. Many systemic diseases occur with symptoms, which manifest in the orofacial region. The mouth can also be affected by gastrointestinal and cutaneous conditions. The treatment of these involves restorative, prosthetic, endodontic and periodontal treatments and therapies. The diagnosis and examination of the oral cavity is done through radiographs or X-rays. Dentists can perform oral surgery procedures like dental implant placement and prescribe local anesthetics, antibiotics, fluorides, painkillers, sedatives/hypnotics and other medications for the treatment of various conditions of the neck and the head. This book aims to shed light on some of the unexplored aspects in the diagnosis and treatment of oral diseases and the recent researches in dentistry. The objective is to give a general view of the different techniques of dentistry and their applications. This book will prove to be immensely beneficial to students and researchers in this field.

I hope that this book, with its visionary approach, will be a valuable addition and will promote interest among readers. Each of the authors has provided their extraordinary competence in their specific fields by providing different perspectives as they come from diverse nations and regions. I thank them for their contributions.

Editor

Spindle Cell Hemangioma in the Mucosa of the Upper Lip

Kazuhiro Murakami ⓘ, **Kazuhiko Yamamoto** ⓘ, **Tsutomu Sugiura, and Tadaaki Kirita**

Department of Oral and Maxillofacial Surgery, Nara Medical University, Kashihara, Nara, Japan

Correspondence should be addressed to Kazuhiro Murakami; murakami@naramed-u.ac.jp

Academic Editor: Yuk-Kwan Chen

Spindle cell hemangioma (SCH) is a unique benign vascular lesion. We present a case of SCH in the upper lip of a 41-year-old woman. A submucosal nodular mass 30×20 mm in size was observed in the left upper lip. The mass developed 5 years earlier and enlarged after repeated ethanol injections. The mass was elastic firm, mobile, bluish in color, and well demarcated in magnetic resonance imaging. Under the clinical diagnosis of hemangioma, surgical excision was performed under local anesthesia. Microscopically, the lesion was composed of irregular cavernous spaces and multiple solid cellular areas. Cavernous spaces were filled with a mix of erythrocytes and organizing thrombi. The solid areas showed proliferation of spindle-shaped cells arranged haphazardly or in short interlacing fascicles. Immunohistochemically, most cells strongly reacted with vimentin. CD31, CD34, factor VIII, smooth muscle actin, and Wilms tumor-1 reacted with endothelial cells lining the cavernous spaces. The cells within solid areas consisted of mixed cell population with variable reaction for the markers except for factor VIII. From these findings, the diagnosis of SCH was made. Two years after surgery, no recurrence was noted. A review of SCH in the head and neck region is made.

1. Introduction

Spindle cell hemangioma (SCH) is a unique vascular lesion, which almost exclusively affects the dermis and subcutaneous tissues of the distal extremities. Perkins and Weiss named a solitary single tumor SCH and multifocal lesions crowded within the same region "spindle cell hemangiomatosis" [1]. More than 200 cases have been reported in the English literature until 2017; however, only 12 cases have been reported to have occurred in the soft tissues of the head and neck region in detail [1–12].

We present an additional case in the mucosa of the upper lip of a 47-year-old woman and review of the literature on SCH of the head and neck region.

2. Case Report

A 41-year-old woman presented with a mass on the left upper lip and difficulty in pronunciation. The mass developed after she bit the upper lip 5 years earlier. The volume of mass was not reduced; however, the patient complained of pain. One year after the development, she visited an otolaryngologist.

The mass was diagnosed as mucocele and aspirated. However, only blood was aspirated from this lesion, and the lesion's size was not reduced. Two years after aspiration, the size of mass increased, and she visited a plastic surgeon. The lesion was diagnosed as hemangioma by magnetic resonance imaging (MRI). Ethanol was injected into the lesion twice. Although the lesion was slightly reduced at the first injection, it did not change at the second. She consulted a dental clinic two years after the second injection and then was referred to our department.

Oral examination revealed a circumscribed submucosal single nodule, approximately 30×20 mm in size in the left upper lip. The overlying mucosa was smooth, with bluish discoloration. On palpation, the nodule was elastic firm and mobile (Figure 1). Cervical lymph nodes were not palpable. MRI revealed a relatively well-demarcated lesion in the left upper lip. The lesion showed low signal intensity on T1-weighted images; however, it had a high signal area suspecting the subacute bleeding image in the centre of tumor. The lesion showed mostly high signal intensity on T2-weighted images (Figure 2). Under the clinical diagnosis of hemangioma, surgical enucleation was performed under local anesthesia. The tumor

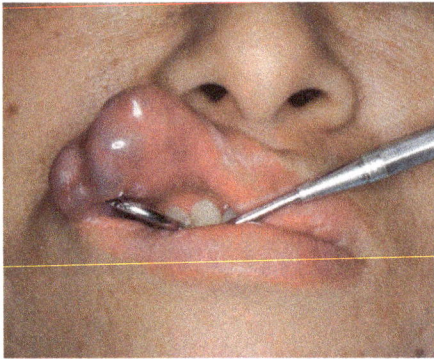

FIGURE 1: Clinical finding before surgery.

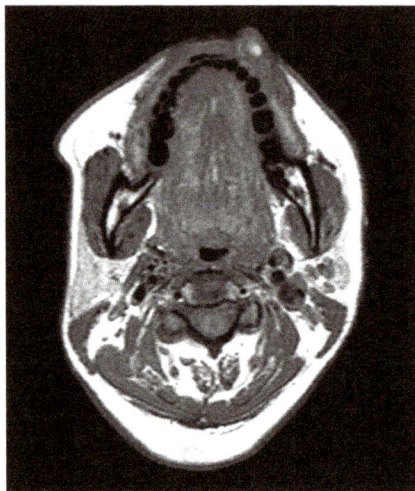

(a)

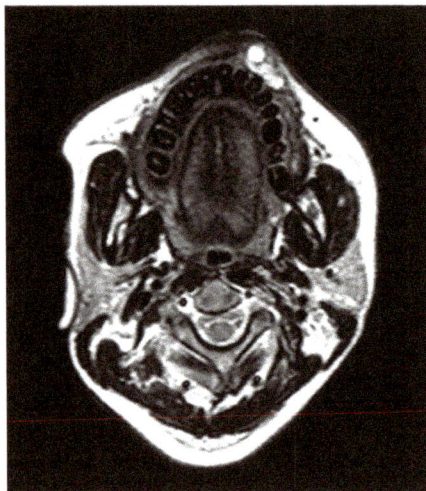

(b)

FIGURE 2: MRI findings. (a) T1-weighted image. (b) T2-weighted image.

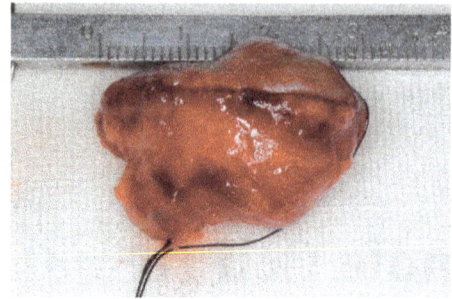

FIGURE 3: Excised tumor: lateral view.

The size of excised the lesion was 30×20 mm. The specimen had reddish brown surfaces covered by thin-walled capsule including the mucosa of partial lower lip and inflow blood vessels which were well demarcated. Microscopically, the lesion was a well-circumscribed mass surrounded by fibrous connective tissue and showed a variety of cellularity imparting a lobular architecture in low power (Figures 5(a)–5(c)). The lesion was characterized by irregular cavernous spaces and solid cellular areas. The cavernous spaces contained erythrocytes and were lined by a single layer of flattened endothelial cells. Large cavernous spaces were filled with a mix of erythrocytes and organizing thrombi. The solid areas showed proliferation of spindle cells arranged haphazardly or in short interlacing fascicles. Epithelioid cells were also seen, some of which contained large cytoplasmic vacuole.

Immunohistochemically, most endothelial cells lining the cavernous spaces, spindle cells within solid areas, and epithelioid cells within both areas strongly reacted with vimentin (Figures 6(a) and 6(b)). The endothelial cells lining the cavernous spaces reacted strongly with CD34 (Figure 7(a)), CD 31, factor VIII, smooth muscle actin (SMA) (Figure 8(a)), and Wilms tumor-1 (WT-1) (Figure 9(a)). The spindle cells within solid areas focally reacted with CD34 (Figure 7(b)), CD31, SMA (Figure 8(b)), and WT-1 (Figure 9(b)), whereas epithelioid cells were positive for SMA (Figure 8(b)), WT-1 (Figure 9(b)) and negative for CD34 (Figure 7(b)), CD31. S100 protein, AE1/AE3, D2-40, and EMA were negative in endothelial cells, epithelioid cells, and spindle cells. From these findings, the lesion was diagnosed as SCH.

3. Discussion

SCH has been diagnosed as various entities including mucocele, hemangioma, pyogenic granuloma, synovial sarcoma, and enchondroma (Table 1) [1–12]. In 1986, Weiss and Enzinger [13] described a unique vascular tumor as hemangioendothelioma with combined features of cavernous hemangioma and Kaposi's sarcoma. The tumor was considered to be an intermediate- or low-grade malignancy, with a biologic behavior between a hemangioma and an angiosarcoma. Fletcher et al. [14] proposed that hemangioendothelioma is caused by abnormalities of blood flow due to an arteriovenous shunt at the affected area, a view shared by some authors [15] and disputed by others [2]. Imayama et al. [16] suggested that hemangioendothelioma is

was removed with ligation and ablation of the inflow blood vessels. The overlying mucosa was partly removed, and the wound was closed by sutures (Figure 3). Postoperative course was uneventful. The patient was free of recurrence 2 years after surgery (Figure 4).

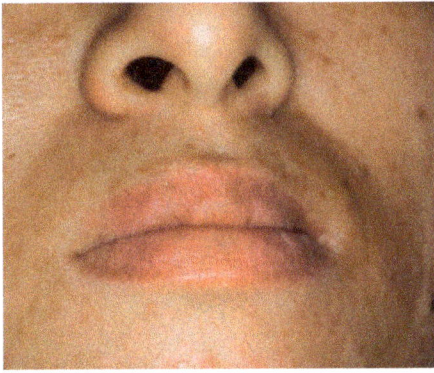

FIGURE 4: Clinical finding 6 months after surgery.

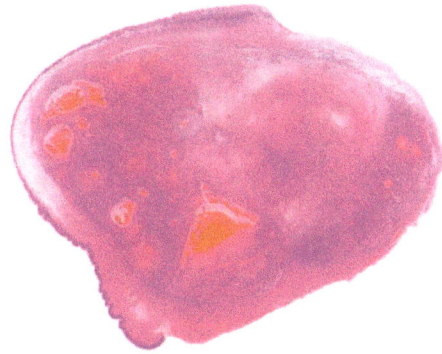

(a)

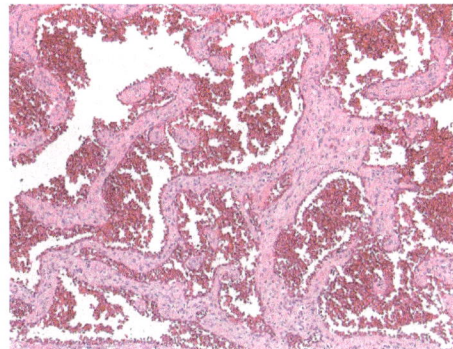

(b)

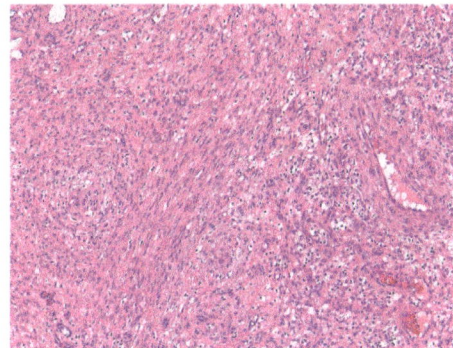

(c)

FIGURE 5: (a) Well-defined submucosal mass with cavernous spaces, solid areas, and number of thrombi. (hematoxylin and eosin stain, original magnification ×5). (b) Irregular cavernous spaces lined by flat endothelial cells. (hematoxylin and eosin stain, original magnification ×100). (c) The spindle-shaped cells in solid areas. (hematoxylin and eosin stain, original magnification ×100).

a reactive process associated with vascular damage. They also hypothesized that the behavior of the endothelium may facilitate thrombosis and that a cyclical process of repeated thrombosis and thrombus organization with new vascular proliferation may explain the pathogenesis of the lesion. Later, Perkins and Weiss [17] proposed the terms SCH for solitary lesions and "spindle cell hemangiomatosis" for multifocal lesions. Since then, SCH has been used for solitary lesions.

Approximately 10% of cases are associated with other developmental anomalies or syndromes, including early-onset varicose veins, lymphedema, Klippel-Trenaunay-Weber syndrome, Maffucci syndrome, epithelioid hemangioendothelioma, and superficial cutaneous lymphatic malformations [8].

SCH is relatively uncommon. Only 12 cases have been reported in the soft tissues of the head and neck region (Table 1) [1–12]. Most cases were clinically diagnosed as intraoral vascular neoplasms, which are benign entities, including pyogenic granuloma, fibroma, peripheral giant cell granuloma, peripheral ossifying fibroma, inflammatory fibrous hyperplasia, and necrotizing ulcerative gingivitis [18]. In the majority of cases, the symptoms were not remarkable [18]. Most SCH lesions were fewer than 2 cm in size [3, 5, 7, 9, 11]. Only four cases in the head and neck region were more than 30 mm, including the present case, which was the only case of the oral lesion more than 30 mm. SCH may arise after trauma, such as repeated injections or surgical excision [17]. In the present case, the lesion developed by biting and enlarged by aspiration and repeated ethanol injection. MRI findings were consistent with those of any other hemangiomatous lesion. The lesion showed low signal intensity on T1-weighted images and high signal intensity in the majority of T2-weighted images. However, on T1-weighted image, high signal intensity was observed in the lesion's centre. The high signal intensity area is considered thrombi. The present case was diagnosed as hemangioma by clinical and MRI findings at first. The final diagnosis of SCH was made by histopathologic findings.

Histologically, SCH shows variable cellularity imparting a lobular architecture on low power. Large, ectatic, vascular spaces lined by flattened endothelial cells are frequently present. The cavernous spaces may contain calcified thrombi, referred to as phleboliths. Between the dilated vascular spaces, there is proliferation of spindle cells composed of endothelial cells, pericytes, and fibroblasts. The endothelial cells often have focal epithelioid features and show focal cytoplasmic vacuolization. Mitotic activity and atypia are low [11, 13].

SCHs resemble the features of Kaposi's sarcoma, such as male predominance and occasional multifocal growth. But Kaposi's sarcoma rarely contains cavernous vessels with thrombi and phleboliths and lacks epithelioid cells, and their spindle cells react for the endothelial marker CD34. On the other hand, SCH does not present the hyaline globules seen in Kaposi's sarcoma or express human herpes virus 8 latent nuclear antigen-1 [1, 17].

(a)

(b)

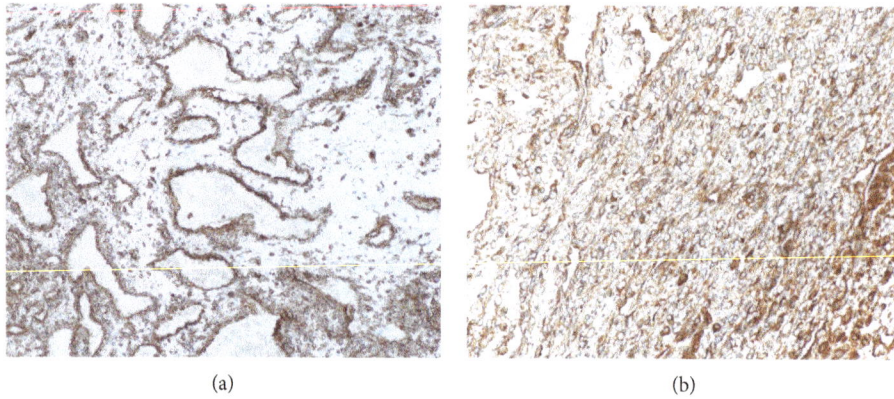

FIGURE 6: (a) Cavernous area (vimentin, original magnification ×100). Most endothelial cells around blood vessels in cavernous area strongly reacted. (b) Solid area (vimentin, original magnification ×200). Spindle cells and epithelioid in solid area are strongly positive.

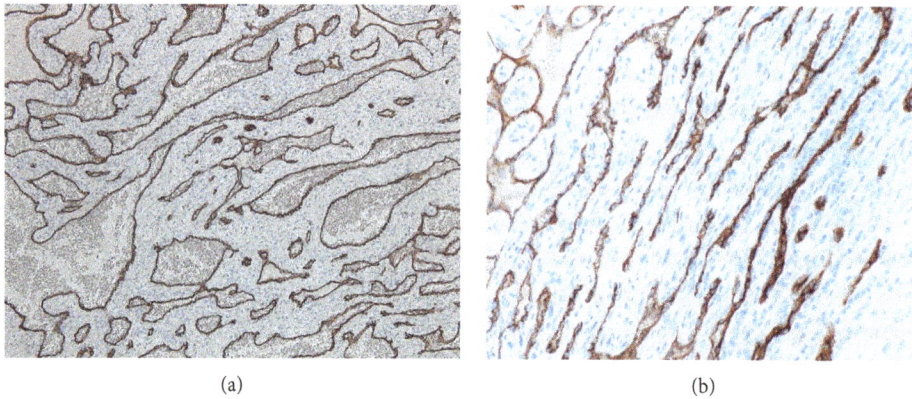

(a)

(b)

FIGURE 7: (a) Cavernous area (CD34, original magnification ×100). Most endothelial cells around vessels in cavernous space are positive. (b) Solid area (CD34, original magnification ×200). Spindle cells in solid area are focally positive.

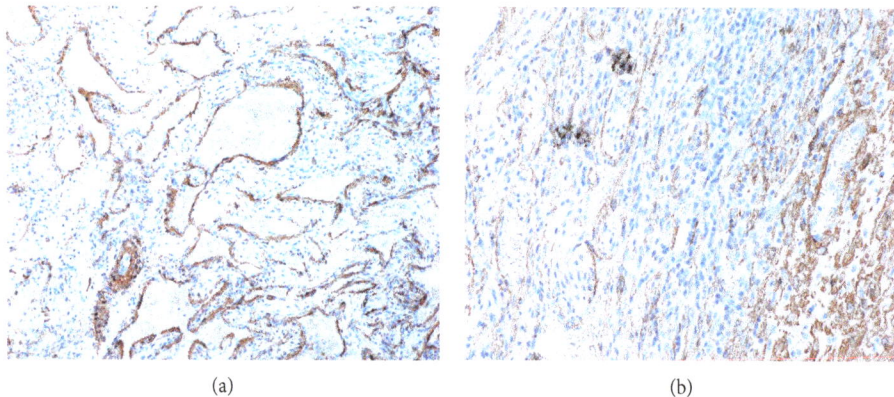

(a)

(b)

FIGURE 8: (a) Cavernous area (SMA, original magnification ×100). Most endothelial cells around vessels are positive. (b) Solid area (SMA, original magnification ×200). Spindle cells in solid area are focally positive.

Immunohistochemically, the cells lining the cavernous space and vacuolated epithelioid cells are positive for vimentin, CD31, CD34, and factor-VIII-related antigen, supporting the endothelial nature [1–3, 5, 7–9, 11, 12, 15]. Weiss and Enzinger [13], Tosios et al. [1], Ide et al. [5], and Cai et al. [9] reported that the lining cells and vacuolated epithelioid cells are positive for vimentin, CD31, CD34, and factor VIII, and in contrast, spindle cells are negative for endothelial markers. However, Sheehan et al. [7] and Chavva et al. [8] reported that spindle cells are positive for these markers. In the present case, spindle cells are focally positive for these markers, (Table 2) suggesting that the tumor's solid area is composed of a mixed cell population with CD31-, CD34-, and factor-VIII-related antigen-negative cells as well

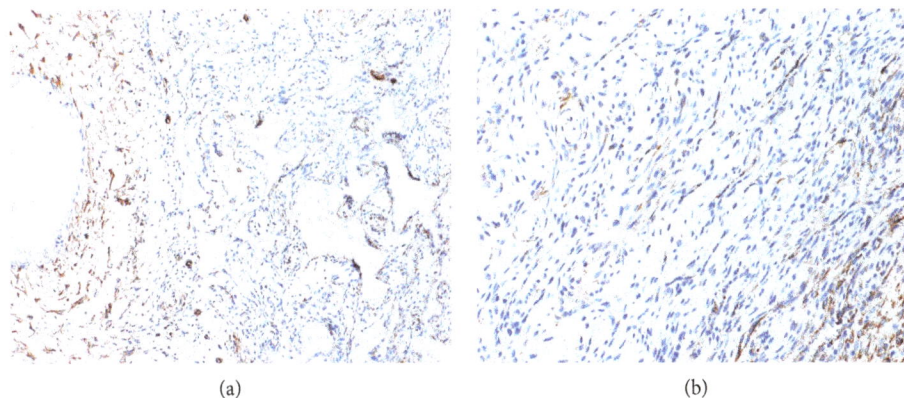

FIGURE 9: (a) Cavernous area (WT-1, original magnification ×100). Endothelial cells are strongly positive in cavernous area. (b) Solid area (WT-1, original magnification ×200). Spindle cells in solid area are focally positive.

TABLE 1: Main clinical features of 13 cases of spindle cell hemangioma of the head and neck.

Author	Age	Gender	Duration (months)	Site	Maximum size (cm)	Clinical diagnosis	Follow-up (months)
Tosios et al. [1]	29	Female	12	Upper lip	1	Mucocele	36FOD
Scott and Rosai [2]	70	Male	RP	Ear	NA	Cavernous hemangioma	NA
Tosios et al. [3]	12	Female	NA	Mandibular vestibule	1	Hemangioma or pyogenic granuloma	LFU
Baron et al. [4]	1.5	Male	13	Lateral nasal side wall	1	Hemangioma	24 recurrence
Ide et al. [5]	55	Male	3	Palate	1.2	Pyogenic granuloma	12FOD
Lade et al. [6]	25	Male	6	Posterior pharyngeal wall	6	Synovial sarcoma	48FOD
Sheehan et al. [7]	44	Male	NA	Buccal mucosa	1	Vascular tumor	13FOD
Chavva et al. [8]	33	Male	8	Oral floor	1	Minor salivary gland tumor	6FOD
Cai et al. [9]	34	Female	24	Lower lip	2	Enchondromas (Maffucci syndrome)	NA
Minagawa et al. [10]	67	Female	4	Temporal muscle	4	Vascular tumor	24FOD
French et al. [11]	52	Female	6	Tongue	2	Polypoid haemangiomatous lesion	24FOD
Gbolahan et al. [12]	9	Female	12	Orbit	8	Tumor in the inferolateral orbit	21FOD
Present case	41	Female	60	Upper lip	3	Hemangioma	24FOD

RP: recent presentation; NA: not available; FOD: free of disease; LFU: lost to follow-up.

as antigen-positive cells. SMA-positive pericytes reacted for both endothelial cells and spindle cells in all four reports including the present case which underwent this staining (Table 2). All cases which underwent staining with CD31, CD34, vimentin, and SMA (7, 8, 3, and 4 of 10 cases) were positive for endothelial cell, and all cases stained by vimentin and SMA were positive for both endothelial cells and spindle cells in (Table 2). Four of six cases stained by CD31 and five of seven cases stained by CD34 were positive for spindle cell. From these results, these markers were considered extremely sensitive markers in diagnosing SCH in the head and neck. S100, AE1/AE3, and EMA epithelial markers were negative in both cavernous and solid areas of two cases [9], including the present case; therefore, these makers may be not useful (Table 2). Tosios et al. [1] reported that CD 68, macrophage marker was positive; however, it was negative in the present case, and this marker's usefulness was not demonstrated (Table 2). Wang et al. [19] reported that SCH is a lymphatic malformation because D2-40 and Prox1 reacted in SCH. However, in the present case, D2-40 was negative, and Prox1 staining was impossible to conduct at our facility (Table 2).

From this result, we could not determine if SCH is a lymphatic malformation. The proliferating epitheloid and round endothelial cells were negative for WT-1, a marker for differentiating vascular neoplasia from vascular malformation, whereas the spindle cells were focally positive in Wang's cases. However, in the present case, WT-1 was focally positive at both endothelial cells in cavernous areas and spindle cells in solid areas. Although Wang et al. suggested that SCH is primarily a lymphatic malformation, we consider that SCH is a vascular lesion arising from a vascular malformation, composed of mixed cells, such as vascular and lymphatic cells from the immunochemical result of all the markers performed in this case and other literatures [1, 5, 7, 9, 11, 15, 17, 19].

Surgical excision is the standard treatment for SCH, with excellent prognosis. Although more than 50% of patients may develop new lesions in the same anatomic region several years after initial excision [1], these are not considered a recurrence but new primaries or continuous multifocal intravascular growth. Postoperative radiotherapy and administration of low-dose interferon α-2b and recombinant

TABLE 2: Immunohistochemical analysis of the SCH cases in head and neck in the literature.

Author	CD34		CD31		VIMENTIN		SMA		Factor VIII		CD68		S100		EMA		AE1/AE3		D2-40		WT-1	
	C	S	C	S	C	S	C	S	C	S	C	S	C	S	C	S	C	S	C	S	C	S
Tosios et al. [1]	+	+					+	+	+	+	+	+										
Scott and Rosai [2]	+		+						+	+												
Tosios et al. [3]					+	+																
Ide et al. [5]	+	–	+	–			+	+	+	–												
Sheehan et al. [7]	+	+	+	+																		
Chavva et al. [8]	+	+	+	+	+	+	+	+														
Cai et al. [9]	+	–	+	–	+		+	+					–	–			–	–	+			
French et al. [11]			+	+																–		
Gbolahan et al. [12]	+	+																				
Present case	+	+	+	+	+	+	+	+	+	–	–	–	–	–	–	–	–	–	–	–	+	+

C: cavernous area; S: solid area; (+): immunopositivity; (–): immunonegativity.

interleukin-2 were reported to be successful in inaccessible lesions [1]. On the contrary, Chavva et al. [8] reported that radiation therapy is contraindicated due to the danger of malignant transformation. The literature contains no reports of patient mortality or metastasis from SCH. Spontaneous regression has been reported [14]. In the present case, the lesion was surgically removed, and no recurrence was observed 2 years after surgery.

4. Conclusion

SCH is considered an unusual vascular lesion in the oral cavity. Awareness of clinical, histologic, and histochemical features is important for differential diagnosis of the lesion from more aggressive vascular tumors to avoid unnecessary treatment. Although the common size of SCH is less than 20 mm, the size of it is guessed to be increased to more than 30 mm by frequent stimulation. In the diagnosis of SCH in head and neck, it is considered CD 31, CD 34, vimentin, and SMA are beneficial. We suppose the surgical removal of SCH is appropriate treatment with good clinical outcome.

Acknowledgments

The authors thank Dr. Shuhei Yamashita, the president of Hattori memorial hospital, for perioperative management of the patient and Dr. Motokatsu Tsuyuki, the vice president of Hattori memorial hospital for histological examination.

References

[1] K. Tosios, I. Gouveris, A. Sklavounou, and I. G. Koutlas, "Spindle cell hemangioma (hemangioendothelioma) of the head and neck: case report of an unusual (or underdiagnosed) tumor," *Oral Surgery, Oral Medicine, Oral Pathology, Oral Radiology, and Endodontology*, vol. 105, pp. 216–221, 2008.

[2] G. A. Scott and J. Rosai, "Spindle cell hemangioendothelioma: report of seven additional cases of a recently described vascular neoplasm," *American Journal of Dermatopathology*, vol. 10, pp. 281–288, 1988.

[3] K. Tosios, I. G. Koutlas, N. Kapranos, and S. I. Papanicolaou, "Spindel-cell hemangioendothelioma of the oral cavity. A case report," *Journal of Oral Pathology and Medicine*, vol. 24, pp. 379–382, 1995.

[4] J. A. Baron, J. Raines, J. Bangert, and R. C. Hansen, "Persistent nodule on the nose," *Archives of Dermatology*, vol. 138, pp. 259–264, 2002.

[5] F. Ide, K. Obara, K. Enatsu, K. Mishima, and I. Saito, "Rare vascular proliferations of the oral mucosa," *Oral Surgery, Oral Medicine, Oral Pathology, Oral Radiology, and Endodontology*, vol. 97, pp. 75–78, 2004.

[6] H. Lade, N. Gupta, P. P. Singh, and G. Dev, "Spindle-cell hemangioendothelioma of the posterior pharyngeal wall," *Ear Nose Throat Journal*, vol. 84, pp. 362–365, 2005.

[7] M. Sheehan, S. O. Roumpf, D. J. Summerlin, and S. D. Billings, "Spindle cell hemangioma: report of a case presenting in the oral cavity," *Journal of Cutaneous Pathology*, vol. 34, pp. 797–800, 2007.

[8] S. Chavva, M. H. Priya, K. Garlapati, G. S. P Reddy, and A. Gannepalli, "Rare case of spindle cell haemangioma," *Journal of Clinical and Diagnostic Research*, vol. 9, pp. Z19–Z21, 2015.

[9] Y. Cai, R. Wang, X. M. Chen, Y. F. Zhao, Z. J. Sun, and J. H. Zhao, "Maffucci syndrome with the spindle cell hemangiomas in the mucosa of the lower lip: a rare case report and literature review," *Journal of Cutaneous Pathology*, vol. 40, no. 7, pp. 661–666, 2013.

[10] T. Minagawa, T. Yamao, and R. Shioya, "Spindle cell hemangioendothelioma of the temporal muscle resected with zygomatic osteotomy: a case report of an unusual intramuscular lesion mimicking sarcoma," *Case Reports in Surgery*, vol. 2011, Article ID 481654, 4 pages, 2011.

[11] K. E. M. French, M. Felstead, N. Haacke, J. Theaker, P. A. Brennan, and S. D. Colbert, "Spindle cell haemangioma of the tongue," *Journal of Cutaneous Pathology*, vol. 43, pp. 1025–1027, 2016.

[12] O. O. Gbolahan, O. Fasina, A. O. Adisa, and O. A. Fasola, "Spindle cell hemangioma: unusual presentation of an uncommon tumor," *Journal of Oral and Maxillofacial Pathology*, vol. 19, p. 406, 2015.

[13] S. W. Weiss and F. M. Enzinger, "Spindle cell hemangioendothelioma: a low grade angiosarcoma resembling a cavernous haemangioma and Kaposi's sarcoma," *American Journal of Surgical Pathology*, vol. 10, no. 8, pp. 521–530, 1986.

[14] C. D. M. Fletcher, A. Beham, and C. Schmid, "Spindle cell haemangioendothelioma: a clinicopathological and immunohistochemical study indicative of nonneoplastic lesion," *Histopathology*, vol. 18, no. 4, pp. 291–301, 1991.

[15] C. A. Harrison, J. R. Srinivasan, J. L. Stone, and R. E. Page, "Spindle cell haemangioendothelioma in an arteriovenous fistula of the ring finger after blunt trauma," *British Journal of Plastic Surgery*, vol. 56, no. 8, pp. 822–824, 2003.

[16] S. Imayama, Y. Murakami, H. Hashimoto, and Y. Hori, "Spindle hemangioendothelioma exhibits the ultrastructural features of reactive vascular proliferation rather than angiosarcoma," *American Journal of Clinical Pathology*, vol. 97, no. 2, pp. 279–287, 1992.

[17] P. Perkins and S. W. Weiss, "Spindle cell hemangioendothelioma: an analysis of 78 cases with reassessment of its pathogenesis and biologic behavior," *American Journal of Surgical Pathology*, vol. 20, no. 10, pp. 1196–1204, 1996.

[18] M. A. Grodon-Nunez, L. M. M. Silva, M. F. Lopes, S. F. Oliveria-Neto, A. P. Maia, and H. C. Galvao, "Intraoral epithelioid hemangioendothelioma: a case report and review of the literature," *Medicina Oral Patología Oral y Cirugia Bucal*, vol. 15, no. 2, pp. e340–346, 2010.

[19] L. Wang, T. Gao, and G. Wang, "Expression of Prox1, D2-40, and WT1 in spindle cell hemangioma," *Journal of Cutaneous Pathology*, vol. 41, no. 5, pp. 447–450, 2014.

Bite Reconstruction in the Aesthetic Zone Using One-Piece Bicortical Screw Implants

Stefan Ihde,[1] Łukasz Pałka (ID),[2] Maciej Janeczek (ID),[3] Piotr Kosior,[4] Jan Kiryk,[5] and Maciej Dobrzyński (ID)[4]

[1]Dental Implants Faculty, International Implant Foundation, 116 Leopold Street, 80802 Munich, Germany
[2]Reg-Med Dental Clinic, Rzeszowska 2, 68-200 Żary, Poland
[3]Department of Biostructure and Animal Physiology, Wroclaw University of Environmental and Life Sciences, Kożuchowska 1, 51-631 Wroclaw, Poland
[4]Department of Conservative Dentistry and Pedodontics, Wroclaw Medical University, Krakowska 26, 50-425 Wroclaw, Poland
[5]Private Dental Clinic Maciej Kozłowski, Spokojna 23, 56-400 Oleśnica, Poland

Correspondence should be addressed to Maciej Dobrzyński; maciej.dobrzynski@umed.wroc.pl

Academic Editor: Sukumaran Anil

The aim of this article was to present the clinical application of a new, smooth surfaced one-piece bicortical screw implant with immediate loading protocol. An 18-year-old, healthy male patient with a history of total dislocation and replantation of teeth 11 and 21 in early childhood was admitted to the clinic. Teeth 11 and 21 were extracted, and two long one-piece implants were inserted at extraction sockets in one surgical session under local anesthesia. Temporary composite crowns were placed in the patient on the same day. After 3 months, the single-phase two-layer impression was made and the composite crowns were replaced with metal-ceramic crowns. After 12 months, satisfactory aesthetic and functional results were obtained.

1. Introduction

Recently, immediate implant placement after tooth extraction with early loading has become a more common procedure, especially when the anterior teeth are missing. The advantages of this procedure include fewer surgical interventions, reduction in overall treatment time, reduced soft and hard tissue loss, and psychological satisfaction to the patient.

The aim of this article was to present the clinical application of a new, smooth surface, one-piece bicortical screw implant with immediate loading protocol. With its new design, it is now very simple to achieve durable reconstruction of function and a very good aesthetics [1]. The implant neck is bendable and the head can be ground, so there are no complications regarding the parallelism of the abutments. The paper reports the successful clinical case of immediate replacement of two frontal incisors with active fistula and periodontitis. The complete treatment

was conducted without bone or soft tissue augmentations and with minimal risk of peri-implantitis.

2. Case Report

An 18-year-old, healthy male patient with a history of total dislocation and replantation of teeth number 11 and 21 in early childhood was reported to the clinic. Due to heavy root resorption, active fistula, and severe atrophy of the alveolar ridge, mostly related to the vestibular cortical plate, a decision was made to extract the teeth and to use one-piece immediate loading smooth surface bicortical screw implants (Figure 1) [2–4]. Following soft tissue cleaning with antiseptic 5% Betadine® solution, teeth 11 and 21 were extracted under local anesthesia (citocartin 100 solution and articaine 4% with Adrenaline 1 : 100000). The procedure was performed atraumatically with the careful use of luxators (SDI®) and periotomes (Medessa®) to avoid damage of the continuity of the alveolar ridge. Extraction sockets were

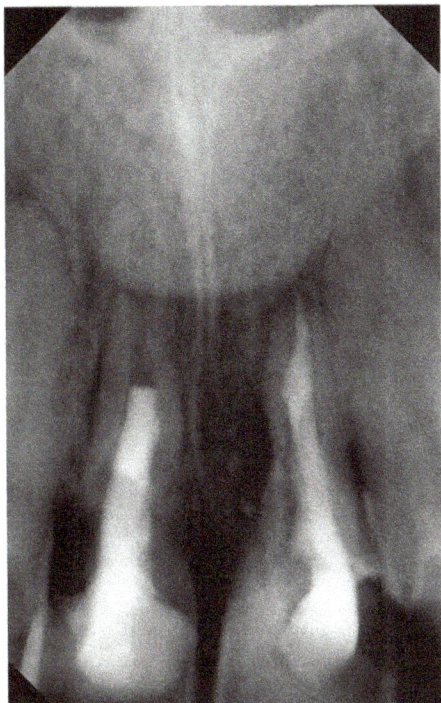

FIGURE 1: X-ray presenting severe root resorption of teeth 11 and 21.

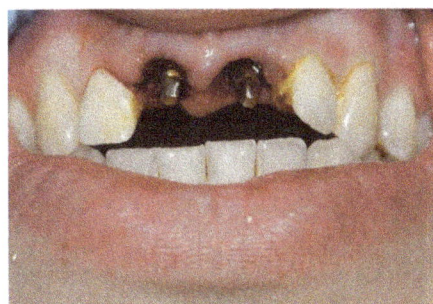

(a)

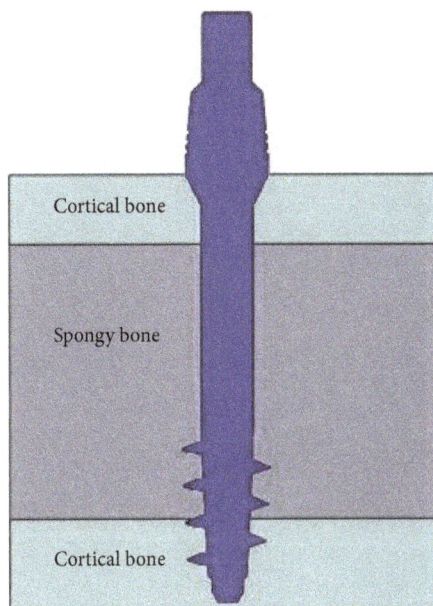

Cortical bone

Spongy bone

Cortical bone

(b)

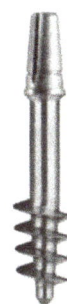

BCS®   IHDEDENTAL

(c)

FIGURE 2: Immediate implant placement after tooth extractions: (a) the photo of immediate implants in the mouth right after placement, (b) the scheme of immediate implant placement, and (c) the photo of immediate implant.

thoroughly debrided and granulation tissue removed. The edges of the gingival garlands were aligned using a scalpel. The preparation of osteotomy sites was carried out using the sequential order of calibrated drills recommended by the manufacturer, cooled with saline solution in external mode at a speed of 800 rpm. The implant beds were prepared with the use of a 2.0 mm drill (30 mm long) on a straight handpiece. Two long one-piece implants with a diameter of 3.5 and a length of 22 mm were placed and anchored in the second cortical in the floor of the nose with a perfect primary stability (Figures 2(a)–2(c)) [5]. The implants were inserted into the bone (with insertion torque of 35–40 Ncm) using hand tools to achieve primary stabilization. Postoperative intraoral periapical radiograph was taken, confirming the accuracy of placement of implants. The extraction socket and space between the implant and the bone was filled with collagen sponge (Spongostan). Abutments were attached to the implant body and prepared for parallelism and adequate space. At the same day, provisional composite crowns were placed in the patient for immediate replacement of the missing front teeth due to functional and aesthetic requirements (Figure 3) [6].

After 3 months, when the peri-implant tissues have healed, the single-phase two-layered impression (Panasel transfer polyvinyl siloxane mass, Kettenbach®) of implant transfers was made with closed tray technique. The composite crowns were replaced with metal-ceramic crowns and cemented with Fuji IX cement (Figures 4 and 5) [7]. Follow-up was done after 3-, 6-, and 12-month intervals. Comparison of pre- and postprocedure radiographs clearly revealed elevated peri-implant marginal bone in response to the action of loading forces [8, 9]. Very good aesthetic

result of this treatment was achieved by the preservation of gingival papillae (Figure 6).

3. Discussion

If chosen, in presented clinical case, conventional two-stage implantation (with or without immediate implant placement)

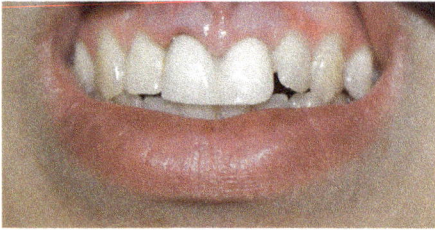

FIGURE 3: Temporary composite crown delivered on the same day. Still visible active fistula over tooth 11.

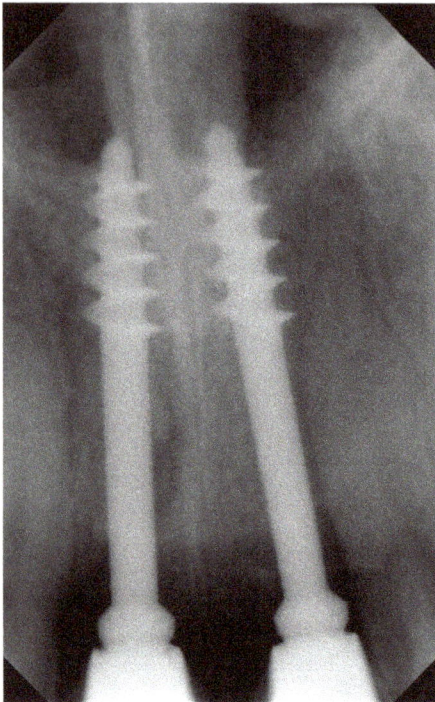

FIGURE 6: Good aesthetic after 12 months with papilla preservation.

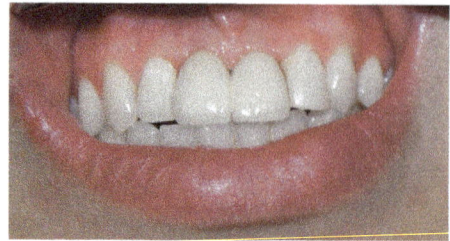

FIGURE 4: X-ray after 3 months with try-in metal-ceramic crowns.

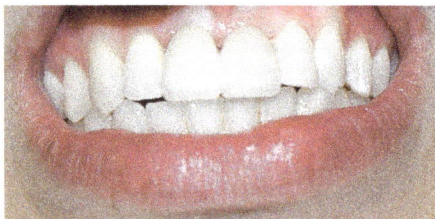

FIGURE 5: Metal ceramic crowns after cementation.

would require bone augmentation following teeth extraction. The aforementioned implant can be loaded after a minimum of 6 to 9 months. The main drawback of this treatment option is lack of predicting the bone modeling process after extraction as well as implant placement. The use of biomaterials for bone regeneration is highly risky because of ongoing active inflammation; it is time-consuming and expensive. Thinking of the long-term outcome, we particularly need to consider the possible direction of physiological atrophy of the maxillary alveolar bone and complications in a case

of implant surface exposure and its subsequent bacterial contamination [2].

The bicortical implant anchorage is an excellent treatment option, which allows us to predict the outcome of our treatment due to an anatomically stable position of at least one cortical bone (second or third). This type of bone does not undergo typical physiological changes and if damaged, its continuity will always be restored. The thin neck, penetrating the mucosa and polished surface of an implant, prevents bacterial contamination and peri-implantitis [2, 3, 10]. The transmission of load on the thread anchorage in the highly mineralized bone allows bone regeneration and (what is reserved only for bicortical, polished implants) regaining stabilization in case of sterile loosening of the implant. Even in case of bone resorption around the implant, it is possible to cutoff the head and replace it with a newly cemented abutment on the remaining implant neck.

According to the comparative studies of implantation using bicortical screws and two-phase implants (Integral Systems), patients experienced less postoperative discomfort in the case of the bicortical screws (less invasive treatment and no preparation of the periosteal flap) [11]. In clinical cases which did not require teeth extractions, patients were immediately provided (up to 3 days from the implantation procedure) with final prosthetic restorations of all types available on the market (metal-ceramic, metal-composite, and zirconium).

4. Conclusions

Clinical and radiographic evaluations after 12 months showed satisfactory preservation of marginal bone structure and peri-implant soft tissues condition as well as excellent aesthetic rehabilitation which is highly accepted by the patient. Our study revealed that final results and long-term success of immediately loaded one-piece implants were not different from conventional two-stage screw implants. The unquestionable benefits of bicortical implant use are the reduction of the number of visits, nonexistent need for regeneration procedures (and consequently costs reduction), and the possibility of immediate loading of the implanted screws due to optimal primary stabilization, which is obtained by placing the implants in the cortical bone. Regenerative procedures (including simultaneous implantation) are not required for this type of implants, but they can be implemented due to aesthetic or functional purposes. Despite the advantages of the use of bicortical implants allowing to achieve the immediate aesthetic rehabilitation, the risk of gingival recession and bone atrophy still exists. A sine qua non condition for a long-term prosthetic reconstruction based on bicortical implants, as well as for other types of restorations, is very good oral hygiene [3].

Acknowledgments

This work was supported by statutory research and development activity funds assigned to the Faculty of Veterinary Medicine, Wrocław University of Environmental and Life Sciences.

References

[1] S. Ihde, Ł. Pałka, E. Bryła, and M. Dobrzyński, "Całkowita rehabilitacja implantoprotetyczna szczęki i żuchwy za pomocą implantów bikortykalnych o natychmiastowym protokole obciążenia – opis przypadku," *Gerontologia Współczesna*, vol. 4, no. 1, pp. 15–18, 2016.

[2] F. Rossi, M. E. Pasqualini, L. Dal Carlo, M. Shulman, M. Nardone, and S. Winkler, "Immediate loading of maxillary one-piece screw implants utilizing intraoral welding: a case report," *Journal of Oral Implantology*, vol. 41, no. 4, pp. 473–475, 2015.

[3] C. L. Dal, S. Rossi, M. E. Pasqualini et al., "Intraoral welding and lingialized (lingual contact) occlusion: a case report," *Implants CE Magazine*, vol. 2, pp. 4–7, 2015.

[4] M. E. Pasqualini, D. Lauritano, F. Rossi et al., "Rehabilitations with immediate loading of one-piece implants stabilized with intraoral welding," *Journal of Biological Regulators and Homeostatic Agents*, vol. 32, no. 2, Supplement 1, pp. 19–26, 2018.

[5] K. Kirstein, M. Dobrzyński, P. Kosior et al., "Infrared thermographic assessment of cooling effectiveness in selected dental implant systems," *BioMed Research International*, vol. 2016, Article ID 1879468, 8 pages, 2016.

[6] G. M. Raghoebar, B. Friberg, I. Grunert, J. A. Hobkirk, G. Tepper, and I. Wendelhag, "3-year prospective multicenter study on one-stage implant surgery and early loading in the edentulous mandible," *Clinical Implant Dentistry and Related Research*, vol. 5, no. 1, pp. 39–46, 2003.

[7] L. Linkow, *The Legends of Implant Dentistry*, Jaypee Brothers Medical Publishers LTD, New Delhi, India, 2010.

[8] F. Ivanjac, V. S. Konstantinović, V. Lazić, I. Dordević, and S. Ihde, "Assessment of stability of craniofacial implants by resonant frequency analysis," *Journal of Craniofacial Surgery*, vol. 27, no. 2, pp. e185–e189, 2016.

[9] F. R. Verri, R. S. Cruz, C. A. A. Lemos et al., "Influence of bicortical techniques in internal connection placed in premaxillary area by 3D finite element analysis," *Computer Methods in Biomechanics and Biomedical Engineering*, vol. 20, no. 2, pp. 193–200, 2017.

[10] H. C. Han, H. C. Lim, J. Y. Hong et al., "Primary implant stability in a bone model simulating clinical situations for the posterior maxilla: an in vitro study," *Journal of Periodontal & Implant Science*, vol. 46, no. 4, pp. 254–265, 2016.

[11] M. Grotowska and T. Grotowski, "Ocena wyników leczenia implantoprotetycznego z zastosowaniem śruby bikortykalnej Garbaccia w badaniach 10-letnich część I," *Magazyn Stomatologiczny*, vol. 11, pp. 46–54, 2009.

3

Preaugmentation Soft Tissue Expansion: A Report of Four Pilot Cases

Farah Asa'ad [iD],[1] **Gionata Bellucci** [iD],[1] **Luca Ferrantino** [iD],[1] **Davide Trisciuoglio,**[1] **Silvio Taschieri** [iD],[2] **and Massimo Del Fabbro**[2]

[1]*Department of Biomedical, Surgical and Dental Sciences, Foundation IRCCS Ca' Granda Polyclinic, University of Milan, Milan, Italy*
[2]*Department of Biomedical, Surgical and Dental Sciences, IRCCS Galeazzi Orthopaedic Institute, University of Milan, Milan, Italy*

Correspondence should be addressed to Farah Asa'ad; farahasaad83@gmail.com

Academic Editor: Gerardo Gómez-Moreno

This pilot study aimed at investigating the safety and feasibility of pre-augmentation soft tissue expansion (STE). Tissue expanders of different sizes (from 240 to 1300 mm^3) were implanted subperiosteally in four patients requiring vertical and/or horizontal bone augmentation, and left in situ for 20–60 days, according to the expander size. Guided bone regeneration was carried out after STE completion. Horizontal and vertical bone gains were analyzed through CBCT. Optical scanning and superimposition of cast models were used for volumetric analysis. The mean soft tissue volume increase was 483.8 ± 251.7 mm^3. Horizontal bone gain averaged 3 mm in two successfully expanded sites while one case had a vertical bone gain of 8 mm. Despite promising outcomes in bone and soft tissue gain, the present technique needs improvement before being applied routinely in everyday dental practice.

1. Introduction

In modern dental practice, placement of endosseous implants is constantly increasing, as many patients are seeking replacement of lost teeth with this modality of treatment. Since the overall success of dental implant therapy depends on the presence of adequate bone volume at implant sites [1], sufficient vertical and horizontal amounts of alveolar ridge prior to dental implant placement are essential.

Bone augmentation can be performed using different techniques: bone blocks and/or guided bone regeneration (GBR) are applied for horizontal bone augmentation [2]. Vertical bone augmentation employs more challenging and technique-sensitive methods: vertical GBR, onlay grafting, inlay grafting, and distraction osteogenesis [3, 4], and is frequently associated with high complication rates such as soft tissue dehiscence and subsequent exposure of bone grafts into the oral cavity [5].

Consequently, soft tissue expanders have been introduced in implant therapy, as pre-augmentation devices, to avoid the complications associated with bone-grafting procedures [6–9]. The currently used soft tissue expanders made of hydrogel, which is the same material used to fabricate contact lenses, are designed and manufactured since 1999 under the name of Osmed® (Ilmenau, Germany), which is the first commercially available self-inflatable osmotic expander and has been FDA-approved since 2001.

Up to date, there is scarce clinical evidence describing soft tissue expansion (STE) prior to bone augmentation procedures: only two case series [6, 8] and one randomized controlled clinical trial [7] are available in literature. These studies have evaluated the outcomes of bone regeneration, but neither has provided clear technical guidelines on the intraoral clinical utilization of these devices nor volumetric analysis of soft tissues. Only post-expansion changes in the profile of the attached gingiva was evaluated in one randomized controlled clinical trial [7]. The authors did not measure the total volume change of soft tissues, as they only aimed to determine the overall stability of the expanded soft tissues by evaluating their profile changes over time.

Based on these observations, we present a report of four pilot cases on preaugmentation soft tissue expansion, utilizing Osmed® expanders (Osmed GmbH, Ilmenau, Germany), to gain insight into the safety and effectiveness of this approach. We also performed volumetric analysis by optic scanning to evaluate the changes in soft tissue volume post-expansion.

2. Materials and Methods

This clinical study was conducted in the period between May 2016 and September 2017.

2.1. Study Participants and Inclusion Criteria. From the pool of patients attending the Dental Clinic of the Ospedale Maggiore Policlinico, University of Milan, Milan, Italy, four participants requiring alveolar bone augmentation and dental implant placement were included in this clinical investigation. All patients were enrolled into the study after explaining its objectives and obtaining their verbal and written informed consent. All patients were treated according to the principles enunciated in the Helsinki Declaration of 1980 for biomedical research involving human subjects.

Study participants fit the following inclusion criteria:

(1) Patients in need for bone augmentation procedures in vertical and/or horizontal dimensions, either in the maxilla or mandible, prior to dental implant placement.

(2) The edentulous area of interest had insufficient amount of soft tissues.

(3) In partially edentulous areas, neighboring teeth should have had no clinical signs of caries, periapical infections, or periodontal inflammation. If active periodontal disease was present, the periodontal condition had to be stabilized first.

(4) Patients without any systemic diseases (ASA-1 or ASA-2 according to the classification of the American Society of Anaesthesiologists).

(5) Non-smokers or ex-smokers who have quit smoking since at least one-year prior to enrollment in the study.

The exclusion criteria were the following:

(1) Self-declaration of pregnancy

(2) Patients on medications that would adversely affect the outcomes of implant therapy and bone regeneration procedures (e.g., bisphosphonates and antiresorptive drugs)

3. Case Presentation

3.1. Case 1. A 44-year-old female patient of Caucasian origin visited the dental clinic seeking replacement of missing teeth in the lower right mandible. Clinical examination revealed missing right mandibular 1st, 2nd, and 3rd molars. Severe bone resorption was evident, accompanied by inadequate amounts of soft tissue. Radiographic evaluation on cone beam computed tomography (CBCT) scans revealed severe vertical bone resorption. Based on these findings, pre-augmentation soft tissue expansion (STE) was scheduled, followed by vertical bone augmentation and placement of dental implants.

3.2. Case 2. A 53-year-old male patient of Caucasian origin visited the dental clinic to substitute a removable acrylic partial denture that he has been wearing for over five years with a fixed prosthesis in the lower jaw. After the patient was asked to remove the denture, clinical examination revealed that all lateral and central incisors were missing. Signs of bone resorption and inadequate amounts of soft tissue were clearly visible. CBCT scan revealed severe horizontal bone resorption. In order to install implant-supported fixed prosthesis, pre-augmentation STE was planned as the first step, followed by horizontal bone augmentation and dental implant placement.

3.3. Case 3. A 58-year-old female patient of Caucasian origin visited the dental clinic to replace a missing lower mandibular first molar. Dental history revealed that the missing tooth was already restored with a dental implant one year ago, but the implant has failed and was removed few months ago. Signs of bone resorption and inadequate soft tissue amount were obvious upon clinical examination. CBCT scan revealed severe horizontal bone resorption. Preaugmentation STE was scheduled, followed by horizontal bone augmentation and dental implant placement.

3.4. Case 4. A 60-year-old female patient of Caucasian origin visited the dental clinic to replace missing teeth in the upper right and left posterior maxillae. Clinical examination of the upper right posterior maxilla revealed missing 2nd premolar and 1st molar, while all the posterior maxillary teeth were completely missing in the left side (i.e., 1st and 2nd premolars and 1st, 2nd, and 3rd molars). Soft tissue amount was inadequate in both areas. CBCT scan showed a moderate horizontal bone loss in both sides. Therefore, STE in the right and left maxillary sides followed by horizontal bone augmentation and dental implant placement were planned.

All the photos present in this report represent the left maxillary side of Case 4.

3.5. Implantation of Soft Tissue Expanders. Based on the extension and location of the edentulous area, intraoral cupola expanders (final volume: 0.35 ml) or cylinder expanders (final volumes: 0.24 ml, 0.7 ml, and 1.3 ml) were applied (Osmed expanders, Osmed GmbH, Ilmenau, Germany). Expanders were left in situ for 20, 40, or 60 days, depending on the final volume of the utilized expander. The appropriate expander was selected using a specific surgical

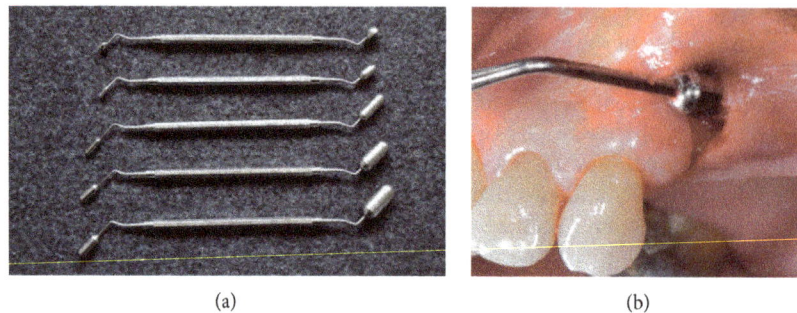

(a)   (b)

FIGURE 1: (a) Specific surgical templates used to choose the appropriate soft tissue expander. Each template has two ends that reflect the initial and final expander volumes. Courtesy of Osmed GmbH (Ilmenau, Germany). (b) Subperiosteal pouch prepared under local anesthesia and controlled with the surgical template.

template corresponding to the initial and final volumes of the expander (Figure 1(a)).

Expanders were inserted using the same surgical technique previously described in literature [8]. Briefly, expanders were inserted in a subperiosteal pouch prepared under local anesthesia and controlled with the specific surgical template (Figure 1(b)) to ensure the device is easily fit without tension into the prepared pouch. The expander was handled carefully by holding its flat end with tweezer. To prevent any dislocation or potential migration, expanders were fixed with a bone fixation screw (Figure 2), at the flat end, which does not have an expansion capability. In all cases, the surgical site was closed utilizing a mattress suture. No antibiotics were prescribed, and sutures were removed 10 days after expander insertion. Any complications, such as expander expulsion, and soft tissue changes in terms of color, inflammation, and bleeding were documented throughout the expansion period.

3.6. Expander Removal and Bone Augmentation.

When the expansion phase was successfully completed, expander removal and bone augmentation were scheduled at the same appointment. Depending on the dimension of alveolar bone resorption, vertical and/or horizontal bone augmentation was performed.

Under local anesthesia, a midcrestal incision was done and a full mucoperiosteal flap was released, and the expander and its fixing screw were removed. Bone surface was carefully examined for any signs of potential resorption due to pressure from the expander (Figures 3(a)–3(c)).

In all cases, bone augmentation was performed using particulate autogenous bone harvested with bone scraper from the surgical site, mixed with xenograft (Bio-Oss®, Geistlich Pharma, Wolhusen, Switzerland). In case of vertical bone augmentation, the graft was covered with titanium reinforced PTFE high-density membrane (Cytoplast® Ti-250, Osteogenics Biomedical Inc., Lubbock, TX, USA), while collagen membrane was used (Bio-Gide®, Geistlich Pharma, Wolhusen, Switzerland), in the case of horizontal bone augmentation (Figures 4(a) and 4(b)). Tension-free primary closure was achieved in all cases without utilizing deep periosteal and/or vertical releasing incisions (Figure 4(c)).

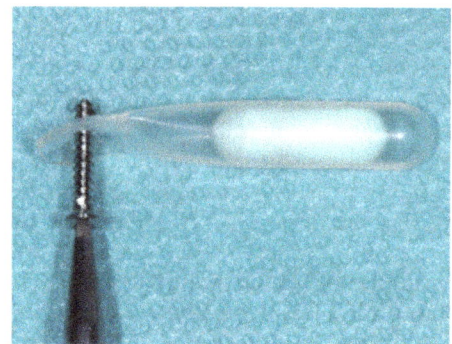

FIGURE 2: Insertion of bone fixation screw at the flat end to prevent potential expander migration.

For all patients, administration of antibiotics started one hour before the augmentation surgery (amoxicillin/calvulanic acid, 2 g) and continued for 7 days every 12 hours. Chlorhexidine mouthwash (0.2%) was recommended for daily use (3 times/day for 14 days). Ketoprofen (50 mg) was prescribed as an analgesic. Patients were followed up weekly, and sutures were removed two weeks after surgery. Any complications such as soft tissue dehiscence, membrane exposure, and bone graft expulsion were documented throughout the bone healing period.

3.7. Dental Implant Placement.

In patients that completed the study, dental implants (MegaGen Implant Co., Ltd., Gyeongbuk, South Korea) were placed 6 months following bone augmentation (Figure 5(a)). All implants were submerged, and sutures were removed 7–14 days later.

3.8. Radiographs.

Cone beam computed tomography (CBCT) scans were taken for all patients, before placement of soft tissue expanders and 4–6 months following bone augmentation procedures.

Soon after dental implant placement, intraoral radiographs with standardized, appropriate parameter settings, using the parallel technique and the proper film holders to ensure reproducibility, were taken for Case 1 and Case 3, while a panoramic radiograph was taken only for Case 4 (Figure 5(b)) as the patient in this case underwent dental implant placement in the left and right posterior maxillae at the same time.

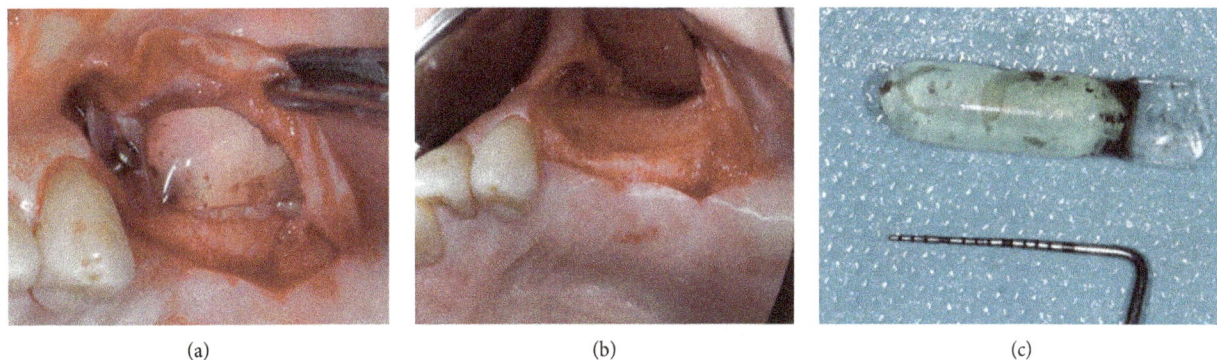

FIGURE 3: (a) Full-thickness flap was elevated to expose the expander and its fixation screw for removal. (b) Expander was removed, and signs of bone resorption due to expansion pressure are evident. (c) Cylinder expander of 0.7 ml final volume is removed. Fluid inside the expander is evident.

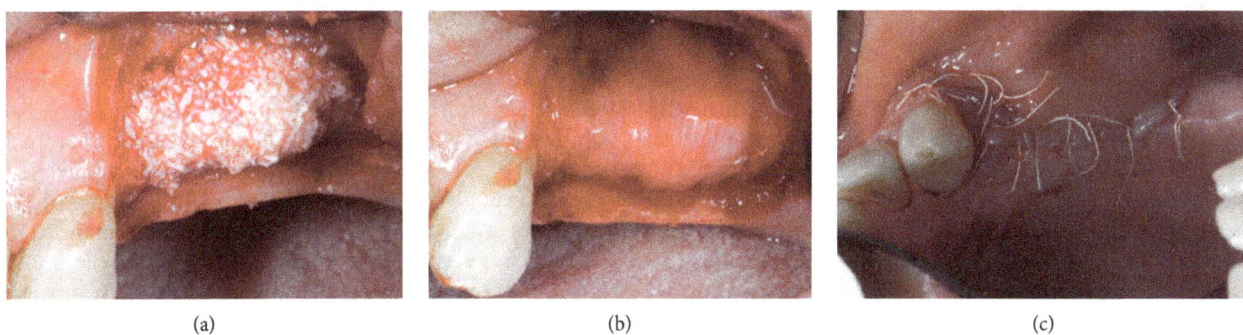

FIGURE 4: (a) Horizontal augmentation was done in this case, utilizing xenograft with autogenous bone. (b) Bone graft was covered with collagen absorbable membrane. (c) Primary, passive wound closure was achieved without deep periosteal releasing incisions.

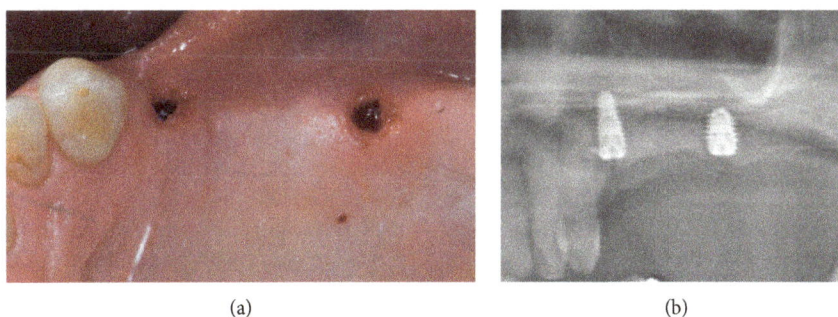

FIGURE 5: (a) Dental implant placement at the area that was expanded and augmented. (b) Section from panoramic radiograph representing the target site after dental implant placement.

Vertical and horizontal bone gains were calculated on CBCT scans, as previously described [6]. Briefly, subtraction of bone height or width "before augmentation" from bone height or width "before placement of dental implants" was performed at landmark sites using the CBCT software.

3.9. *Volumetric Analysis by Optic Scanning.* Volumetric analysis was performed using previously described methods [10, 11] with some modifications. First, alginate impressions were taken for each patient, one immediately before expander insertion and one when the expansion phase was successfully completed, that is, on the appointment of the

expander removal and simultaneous bone augmentation. Then, two master casts, made of dental stone, were fabricated for each patient, based on the pre-expansion and post-expansion alginate impressions.

Next, volumetric changes of the soft tissues were assessed by using an optic scanner and two computer-aided design (CAD) software applications as follows: all the master casts were optically scanned with a 3D camera (Cerec 3D, Sirona Dental Systems GmbH, Bensheim, Germany) and digitalized creating STL files (Standard Tessellation Language). The STL files of pre- and postexpansion models were imported into CAD software (Geomagic Studio® 2013, Raindrop

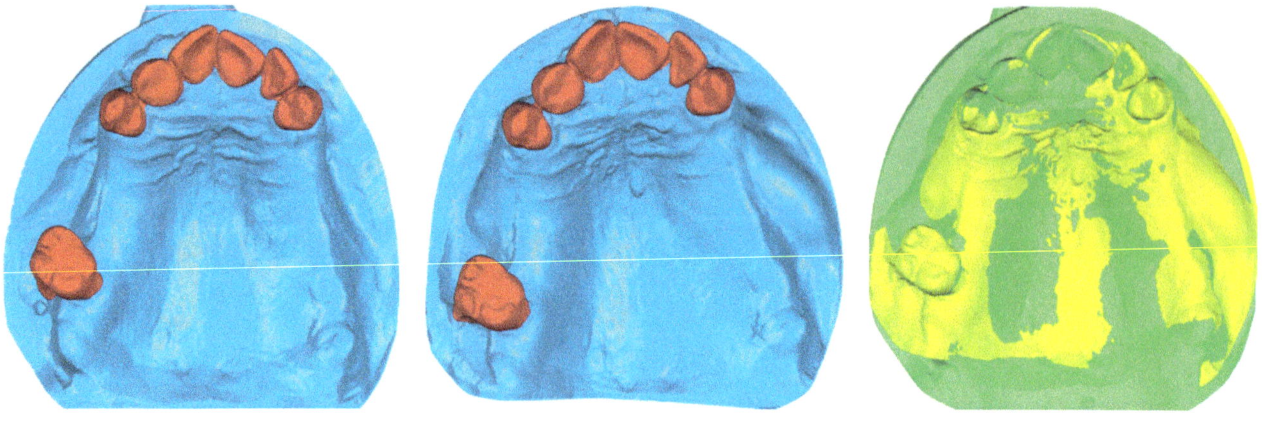

(a)   (b)   (c)

FIGURE 6: Volumetric analysis in the upper left maxilla. (a) Optically scanned preexpansion model. (b) Optically scanned postexpansion model. (c) Superimposed pre- and postexpansion models. Software used: Geomagic Studio 2013, Raindrop Geomagic, NC, USA.

Geomagic, NC, USA) (Figures 6(a) and 6(b)). After being imported, files of pre- and postexpansion models for each patient were accurately superimposed, by using the buccal surface of adjacent teeth as a reference point (Figure 6(c)), applying the best-fit algorithm. After the superimposition was completed, by merging the pre- and postexpansion files into a one unique file, volume changes in the expansion area were calculated using another CAD software (Catia V5, Rand Worldwide Inc., Maryland, USA). The expanded tissues were highlighted with this CAD software, allowing for volume change calculation (Figure 7(a)). After completing the calculations, the expanded area was then extracted into STL format, allowing for superimposition of this area over the original pre-expansion STL file for further confirmation (Figures 7(b) and 7(c)). Volume analysis was done by the same calibrated examiner (FA).

4. Results

Four patients (3 females, 1 male, mean age = 53.6 ± 7.1 years, age range = 44–60 years) were included in this clinical pilot investigation. Expanders were placed at five surgical sites (in Case 4, two different expanders were placed in the same patient). One patient dropped out after soft tissue expansion has failed (Case 2); therefore, only three patients completed the scheduled treatment.

During the expansion period, healing was uneventful in 2 patients ("Case 1 and Case 4" at 3 surgical sites) and the soft tissues undergoing expansion did not show any signs of inflammation or bleeding during or after expansion was completed, while the expansion procedure failed in two patients ("Case 2 and Case 3" at 2 surgical sites) due to perforation of the expanders through the mucosa.

In one of these two sites, the expander was expelled due to crack formation of the silicon shell as a result of handling the body of the expander with the dental tweezer (Figures 8(a)–8(c), "Case 2"). It must be noted that the patient was wearing a removable partial denture during the expansion period despite being advised not to do so. Therefore, taking into consideration the patient's needs, the base of the denture was relieved to accommodate soft tissue expansion in the area. Nevertheless, it seems that wearing a denture, even if relieved, might have contributed to crack propagation in the silicon shell, eventually creating a perforation within the shell and subsequently causing expulsion of the expander at a very late stage of STE.

In the other failed site (Case 3), a cupola expander was inserted in a very tight mucosal pouch due to the anatomical location of the expansion site, which was the first molar. In this case, insertion of the expander in the classical horizontal direction was not possible due to the necessity to fix the expander at the flat end close to the mental nerve, so the prepared pouch was a bit tight to avoid any nerve injury. The expander was expelled within the first week of insertion.

Neither sites were retreated with expanders; one patient dropped out of the study (Case 2), and the other patient underwent bone augmentation two months after failed expansion.

In three patients, one site underwent vertical augmentation (Case 1) and three sites were regenerated horizontally (Case 3 and Case 4); two of the horizontally regenerated sites were preceded by successful STE (Case 4). Tension-free primary wound closure was easily achieved in the cases that were successfully treated with STE, without the need for periosteal deep incisions and/or vertical releasing incisions. It must be noted that deep periosteal releasing incisions were needed to advance the flap over the bone grafting material in the case of failed expansion (Case 3).

Following bone augmentation procedures, wound healing was uneventful, without any reported soft tissue dehiscence, graft expulsion, and/or membrane exposure.

Six months post-augmentation, CBCT analysis revealed that the vertical bone gain was 8 mm (Case 1), while horizontal bone gain for the two successfully expanded sites was 3 mm (Case 4). For the early failed soft tissue expansion case, horizontal bone gain was 2 mm (Case 3) (Table 1).

All three patients received dental implants in the augmented areas (one patient received one dental implant (Case 3), one patient received two dental implants (Case 1), and one patient received four dental implants (Case 4)). Diameter of placed implants ranged between 3.5 and 4 mm, while length range was 7–10 mm. All seven implants were successfully

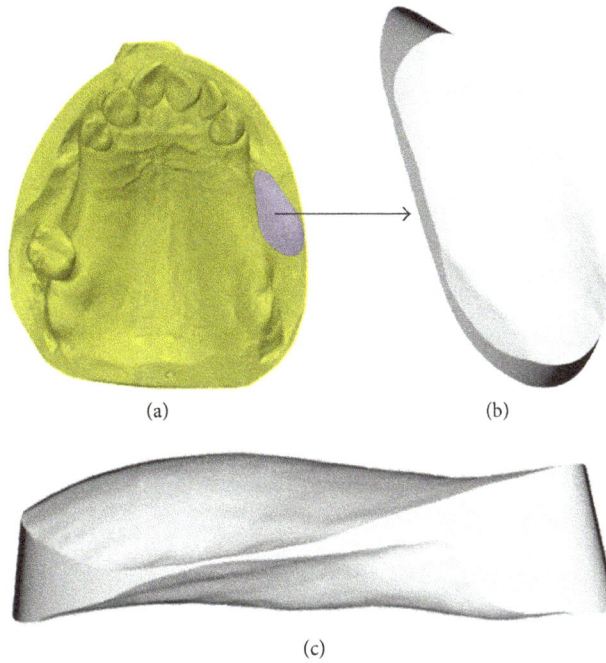

FIGURE 7: Calculation of volumetric changes. (a) Expanded tissues are highlighted with CAD software, and volume change is calculated. (b) The expanded area in STL format (coronal view), which can be superimposed on preexpansion STL file for further confirmation of calculation. (c) The expanded area in STL format (lateral view). Software used: Catia V5, Rand Worldwide Inc., Maryland, USA.

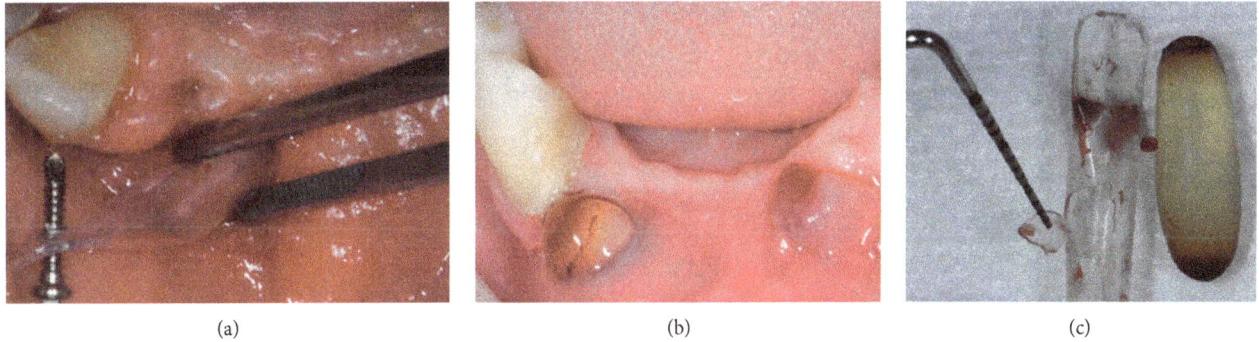

FIGURE 8: (a) The body of the expander was handled with dental tweezer during insertion, creating minor cracks. (b) Late failure of soft tissue expansion as seen by tissue perforation and expulsion of the expander. (c) Perforation of the silicon shell, due to propagation of the crack during expansion.

osseointegrated and scheduled for prosthetic rehabilitation. In those patients, no further soft tissue management was needed, even in terms of soft tissue augmentation.

4.1. Volumetric Analysis Results. Volumetric analysis was done for the three successfully expanded sites (Case 1 and Case 4). Regarding the failed cases, volumetric analysis was only done for the case in which late expansion fail occurred (Case 2), taking into consideration that the postexpansion alginate impression for this case was taken two weeks after failed expander removal.

Results of volumetric analysis are shown in Table 1. For the three successful expansion sites, the soft tissue volume increase was 259.4 mm^2 for the 0.24 ml cylinder expander, 436.1 mm^2 for the 0.7 ml cylinder expander, and 755.9 mm^2

for the 1.3 ml cylinder expander (the mean volume increase of the three successful sites was 483.8 ± 251.7 mm^3).

5. Discussion

In current literature, there are limited available clinical data that describe pre-augmentation soft tissue expansion: two case series [6, 8] and one randomized controlled clinical trial [7].

Kaner and Friedmann [6] were the first to describe the use of osmotic tissue expanders prior to vertical ridge augmentation, reporting a mean vertical bone gain at the time of dental implant placement of 7.5 ± 2.4 mm in twelve patients. In the present report, vertical bone augmentation was performed at one site only, showing a similar high vertical bone gain (8 mm). These findings might suggest that

TABLE 1: Volume gain analysis and bone fill calculations of the study participants.

Expansion zone	Initial expander volume	Final expander volume	Total expansion days	Expansion days as recommended by the manufacturer for the specific final volume	Soft tissue volume gain	Success of expansion	Augmentation dimension	Amount of bone fill in the vertical direction	Amount of bone fill in the horizontal direction
Right posterior mandible (Case 1)	0.25 ml (250 mm^3)	1.3 ml (1300 mm^3)	60 days	60 days	755.9 mm^3	Successful	Vertical	8 mm	N/A
Anterior mandible (Case 2)	0.15 ml (150 mm^3)	0.7 ml (700 mm^3)	38 days	40 days	N/A	Late soft tissue expansion failure	Horizontal	N/A	Patient dropped out of the study after expansion failure
Right posterior mandible (Case 3)	0.05 ml (50 mm^3)	0.35 ml (350 mm^3)	10 days	40 days	N/A	Early soft tissue expansion failure	Horizontal	N/A	2 mm
Left posterior maxilla* (Case 4)	0.15 ml (150 mm^3)	0.7 ml (700 mm^3)	40 days	40 days	436.1 mm^3	Successful	Horizontal	N/A	3 mm
Right posterior maxilla* (Case 4)	0.045 ml (45 mm^3)	0.24 ml (240 mm^3)	20 days	20 days	259.4 mm^3	Successful	Horizontal	N/A	3 mm

N/A: not applicable. *Both sites were in the same patient (Case 4).

vertical bone augmentation preceded by STE could result in predictable vertical bone gain. In fact, a recent systematic review reported that mean vertical bone gain was 4.8 mm with classical bone augmentation procedures [5], which could highlight the importance of pre-augmentation STE.

In the present report, mean horizontal bone gain for successfully expanded sites was 3 mm, which is comparable to other findings in literature regarding bone gain following horizontal bone augmentation without preceding STE [12].

Surplus amount of soft tissues by STE allows for a passive primary closure of the flap minimizing postsurgical complications that would compromise bone fill, such as membrane and/or bone graft exposure. Interestingly, neither of these complications occurred in the current report of cases, and a very low incidence of graft exposure was reported by Kaner and Friedmann [6] (4%). When compared to other studies in literature, higher incidence of bone graft exposure was reported with vertical bone augmentation without preceding soft tissue expansion: 23% [13], 27.3% [14], 25% [15], 33.3% and 50% [16].

Despite the similar findings between the present report and the previously published case series [6], it must be noted that we did not exclusively investigate vertical bone augmentation. Furthermore, the method of expander insertion differed between both studies; we placed the expanders subperiosteally as we hypothesized it might be easier and less demanding surgically, while the submucosal approach has been advocated by Kaner and Friedmann [6] in an attempt to reduce the risk of bone resorption due to pressure exerted on bone surface by the expander. Nonetheless, signs of bone resorption after expander removal were evident on the bone surface at one site in the present report and at two sites in a different clinical study in which subperiosteal implantation of expanders was also employed [8].

In a randomized controlled clinical trial, no signs of bone resorption were reported with the subperiosteal approach which could be due to the much shorter duration of the expansion phase; expansion period of two weeks was chosen by the authors without following the manufacturer's guidelines, in order to avoid the formation of connective tissue capsule around the expander, which might replace the periosteum [7].

Complications related to osmotic tissue expanders reported in the literature have been attributed to different causes: infection, wearing a removable denture, expanding scarred tissues, and perforations either due to utilization of an excessively large expander or due to expander placement too close to the incision line [6–8]. In the present report, one expander failed because it was placed in a tight pouch due to anatomic considerations, and the other expander perforated the tissues at a very late stage into the expansion. Expander perforation into soft tissues at a very advanced stage of expansion has not been previously reported in literature. Therefore, we have looked carefully into the causes that might have contributed to this adverse event at a very late stage of expansion. Clinical photos taken during the surgical procedure revealed that the expander body, and not its flat end, was handled by a sharp instrument (dental tweezer). This might have led to the formation of a minor crack on the shell that propagated during the expansion phase, until the hydrogel body perforated through the crack all the way into the soft tissues.

Up to date, only one clinical study evaluated soft tissue changes during STE. In their randomized controlled clinical trial, Abrahamsson et al. [7] measured soft tissue stability of the attached gingiva at baseline and 6 months after augmentation in control and test groups and additionally at post-expansion in the test group, by using an objective 3D metering device. The mean soft tissue profile gain at the attached gingiva level was 2.9 ± 1.1 mm when compared to baseline, while it decreased to 2.3 ± 2.1 mm at the time of implant placement, when compared with baseline. The control group showed a soft profile change of 1.5 ± 1.4 mm at the time of fixture installation. Even if the test group showed increased gingival dimensions after surgeries, the differences were not statistically significant. The authors did not measure the total volume change in soft tissues, as they only wanted to determine overall stability of created soft tissues by evaluating soft tissue profile changes over time. Although soft tissue profile became less prominent after healing of bone graft when compared to pre-augmentation soft tissue profile, this result was statistically insignificant.

In attempt to evaluate the total volume change, we have done volumetric analysis using previously described methods [10, 11] with some modifications. For the three successful expansion sites, soft tissue volume increase corresponded only to the 0.24 ml (240 mm^3) cylinder expander (volume increase = 259.4 mm^3), while this increase was almost half of the final expander volume for the 0.7 ml (700 mm^3) and 1.3 ml (1300 mm^3) cylinder expanders (volume increase = 436.1 mm^3 and 755.9 mm^3, resp.). These findings suggest that it is difficult to reach a complete volume increase with bigger final volume expanders, probably due to higher pressure distribution to the underlying bone surface. However, this hypothesis needs to be confirmed in future studies, also comparing the volume increase results between different expander insertion approaches, that is, subperiosteal versus submucosal insertion techniques.

To summarize, STE might be a useful pre-augmentation approach specifically for vertical bone augmentation, as it results in high vertical bone gain with minimal post-surgical complications. The ideal clinical scenario for this specific application would be the need of vertical bone augmentation in the posterior mandible with limited amount of present soft tissues, consisting only of alveolar mucosa.

Findings of this report of four pilot cases must be interpreted with caution; volume analysis does not provide information on the actual volume changes in the tissues, as the post-expansion impressions were taken while expanders were still in situ. However, the volumetric analysis still gives an insight into the overall soft tissue volume changes; expansion pressure to the underlying bone surface, with subperiosteal large expanders, might prevent full soft tissue volume increase corresponding to the final expander volume.

The technique investigated in the present pilot cases still requires improvement for being considered predictable. Future clinical studies should also aim at comparing different expander insertion approaches as well.

6. Conclusions

Soft tissue expansion (STE) might be a beneficial pre-augmentation approach, especially in the vertical dimension. The ideal area for this specific application would be the posterior mandible with the presence of alveolar mucosa.

However, the presented technique still requires improvement before being applied routinely in everyday dental practice.

Acknowledgments

The authors would like to thank Mr. Michael Kircheisen from OSMED Company (Ilmenau, Germany) for providing the expanders used in this study. The authors would like to also thank Mr. Angelo Magni for the technical support provided with the volume analysis. This study was self-supported.

References

[1] F. Javed, H. B. Ahmed, R. Crespi, and G. E. Romanos, "Role of primary stability for successful osseointegration of dental implants: factors of influence and evaluation," *Interventional Medicine and Applied Science*, vol. 5, no. 4, pp. 162–167, 2013.

[2] B. S. McAllister and K. Haghighat, "Bone augmentation techniques," *Journal of Periodontology*, vol. 78, no. 3, pp. 377–396, 2007.

[3] I. Rocchietta, F. Fontana, and M. Simion, "Clinical outcomes of vertical bone augmentation to enable dental implant placement: a systematic review," *Journal of Clinical Periodontology*, vol. 35, pp. 203–215, 2008.

[4] M. Esposito, M. G. Grusovin, P. Felice, G. Karatzopoulos, H. V. Worthington, and P. Coulthard, "Interventions for replacing missing teeth: horizontal and vertical bone augmentation techniques for dental implant treatment," *Cochrane Database of Systematic Reviews*, no. 3, p. CD003607, 2009.

[5] S. S. Jensen and H. Terheyden, "Bone augmentation procedures in localized defects in the alveolar ridge: clinical results with different bone grafts and bone-substitute materials," *International Journal of Oral & Maxillofacial Implants*, no. 24, pp. 218–236, 2009.

[6] D. Kaner and A. Friedmann, "Soft tissue expansion with self-filling osmotic tissue expanders before vertical ridge augmentation: a proof of principle study," *Journal of Clinical Periodontology*, vol. 38, no. 1, pp. 95–101, 2011.

[7] P. Abrahamsson, D. Å. Wälivaara, S. Isaksson, and G. Andersson, "Periosteal expansion before local bone reconstruction using a new technique for measuring soft tissue profile stability: a clinical study," *Journal of Oral and Maxillofacial Surgery*, vol. 70, no. 10, pp. e521–e530, 2012.

[8] C. Mertens, O. Thiele, M. Engel, R. Seeberger, J. Hoffmann, and K. Freier, "The use of self-inflating soft tissue expanders prior to bone augmentation of atrophied alveolar ridges," *Clinical Implant Dentistry and Related Research*, vol. 17, no. 1, pp. 44–51, 2015.

[9] F. Asa'ad, G. Rasperini, G. Pagni, H. F. Rios, and A. B. Gianni, "Pre-augmentation soft tissue expansion: an overview," *Clinical Oral Implants Research*, vol. 27, no. 5, pp. 505–522, 2016.

[10] D. Schneider, U. Grunder, A. Ender, C. H. Hämmerle, and R. E. Jung, "Volume gain and stability of peri-implant tissue following bone and soft tissue augmentation: 1-year results from a prospective cohort study," *Clinical Oral Implants Research*, vol. 22, no. 1, pp. 28–37, 2011.

[11] T. Thalmair, S. Fickl, D. Schneider, M. Hinze, and H. Wachtel, "Dimensional alterations of extraction sites after different alveolar ridge preservation techniques–a volumetric study," *Journal of Clinical Periodontology*, vol. 40, no. 7, pp. 721–727, 2013.

[12] B. Elnayef, A. Monje, G. H. Lin et al., "Alveolar ridge split on horizontal bone augmentation: a systematic review," *International Journal of Oral & Maxillofacial Implants*, vol. 30, no. 3, pp. 596–606, 2015.

[13] J. W. Verhoeven, M. S. Cune, M. Terlou, M. A. Zoon, and C. de Putter, "The combined use of endosteal implants and iliac crest onlay grafts in the severely atrophic mandible: a longitudinal study," *International Journal of Oral & Maxillofacial Implants*, vol. 26, no. 5, pp. 351–357, 1997.

[14] M. Chiapasco, E. Romeo, P. Casentini, and L. Rimondini, "Alveolar distraction osteogenesis vs. vertical guided bone regeneration for the correction of vertically deficient edentulous ridges: a 1-3-year prospective study on humans," *Clinical Oral Implants Research*, vol. 15, no. 1, pp. 82–95, 2004.

[15] P. Proussaefs and J. Lozada, "The use of intraorally harvested autogenous block grafts for vertical alveolar ridge augmentation: a human study," *International Journal of Periodontics & Restorative Dentistry*, vol. 25, pp. 351–363, 2005.

[16] M. Roccuzzo, G. Ramieri, M. Bunino, and S. Berrone, "Autogenous bone graft alone or associated with titanium mesh for vertical alveolar ridge augmentation: a controlled clinical trial," *Clinical Oral Implants Research*, vol. 18, pp. 286–294, 2007.

4

Assessment of Occlusal Function in a Patient with an Angle Class I Spaced Dental Arch with Periodontal Disease Using a Brux Checker

Ayako Taira,[1] Shiho Odawara,[2] Shuntaro Sugihara,[3] and Kenichi Sasaguri ⓘ[1]

[1]Department of Dentistry, Oral and Maxillofacial Surgery, Jichi Medical University, 3311-1 Yakushiji, Shimotsuke, Tochigi 329-0498, Japan
[2]Division of Orthodontics, Department of Oral Science, Kanagawa Dental University, 82 Inaoka-cho, Yokosuka, Kanagawa 238-8580, Japan
[3]Division of Periodontology, Department of Oral Function and Restoration, Kanagawa Dental University, 82 Inaoka-cho, Yokosuka, Kanagawa 238-8580, Japan

Correspondence should be addressed to Kenichi Sasaguri; sasaguri@jichi.ac.jp

Academic Editor: Hüsamettin Oktay

Comprehensive and appropriate occlusion reconstruction therapy is necessary for orthodontic treatment of adult patients with malocclusion with periodontal disease associated with occlusal trauma. We report the case of a patient with extensive moderate chronic periodontitis associated with occlusal trauma. The patient was diagnosed with extensive moderate chronic periodontitis associated with occlusal trauma and underwent thorough treatment for periodontal disease, oral management, and 20 months of orthodontic therapy. Moreover, reconstructed occlusion was performed to evaluate occlusal trauma for visualization using Brux Checker (BC) analysis before and after active orthodontic treatment. The patient acquired stable anterior guidance and a functional occlusal relationship. BC findings revealed weakening of the functional contact between the lateral occlusal force of the dentition and the front teeth and alveolar bone regeneration. The laminar dura became clearer, and the periodontal tissue improved. Our results suggest that assessment of occlusion function using BC analysis and periodontal examination was effective in enabling occlusal treatment goal clarification through orthodontic treatment in case of periodontal disease associated with occlusal trauma.

1. Introduction

Orthodontic treatment for adult patients with malocclusion complicated by periodontal disease includes comprehensive and appropriate occlusal reconstruction and ongoing oral management during treatment for periodontal disease and the orthodontic process before starting active treatment [1–3]. In particular, when implementing occlusal reconstruction using orthodontic treatment in patients with suspected occlusal trauma, it is possible to achieve appropriate disclusion in the molar region by providing correct anterior guidance, and it is important to weaken the lateral occlusal force. In this case, the patient was suspected to have extensive, moderate chronic periodontitis [4] associated with occlusal trauma;

therefore, a periodontal disease specialist provided adequate treatment for periodontal disease and oral management before orthodontic treatment commenced. When occlusal reconstruction was performed with orthodontic treatment, occlusion was confirmed at the dental chair side, and night-time parafunction was assessed using a Brux Checker (BC; Rocky Mountain Morita Corporation, Tokyo, Japan) [5, 6]. Further, after the patient had used a retainer for 2 years, she underwent coronally advanced flap repositioning surgery with a connective tissue graft for root coverage of the bilateral maxillary lateral incisors to enable cosmetic and hygiene restoration for gingival recession on the labial side of the tooth cervix of the maxillary bilateral incisors. The patient has made a good recovery.

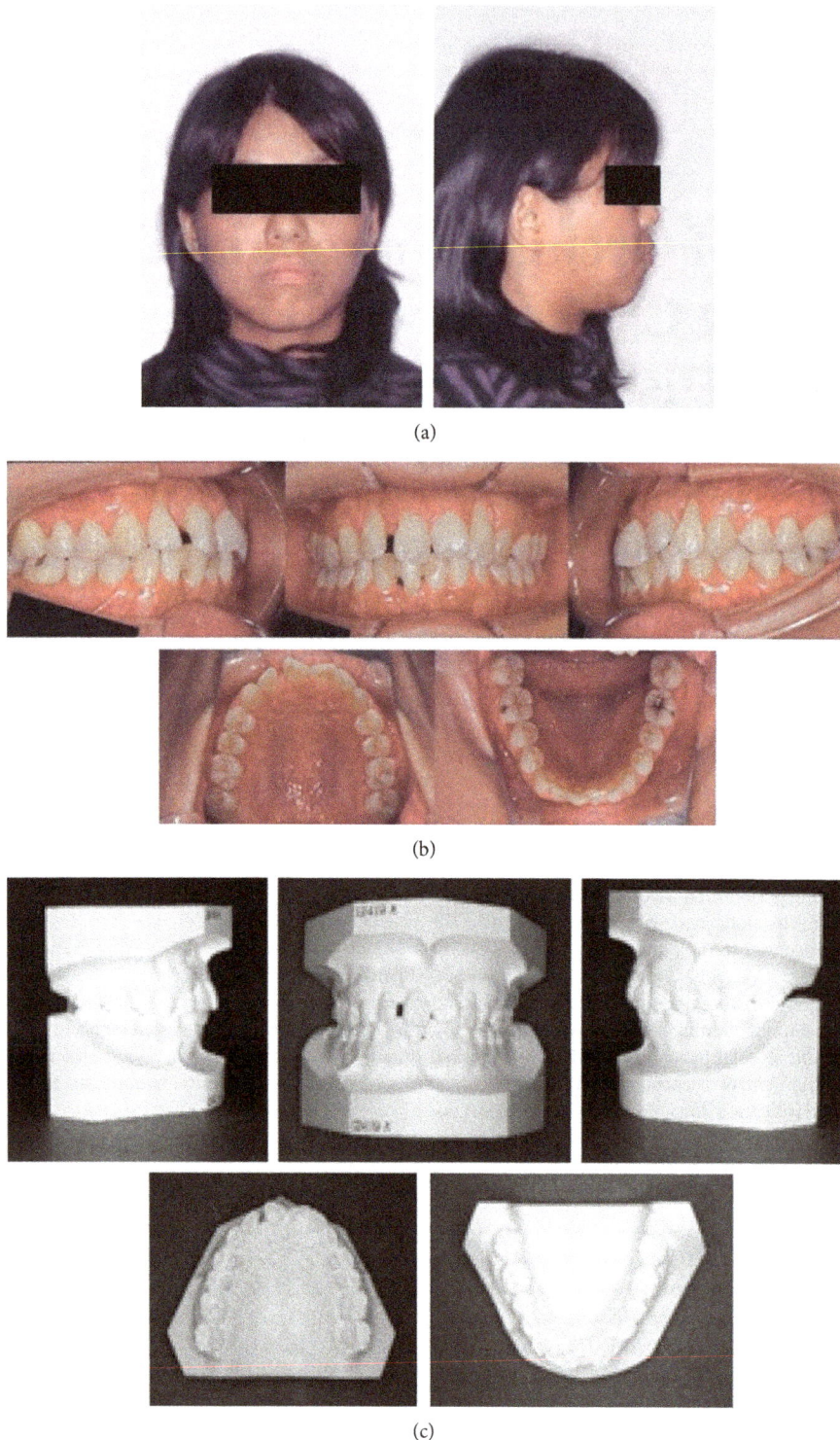

(a)

(b)

(c)

FIGURE 1: Pre-orthodontic treatment facial (a) and intraoral photographs (b) and dental casts (c) are shown.

2. Case Presentation

2.1. Diagnosis. The patient was a woman aged 30 years and 2 months at the initial consultation. She visited the hospital with a chief complaint of severe pain in her maxillary and mandibular front teeth and a spaced dental arch. Her face was bilaterally symmetric, and she had a convex facial profile (Figure 1(a)). The anterior occlusal relationship included an overjet of 2 mm and an overbite of 4 mm; the molar occlusal relationship was bilateral Angle Class I, and the arch length discrepancy was +2 mm for both the maxilla and mandible. The lateral

(a)

(b)

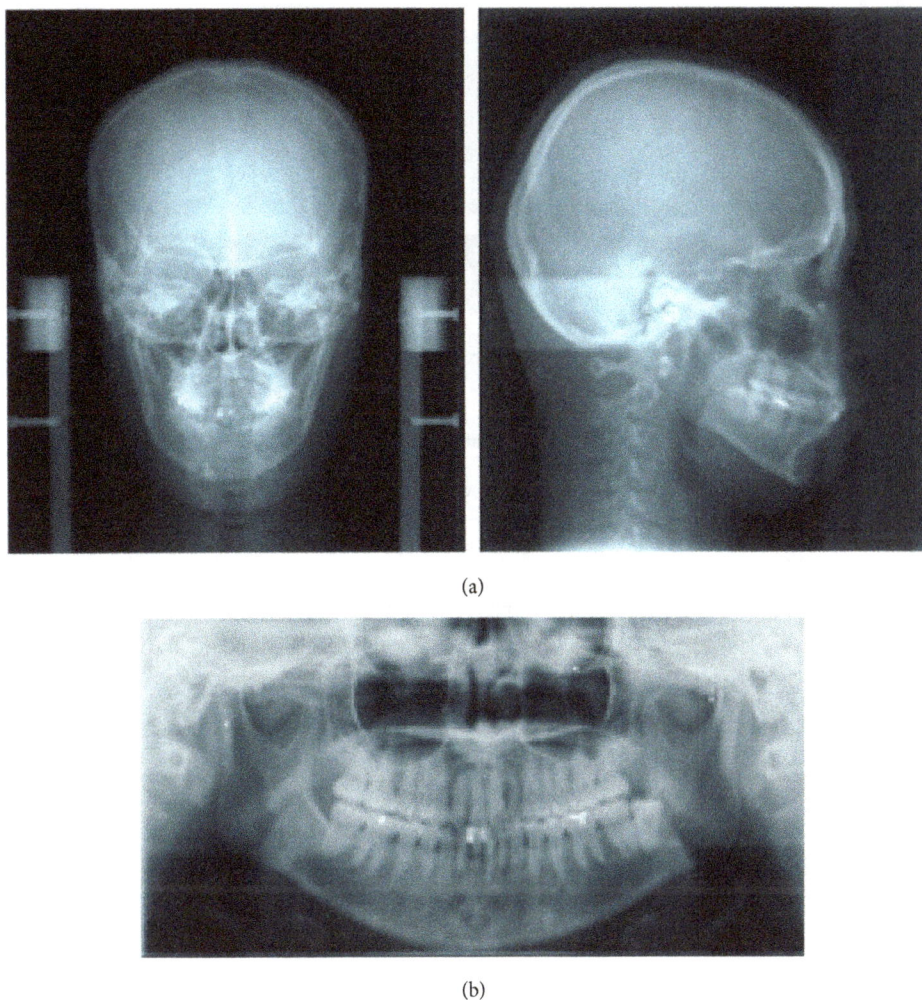

FIGURE 2: Pre-orthodontic treatment cephalograms (a) and panoramic radiograph (b) are shown.

TABLE 1: Summary of the cephalometric findings.

Variables	Japanese norms (adult female)	Pretreatment	Posttreatment	Postretention
SNA (°)	82.3 ± 3.5	85	85	85
SNB (°)	78.9 ± 3.5	79	78	78
ANB (°)	3.4 ± 1.8	6	7	7
FMA (°)	28.8 ± 5.2	30	31	31
IMPA (°)	96.3 ± 5.8	99	102	102
U1 to SN (°)	104.5 ± 5.6	106	99	99
E-line to upper lip (mm)	-2.5 ± 1.90	2	2	2
E-line to lower lip (mm)	0.9 ± 1.90	5	5	5

dentition had relatively good occlusion, but the bilateral maxillary central incisors showed mesial rotation, and her previous dentist had joined the mandibular front teeth with resin, presumably to prevent tooth mobility (Figures 1(b) and 1(c)). Cephalometric analysis showed the following: ANB, 6; FMA, 30; U1-SN, 106; and IMPA, 99 (Figure 2(a) and Table 1). Therefore, the patient's facial type demonstrated a mesofacial pattern, and she was diagnosed orthodontically with an Angle Class I spaced dental arch.

The radiographic findings indicated vertical bone resorption in the mesial portions of the right maxillary and mandibular first molars, and the maxillary and mandibular front teeth showed high-grade bone resorption (Figures 2(b)

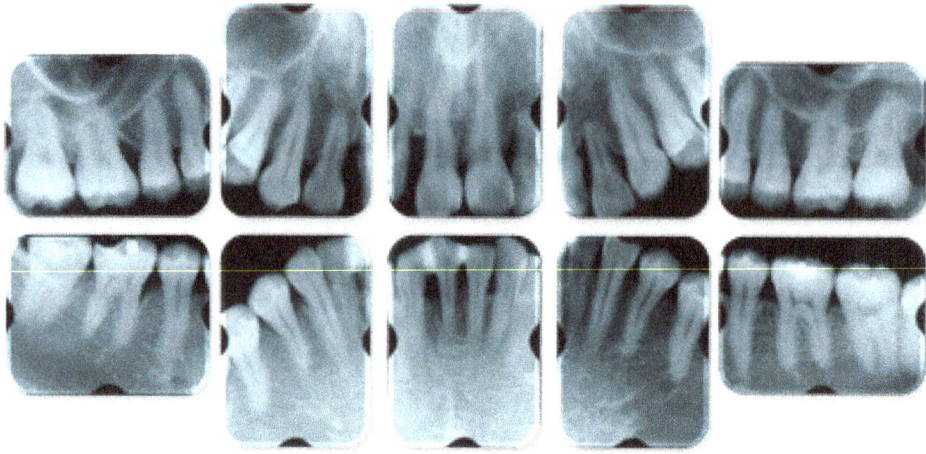

(a)

Tooth		17	16	15	14	13	12	11	21	22	23	24	25	26	27
Maxilla	Furcation														
	Mobility	0	0	0	0	0	0	1	1	1	0	0	0	0	0
	Probing B	3 3 4	4 3 5	4 3 4	3 3 3	3 3 3	3 3 4	5 4 3	3 3 4	5 3 3	2 2 4	3 3 4	3 3 4	3 3 3	3 4 3
	Depth P	3 3 3	4 3 4	4 3 4	3 3 4	3 3 3	3 3 4	5 3 3	3 3 4	5 3 4	4 4 3	4 3 3	4 3 3	4 3 3	4 3 4
Mandibular	Probing L	4 4 4	4 3 2	2 2 2	2 2 2	2 3 3	2 2 4	4 2 2	3 3 3	2 2 2	3 3 3	3 3 3	3 3 3	4 3 3	4 3 4
	Depth B	3 3 3	2 2 5	3 3 3	3 3 3	3 3 3	3 3 4	5 4 2	3 3 3	2 2 3	3 3 3	4 3 3	3 3 3	3 3 3	3 3 3
	Mobility	0	0	0	0	0	0	0	0	0	0	0	0	0	0
	Furcation														
Tooth		47	46	45	44	43	42	41	31	32	33	34	35	36	37

(b)

FIGURE 3: Pre-orthodontic treatment dental radiographs (a) and periodontal examinations (b) are shown. The red color indicates bleeding on probing.

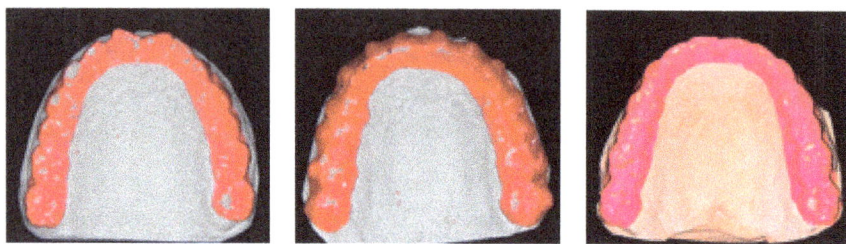

(a)   (b)   (c)

FIGURE 4: Brux Checker findings. (a) Before orthodontic treatment, (b) just before removal of the orthodontic appliance, and (c) at 2 years after retention.

Tooth		17	16	15	14	13	12	11	21	22	23	24	25	26	27
Maxilla	Furcation														
	Mobility	0	0	0	0	0	0	1	1	1	0	0	0	0	0
	Probing B	3 3 2	2 3 4	4 2 3	3 3 3	3 3 3	3 3 2	2 3 3	3 3 3	3 3 4	5 2 3	2 2 2	3 3 2	3 3 3	3 3 3
	Depth P	3 3 3	2 3 3	3 3 3	3 3 2	3 3 3	3 3 2	3 3 3	3 3 4	4 3 3	2 2 3	2 3 3	3 3 3	3 3 3	3 3 3
Mandibular	Probing L	3 3 3	3 3 2	2 2 2	2 2 2	2 3 3	2 2 4	4 2 3	3 3 3	2 2 2	3 3 3	3 3 3	3 3 3	4 3 3	3 3 3
	Depth B	3 3 3	2 2 4	3 3 3	3 3 3	3 3 3	3 3 4	4 3 2	3 3 3	2 2 2	3 3 3	3 3 3	3 3 3	3 3 3	3 3 3
	Mobility	0	0	0	0	0	0	0	0	0	0	0	0	0	0
	Furcation														
Tooth		47	46	45	44	43	42	41	31	32	33	34	35	36	37

FIGURE 5: The periodontal examinations after periodontal treatment are shown. The red color indicates bleeding on probing.

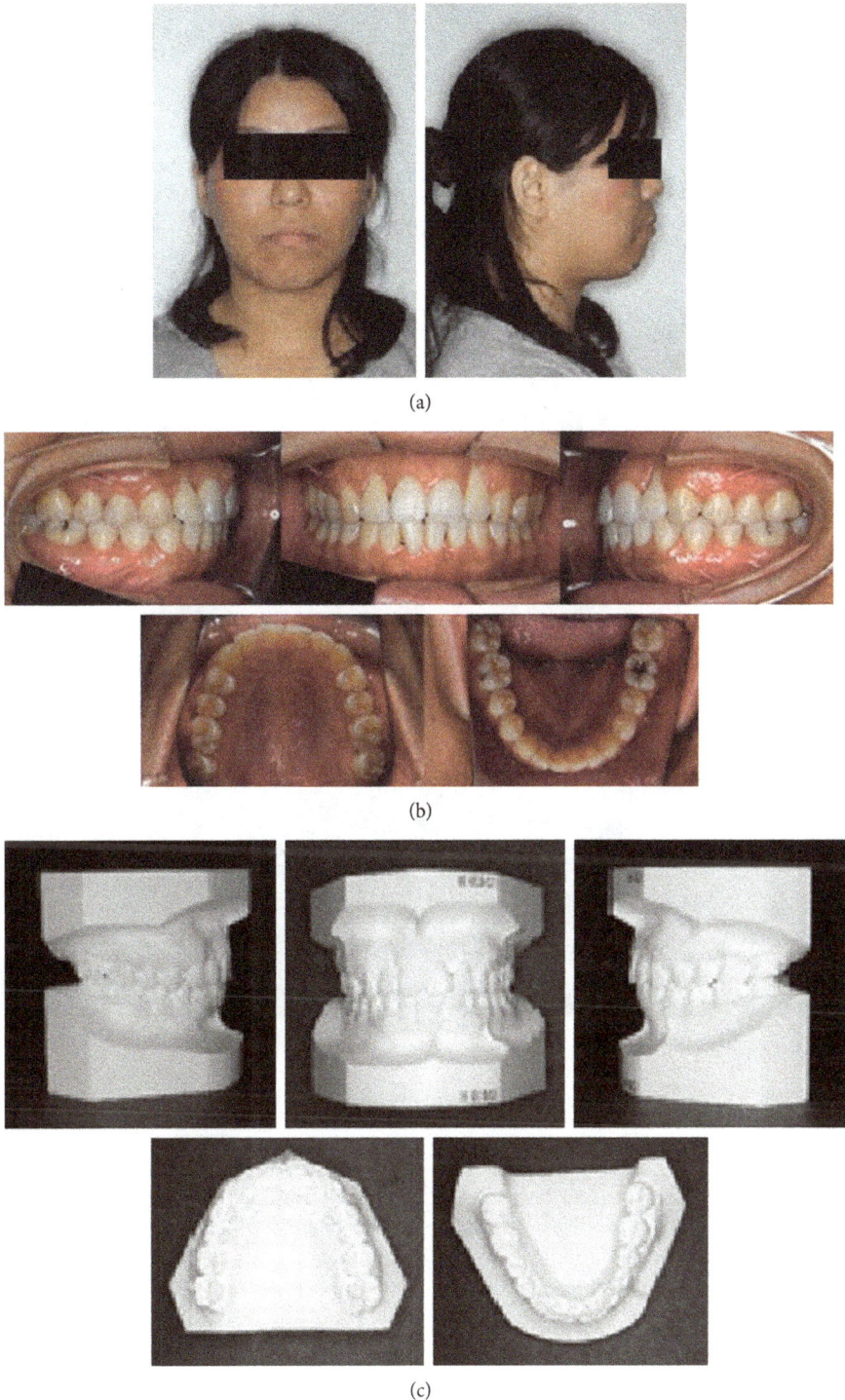

(a)

(b)

(c)

FIGURE 6: Post-orthodontic treatment facial (a) and intraoral photographs (b) and dental casts (c) are shown.

and 3(a)). On the periodontal disease chart, there were swelling of the gingiva in the same location and a periodontal pocket exceeding 4 mm. Bleeding on probing was observed (Figure 3(b)). The front teeth of the lower jaw had been joined with resin at another hospital to prevent tooth mobility. There was also moderate loss of the mesial interdental papilla in the gingival recession area of the bilateral maxillary lateral incisors (Figures 1(b) and 3(a)).

Dental findings showed a reduction in the mesial bone level; therefore, the patient was diagnosed as Class III according to Miller's classification of gingival recession [7]. In this case, given that periodontal lesions were found in the maxillary and mandibular teeth and molar areas, the patient was diagnosed with malocclusion associated with extensive moderate chronic periodontitis. Further, when we examined night-time parafunction using a BC [5, 6], strong functional

(a)

(b)

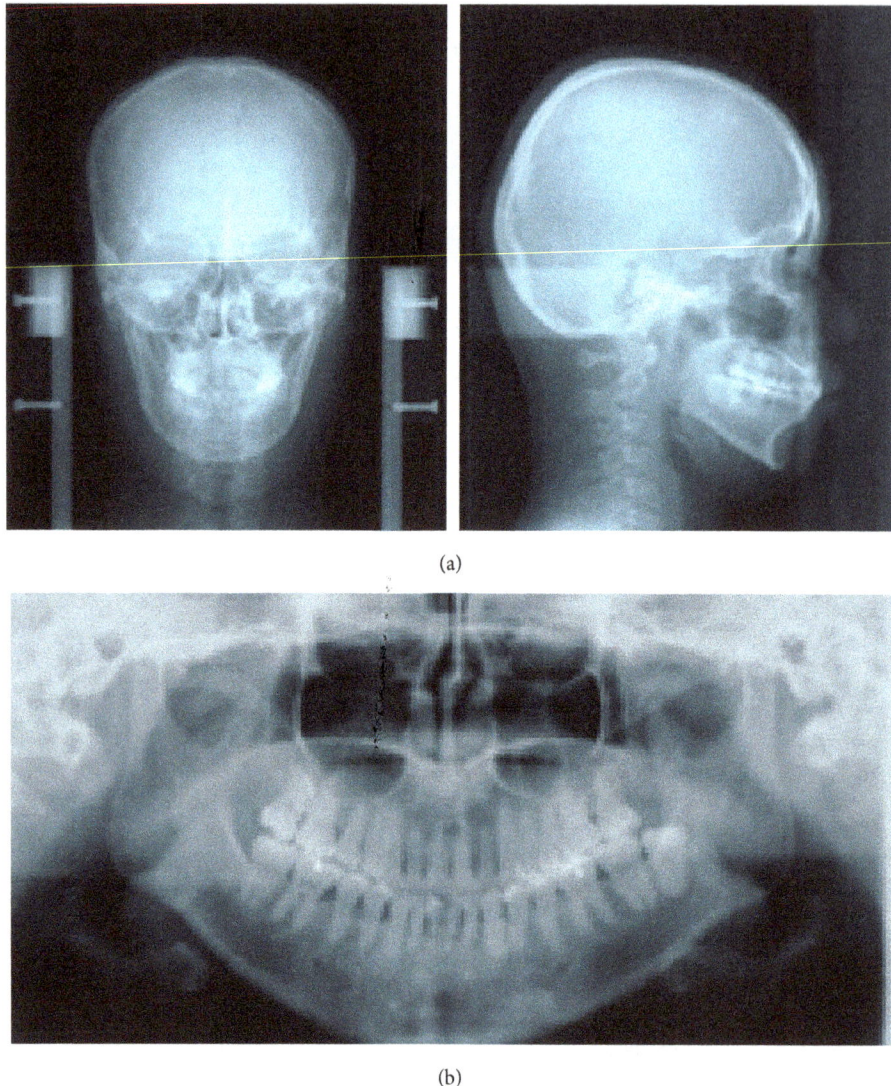

FIGURE 7: Post-orthodontic treatment cephalograms (a) and panoramic radiograph (b) are shown.

contact was noted on the marginal ridges on the mesial side of the bilateral maxillary central incisors and the incisal edges of the bilateral lateral incisors, as well as the right canine, first premolar, and first molar (Figure 4(a)). These locations generally correlated with the locations of the patient's symptoms of periodontal disease according to the periodontal disease chart (Figure 3(b)). The dental findings indicated widening of the periodontal space in the lateral dentition, suggesting that the condition may have been associated with occlusal trauma. Written informed consent was obtained from the subject for publication of this case report and the accompanying photographs, figures, and data.

2.2. Treatment Plan. Based on the above findings, the patient was diagnosed with occlusal trauma and an Angle Class I spaced dental arch associated with extensive moderate chronic periodontitis. The treatment objectives were resolution of the discrepancy, establishing appropriate anterior guidance by capturing the correct tooth axis inclinations for the maxillary and mandibular front teeth, and attenuation of the occlusal trauma. If there were stabilization of functional occlusion after use of a retainer and no progression of periodontal disease, we planned to perform palatal gingival grafting to the tooth cervix of the bilateral maxillary lateral incisors.

2.3. Treatment Progression. A periodontal disease specialist treated the periodontal tissue before orthodontic treatment was commenced. We made the patient aware of the importance of her oral environment and explained the importance of being motivated for the ongoing oral management needed. Approximately 3 months later, there was improvement in the pocket depth, and the bleeding on probing and gingival swelling had resolved, indicating improvement of the periodontal disease (Figure 5). Given that the patient's awareness of the importance of maintaining her oral environment had also improved, we initiated active treatment.

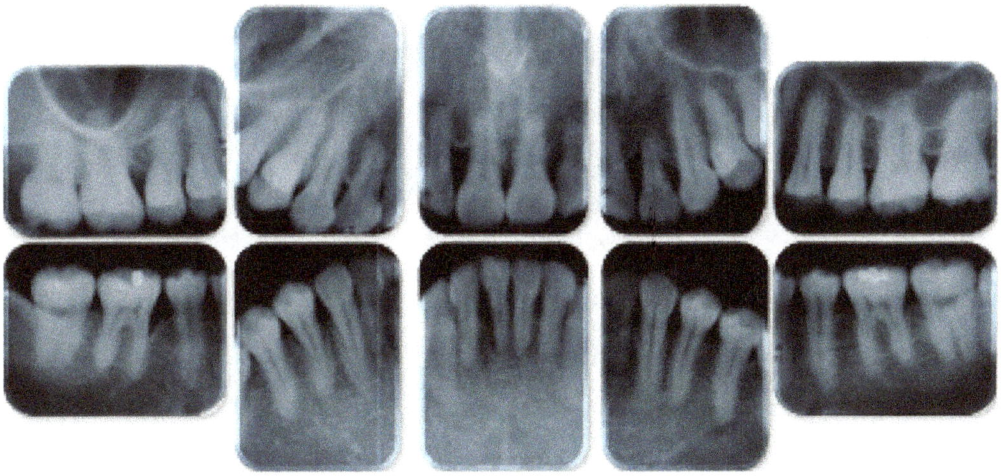

(a)

Tooth		17	16	15	14	13	12	11	21	22	23	24	25	26	27
Maxilla	Furcation														
	Mobility	0	0	0	0	0	0	1	1	1	0	0	0	0	0
	Probing Depth B	3 3 2	2 3 3	3 2 3	3 3 3	3 3 3	3 3 2	2 3 3	3 3 3	4 2 3	2 2 2	3 3 2	3 3 3	3 3 3	3 3 3
	P	3 3 3	2 3 3	3 3 3	3 3 3	3 3 3	3 3 2	3 3 3	3 3 3	3 3 3	2 2 3	2 3 3	3 3 3	3 3 3	3 3 3
Mandibular	Probing Depth L	3 3 3	3 3 2	2 2 2	2 2 2	2 3 3	2 2 3	2 2 2	3 3 3	2 2 2	3 3 3	3 3 3	3 3 3	3 3 3	3 3 3
	B	3 3 3	2 2 4	3 3 3	3 3 3	3 3 3	3 3 3	3 3 2	3 3 3	2 2 3	3 3 3	3 3 3	3 3 3	3 3 3	3 3 3
	Mobility	0	0	0	0	0	0	0	0	0	0	0	0	0	0
	Furcation														
Tooth		47	46	45	44	43	42	41	31	32	33	34	35	36	37

(b)

FIGURE 8: Post-orthodontic treatment dental radiographs (a) and periodontal examinations (b) are shown. The red color indicates bleeding on probing.

For the active treatment, we used a Roth setup with a 0.022-inch slot bracket and started leveling using maxillary and mandibular 0.012-inch round nickel titanium wires. We then increased the wire size sequentially and were using a 016 × 022-inch stainless steel wire after 6 months. We then attached a hook between the maxillary and mandibular lateral incisors and canines and closed the gap using intermaxillary elastics to exert an extremely weak orthodontic force.

The BC showed strong functional contact with the right maxillary lateral dentition before starting active treatment, so construction of appropriate anterior guidance and molar spacing was considered for detailing. At the completion of active treatment, the patient started using a retainer after night-time parafunction was reassessed using the BC (Figure 4(b)). The active treatment lasted 1 year and 8 months (Figures 6–8). A Begg-type retainer plate was used for both the mandible and maxilla. Two years after starting use of the retainers (Figures 9–11), the BC assessment was performed again, and the periodontal disease was reexamined (Figures 11(b) and 4(c)). After the state of occlusion and the periodontal tissue were checked, the patient underwent coronally advanced flap repositioning surgery with a connective tissue graft for root coverage of the labial side of the tooth cervix of the bilateral maxillary lateral incisors using palatal mucosal connective tissue (Figure 12).

2.4. Treatment Results. In a photograph of the oral cavity taken after orthodontic treatment, the maxillary and mandibular spacing had closed, and a continuous and appropriate overbite and overjet were acquired. The findings indicated acquisition of good lateral incisor interdigitation (Figures 6(b) and 6(c)). Panoramic findings indicated good parallelism of the roots of the teeth (Figure 7(b)). Dental findings showed tooth root resorption of the left maxillary lateral incisors, but the lamina dura had become clearer. In addition, the widening of the right maxillary first molar periodontal space had disappeared, and bone regeneration was noted in the mesial area (Figure 8(a)).

The BC findings after completion of treatment indicated weakening of the strong functional contact that was present in the right maxillary lateral dentition and front teeth (Figures 4(a) and 4(b)). In the cephalometric superimposition (Figure 13(a)), the mandible was slightly rotated clockwise, and the patient's profile was virtually unchanged. Dental findings showed slight elongation of the maxillary and mandibular molars, and the angles of the tooth axis inclinations of the maxillary front teeth had lessened (Figures 2(a) and 7(a), Table 1). After 2 years of using the retainer, when the BC assessment was performed again and periodontal disease was reexamined (Figures 4(c) and 9–11), there was no major change from that at the end of active treatment (Figures 7(a), 10(a),

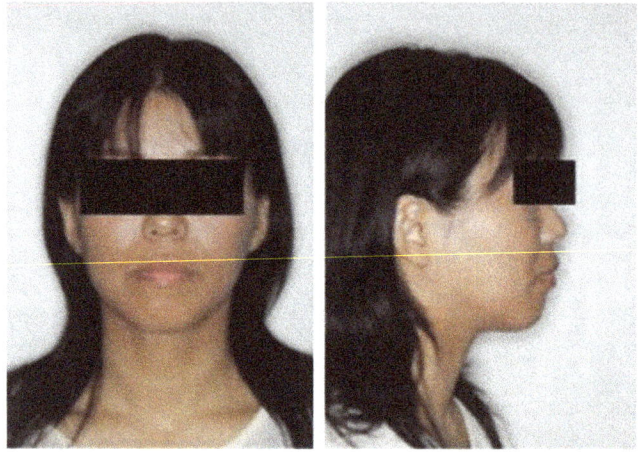

(a)

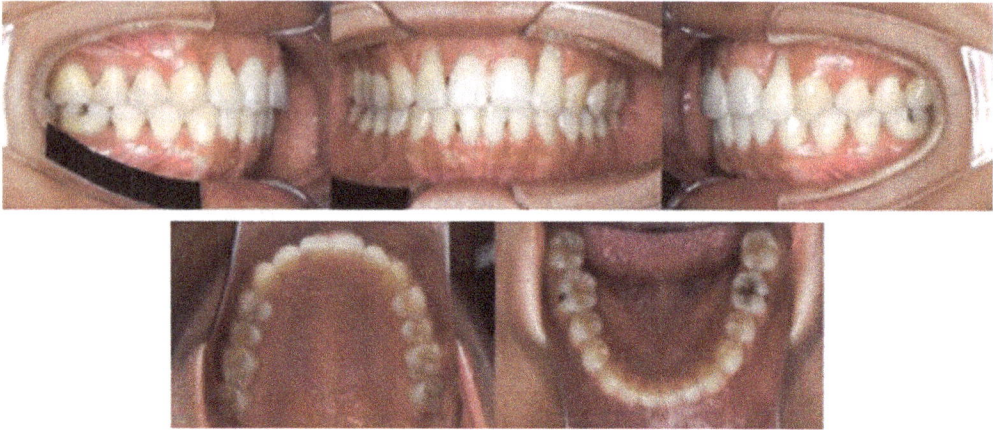

(b)

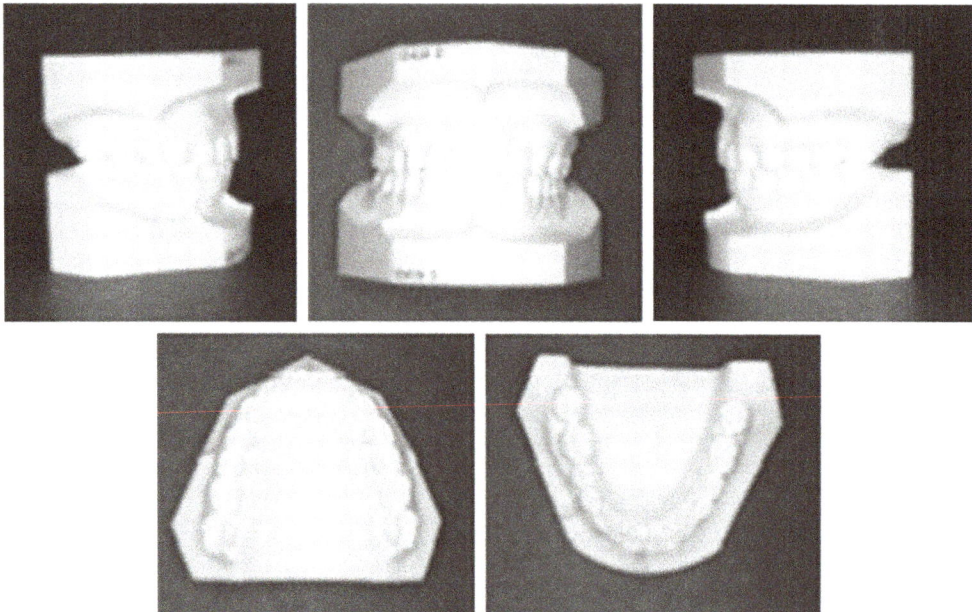

(c)

FIGURE 9: Postretention facial (a) and intraoral photographs (b) and dental casts (c) are shown.

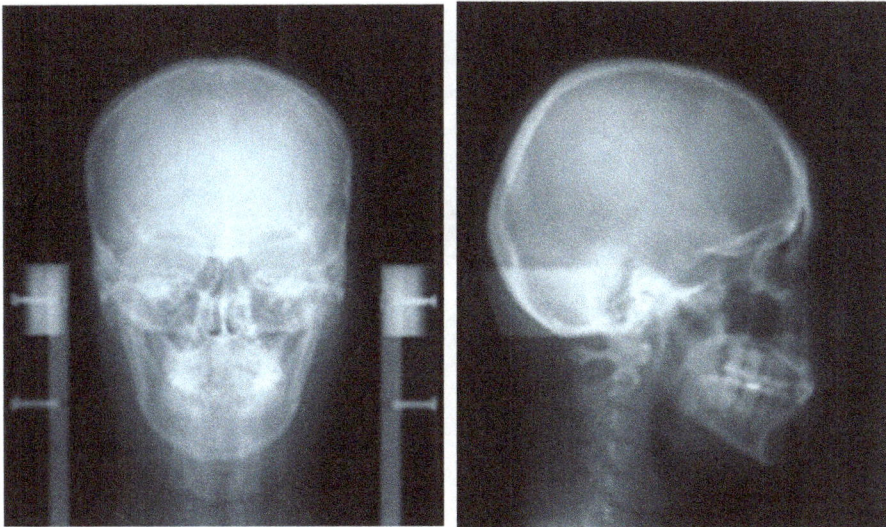

(a)

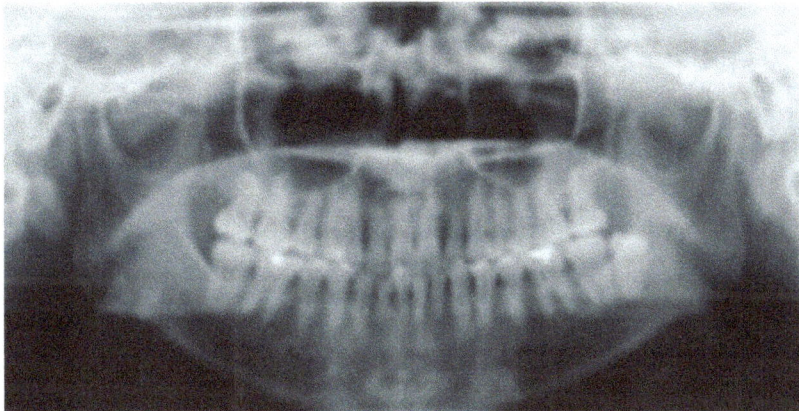

(b)

FIGURE 10: A post-retention cephalograms (a) and panoramic radiographs (b) are shown.

and 13(b) and Table 1). Therefore, the patient underwent coronally advanced flap repositioning surgery with a connective tissue graft for root coverage of the bilateral maxillary lateral incisors. Seventeen months after surgery, the patient had improved oral hygiene, had acquired esthetically good periodontal tissue, had stable functional occlusion, and was satisfied with the outcome (Figure 12(d)).

3. Discussion

From the results of the cephalometric analysis, this patient did not have particularly major dental or skeletal malocclusion, but her facial type was convex, and the distance between the upper lip and the E-line was 2 mm and that from the lower lip to the E-line was 5 mm (Table 1). Therefore, we considered that extraction of the first premolar or the front teeth might improve her profile from lingual movement of the maxillary and mandibular front teeth. However, there was significant alveolar bone resorption in the areas of the maxillary and mandibular

front teeth, so tooth extraction may have caused more significant loss of the supporting tissue, and the patient did not want tooth extraction to improve her profile. Therefore, treatment was commenced without tooth extraction.

In this patient, gingivitis, bleeding on probing, and tooth mobility were located in the maxillary and mandibular first molars and the maxillary and mandibular front teeth (Figures 3(a) and 3(b)), so the patient was diagnosed with Angle Class I extensive moderate chronic periodontitis [4]. Further, there was widening of the periodontal space in the right maxillary lateral dentition, which is a characteristic of occlusal trauma. Therefore, this patient was investigated using the BC with the aim of visualizing and assessing the cause of the occlusal trauma (Figure 4(a)), which is considered to be a factor exacerbating periodontitis [5, 6]. The results of that investigation confirmed that the location of functional contact in night-time parafunction correlated with the location of periodontal lesions on the chart. Thus, the aim of the orthodontic treatment was to close

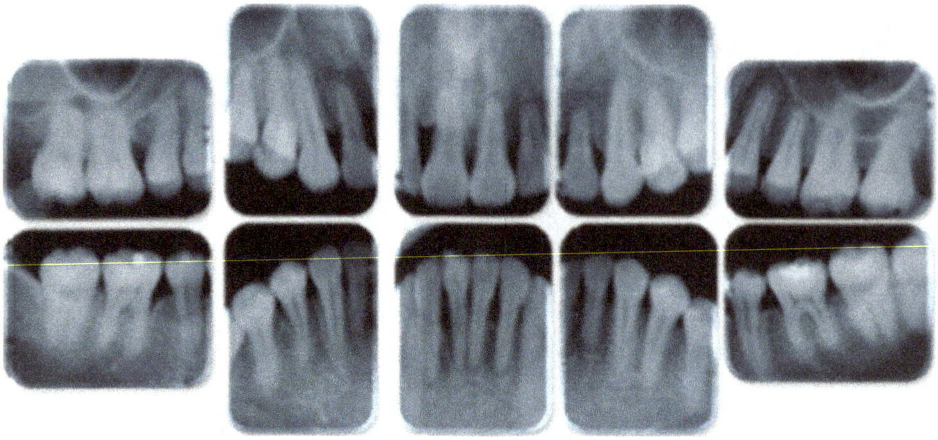

(a)

Tooth		17	16	15	14	13	12	11	21	22	23	24	25	26	27
Maxilla	Furcation														
	Mobility	0	0	0	0	0	0	0	0	0	0	0	0	0	0
	Probing B	3 3 2	2 3 3	3 2 3	3 3 3	3 3 3	3 3 2	2 3 3	3 3 3	4 2 3	2 2 2	3 3 2	3 3 3	3 3 3	3 3 3
	Depth P	3 3 3	2 3 3	3 3 3	3 3 2	3 3 3	3 3 2	3 3 3	3 3 3	3 3 3	2 2 3	2 3 3	3 3 3	3 3 3	3 3 3
Mandibular	Probing L	3 3 3	3 3 2	2 2 2	2 2 2	2 3 3	2 2 3	3 2 2	3 3 3	2 2 2	3 3 3	3 3 3	3 3 3	3 3 3	3 3 3
	Depth B	3 3 3	2 2 4	3 3 3	3 3 3	3 3 3	3 3 3	3 3 2	3 3 3	2 2 3	3 3 3	3 3 3	3 3 3	3 3 3	3 3 3
	Mobility	0	0	0	0	0	0	0	0	0	0	0	0	0	0
	Furcation														
Tooth		47	46	45	44	43	42	41	31	32	33	34	35	36	37

(b)

FIGURE 11: Post-retention dental radiographs (a) and periodontal examinations (b) are shown. The red color indicates bleeding on probing.

the spaced dental arch orthodontically and improve the tooth axes as well as to establish anterior guidance and reduce the functional lateral occlusal force of the lateral dentition as much as possible, thereby reducing occlusal trauma.

Orthodontic treatment for patients with periodontal disease not only exacerbates inflammation of the periodontal tissue with movement of the teeth, but may also promote resorption of diseased alveolar bone [8, 9]. Therefore, before starting active treatment with orthodontics, periodontal disease should be treated appropriately. This is essential to ensure ongoing management of the oral environment during orthodontic treatment. Before starting orthodontic treatment, we ensured that the inflammation was controlled by thorough periodontal treatment from a periodontal disease specialist, that the oral environment was stabilized, and that the patient thoroughly understood the importance of maintaining a stable oral environment (Figure 5). The orthodontic forces were set up to act continuously but as weakly as possible [10]. After leveling was complete, retraction on the maxillary and mandibular front teeth was performed using sliding mechanics with intermaxillary elastics. With detailing, appropriate step bends were performed as needed to achieve disclusion of the lateral dentition as much as possible during forward and lateral movement, and this was checked at each dental visit by moving the jaw in a gliding motion.

The BC was developed in 2006 as a simple way to observe parafunction during sleep [5]. The BC can observe occlusion at night-time to supplement information obtained from the articulator and/or chair side. Reports show that it is possible to observe the pattern, direction, and area of night-time grinding. Further, our own previous research [11] has shown a difference in contact aspects between occlusion observed on oral examination at the chair side and BC observations. We reported that there was less canine contact during night-time parafunction than when the patient was awake and increased contact on the working and nonworking sides of the molar region. The BC findings before removal of the device indicated that the gliding surfaces of the front teeth and the right lateral dentition were decreased in comparison with those before active orthodontic treatment (Figure 4(b)). This was one of the factors in the decision to complete active treatment and start use of a retainer using a plate. In other words, at the completion of active treatment, the lateral occlusal force of the lateral dentition due to night-time parafunction and excess occlusive force from the front teeth had lessened. Because of the synergistic effect of treatment for periodontal disease, there was regeneration of the bone in the mesial right maxillary first molar region. We considered that it might also have worked effectively on recovery of the lamina dura in other locations of bone resorption. Animal models of induction of periodontal disease have shown that if

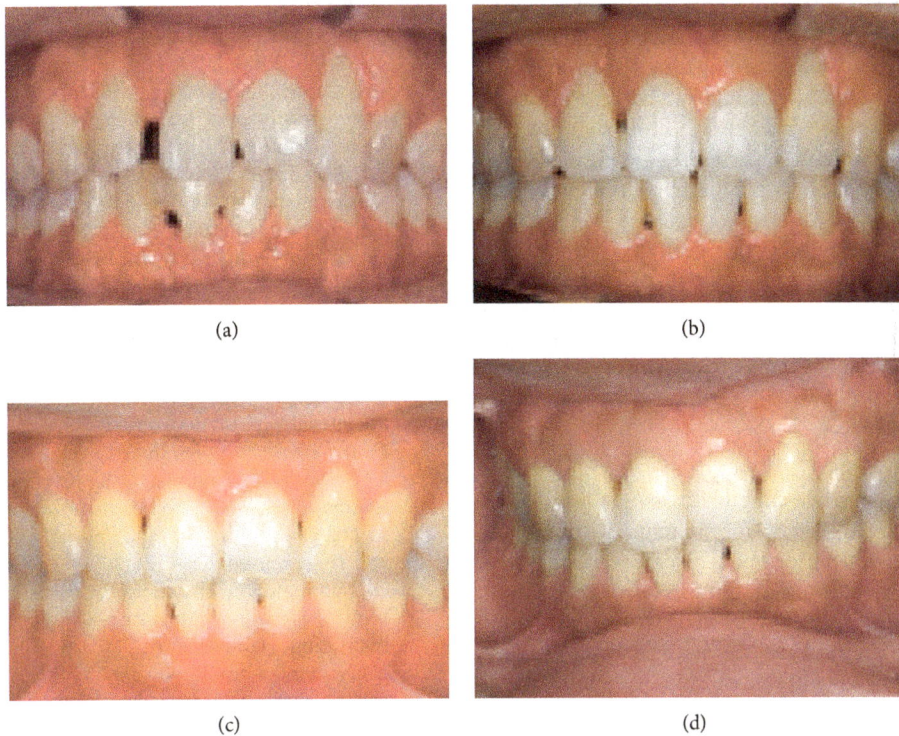

FIGURE 12: Frontal views of intraoral photographs are shown. (a) Before orthodontic treatment, (b) after orthodontic treatment, (c) at 6 months after periodontal surgical treatment, and (d) at 1 year 5 months after periodontal surgical treatment.

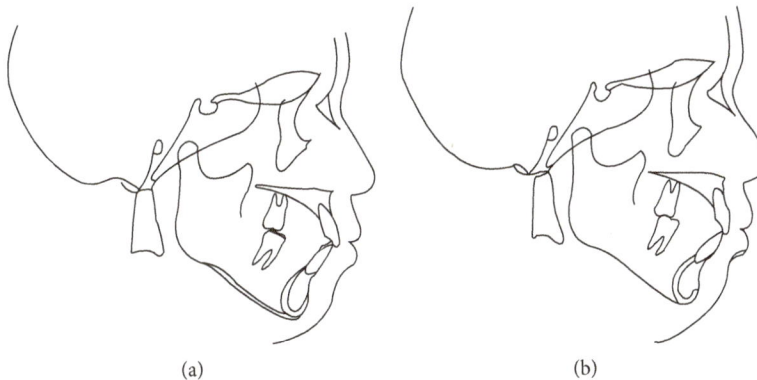

FIGURE 13: A superimposed cephalometric tracing is shown. (a) From pre-orthodontic treatment to post-orthodontic treatment; (b) from post-orthodontic treatment to postretention.

traumatic occlusion is added, there is accelerated loss of attachment, and induction of alveolar bone osteoclasts is activated [12]. Based on this information, investigating this condition based on the results of an assessment of occlusion function with the BC and periodontal examination is considered effective in enabling occlusal treatment goal clarification through orthodontic treatment in cases of periodontal disease associated with occlusal trauma, as in the present case. We believe that an effective technique can be established as a research method for the relationship between periodontal findings and occlusion aspects.

After 2 years of using a retainer and after checking that there was no pathologic function contact on reassessment with the BC (Figure 4(c)), we decided to perform periodontal surgical treatment for the bilateral maxillary lateral incisors. We were able to confirm that the bilateral lateral incisors had clearer lamina dura than that before surgery and that the periodontal tissue was stable (Figures 9(b) and 10(b)). However, there was high-grade gingival recession, which was an esthetic failure. The depth of the gingival recession was more than 3 mm for both teeth, and the width of the keratinized tissue on the root apex side was 2 mm or greater. Therefore, we explained that it may not be possible to completely cover the root surface and performed coronally advanced flap repositioning surgery together with a connective tissue graft for root coverage [13]. The left lateral incisors had significantly more bone resorption than on the right side, which resulted in a lower coverage rate than on the right side. Root surface coverage has been reported in a systematic review by the American Academy of Periodontology in 2015 [14], and the report showed that predictability was high for Classes I and II in Miller's classification, but was low for Classes III and IV. Our patient had similar results, but was satisfied with the results, and after a year of recuperation, she continues to convalesce well (Figure 12).

4. Conclusion

Collaborating with a periodontal disease specialist to manage orthodontic treatment for patients with malocclusion associated with periodontal disease not only ensures a better oral environment, but is also considered effective in motivating patients to maintain a good oral environment. Visualization of night-time parafunction with the BC enables not only an examination of possible occlusal trauma by investigating the results together with the periodontal chart, but also clarification of treatment goals for occlusal reconstruction through orthodontic treatment.

References

[1] Y. Nakamura, K. Gomi, T. Oikawa, H. Tokiwa, and T. Sekiya, "Reconstruction of a collapsed dental arch in a patient with severe periodontitis," *American Journal of Orthodontics and Dentofacial Orthopedics*, vol. 143, no. 5, pp. 704–712, 2013.

[2] Y. Xie, Q. Zhao, Z. Tan, and S. Yang, "Orthodontic treatment in a periodontal patient with pathologic migration of anterior teeth," *American Journal of Orthodontics and Dentofacial Orthopedics*, vol. 145, no. 5, pp. 685–693, 2014.

[3] Y. Ishihara, K. Tomikawa, T. Deguchi et al., "Interdisciplinary orthodontic treatment for a patient with generalized aggressive periodontitis: assessment of IgG antibodies to identify type of periodontitis and correct timing of treatment," *American Journal of Orthodontics and Dentofacial Orthopedics*, vol. 147, no. 6, pp. 766–780, 2015.

[4] L. J. Brown and H. Löe, "Prevalence, extent, severity and progression of periodontal disease," *Periodontology 2000*, vol. 2, no. 1, pp. 57–71, 1993.

[5] K. Onodera, T. Kawagoe, K. Sasaguri, C. Protacio-Quismundo, and S. Sato, "The use of a bruxchecker in the evaluation of different grinding patterns during sleep bruxism," *Cranio*, vol. 24, no. 4, pp. 292–299, 2006.

[6] B. K. Park, O. Tokiwa, Y. Takezawa, Y. Takahashi, K. Sasaguri, and S. Sato, "Relationship of tooth grinding pattern during sleep bruxism and temporomandibular joint status," *Cranio*, vol. 26, no. 1, pp. 8–15, 2008.

[7] P. D. Miller Jr., "A classification of marginal tissue recession," *International Journal of Periodontics and Restorative Dentistry*, vol. 5, no. 2, pp. 8–13, 1985.

[8] J. Lindhe and G. Svanberg, "Influence of trauma from occlusion on progression of experimental periodontitis in the beagle dog," *Journal of Clinical Periodontology*, vol. 1, no. 1, pp. 3–14, 1974.

[9] J. L. Wennström, B. L. Stokland, S. Nyman, and B. Thilander, "Periodontal tissue response to orthodontic movement of teeth with infrabony pockets," *American Journal of Orthodontics and Dentofacial Orthopedics*, vol. 103, no. 4, pp. 313–319, 1993.

[10] M. M. Ong and H. L. Wang, "Periodontic and orthodontic treatment in adults," *American Journal of Orthodontics and Dentofacial Orthopedics*, vol. 122, no. 4, pp. 420–428, 2002.

[11] T. Kawagoe, J. Saruta, S. Miyake, K. Sasaguri, S. Akimoto, and S. Sato, "Relationship between occlusal contact patterns and the prevalence of non-carious cervical lesions," *Journal of Dental Health*, vol. 58, pp. 542–547, 2008.

[12] S. Nakatsu, Y. Yoshinaga, A. Kuramoto et al., "Occlusal trauma accelerates attachment loss at the onset of experimental periodontitis in rats," *Journal of Periodontal Research*, vol. 49, no. 3, pp. 314–322, 2014.

[13] O. Zuhr and M. Hürzeler, *Plastic-Esthetic Periodontal and Implant Surgery: Microsurgical Approach*, Quintessence Publishing, Hanover Park, IL, USA, 2012.

[14] L. Chambrone and D. N. Tatakis, "Periodontal soft tissue root coverage procedures: a systematic review from the AAP Regeneration Workshop," *Journal of Periodontology*, vol. 86, no. 2, pp. S8–S51, 2015.

5

Interceptive Correction of Anterior Crossbite Using Short-Span Wire-Fixed Orthodontic Appliance

S. Nagarajan M. P. Sockalingam ⓘD, Khairil Aznan Mohamed Khan, and Elavarasi Kuppusamy

Centre for Family Oral Health, Faculty of Dentistry, The National University of Malaysia (UKM), Bangi, Malaysia

Correspondence should be addressed to S. Nagarajan M. P. Sockalingam; drnaga67@gmail.com

Academic Editor: Giuseppe Alessandro Scardina

Anterior crossbite is relatively a common presentation in the mixed dentition stage. If left untreated, it can lead to a host of problems and may complicate future orthodontic treatment. One of the major difficulties in performing anterior crossbite correction in young children is treatment compliance. In most cases, poor compliance is due to the unacceptability of the removable appliance used. This article describes three cases of successful correction of anterior crossbite of patients in mixed dentition using short-span wire-fixed orthodontic appliances. This sectional appliance provides an alternative method of correcting anterior crossbite of dental origin and offers many advantages compared to the use of removable appliances.

1. Introduction

Anterior crossbite is defined as an abnormal reversed relationship of a tooth or teeth to the opposing teeth in the buccolingual or labiolingual direction, and it is also known as reverse articulation [1]. The prevalence of anterior crossbite ranges from 4.5% to 9.5% based on the respective studied populations [2–5]. In children with malocclusion, it is reported to be around 27% [6].

Many factors may contribute toward the development of anterior crossbite, and the contributory factors can be categorised based on the nature of the crossbite into skeletal, dental, and functional entities [7]. Skeletal anterior crossbite arises due to either genetic or hereditary influence or discrepancy in the size of the maxilla and mandible. The skeletal entity usually involves a segment of maxillary teeth that are proclined at normal angulation but positioned behind the mandibular incisors. In the anterior crossbite of dental origin, one or two teeth are often involved, and the affected tooth/teeth are either upright or retrocline without any significant maxilla-mandible discrepancy. In the functional-type crossbite, a premature contact between the opposing tooth/teeth could result in the deflection of the mandible to the sides or anteriorly, and this leads to the development of pseudoclass-III [8].

Anterior crossbite may give rise to enamel wear mainly close to the incisal edge due to heavy contact between the opposing tooth/teeth [6]. An abnormal bite between the opposing teeth can also affect periodontal health, and this could lead to the gingival recession with thinning of the alveolar bone and mobility of the opposing mandibular tooth/teeth [6, 9, 10]. Functional crossbite due to the premature contact could lead to a possible jaw deviation and temporomandibular pain dysfunction [6, 11].

Many treatment modalities ranging from simple to complex means are available to correct anterior crossbite; some use removable appliances and others use fixed appliances [7, 12–20]. The appropriate method to treat anterior crossbite will depend on the aetiology of the crossbite, the patient's age and compliance, eruption status of the teeth, space availability, and treatment affordability. A simple method such as tongue blade can be used in the early stages of anterior crossbite development as the tooth/teeth are erupting. Appliances such as Catlan's appliance and removable appliances with z-spring(s) or expansion screw or microscrew(s) are often used to correct anterior crossbite related to dental factors in the preadolescent age group. Crossbite of skeletal origin often requires complex methods, such as rapid maxillary expansion and Frankel III appliances. Occasionally, use of extra-oral devices such as a face mask and a chin cup may be necessary to correct the skeletal-based anterior crossbite [7].

This article highlights three cases of successful correction of anterior crossbite using simple short-span wire-fixed orthodontic appliances. The use of this type of appliance provides an alternative treatment modality to correct anterior crossbite with good patient compliance and minimal disruption of oral functions.

2. Case Report

2.1. Case 1. An 8-year 5-month old boy came with his parents to the Paediatric Dental Clinic of the Dental Faculty at the National University of Malaysia (UKM) with a primary complaint of maligned teeth. Parents noticed that some of their son's upper teeth were behind his lower teeth. The patient has no previous history of dental treatment, and his medical history was noncontributory.

Intraoral examination revealed the patient in mixed dentition stage with the first permanent molars in a Class I relationship. Three of his permanent maxillary teeth, right lateral incisor (tooth 12), left central incisor (tooth 21), and left lateral incisor (tooth 22), were in a crossbite relationship (Figure 1). Slight enamel attrition was noted on the labial surface of tooth 22 close to the incisal edge due to traumatic occlusion. Space analysis using the Moyer's mixed dentition analysis showed the availability of adequate space within the arch for realignment of teeth.

After discussing the treatment modalities with parents, we selected a short-span wire-fixed orthodontic treatment with four preadjusted edgewise brackets with a 0.022″ slot. The brackets were bonded on the labial aspects of the four maxillary permanent incisors. A short-span nickel-titanium (Ni-Ti) 0.014″ round archwire is cut equally on both sides of the centreline and placed into the bracket slots (Figure 2). The wire was stabilised in its position using elastic ties. The patient's bite was raised using 2 mm thickness of glass ionomer cement (GIC) placed on the occlusal aspects of both the mandibular first permanent molars (tooth 36 and tooth 46).

Two weeks later, there was some evidence of anterior movement of the maxillary teeth that were in crossbite. Within a month after the initiation of treatment, the anterior crossbite was corrected successfully. The 0.014″ round Ni-Ti archwire was changed to the 0.016″ round Ni-Ti archwire and retained for further two weeks before debonding of the brackets. At 3-month review, the incisor teeth were still in positive overjet (Figure 3).

2.2. Case 2. A 7-year 2-month old boy was seen in the Paediatric Clinic at the Faculty of Dentistry, National University of Malaysia (UKM), for routine dental assessment. He had previous dental treatment under general anaesthesia two years ago, and his medical history was noncontributory.

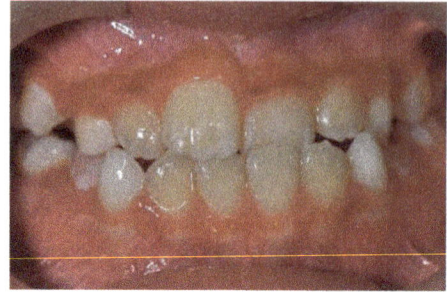

FIGURE 1: Pretreatment photograph of tooth 12, 21, and 22 in crossbite.

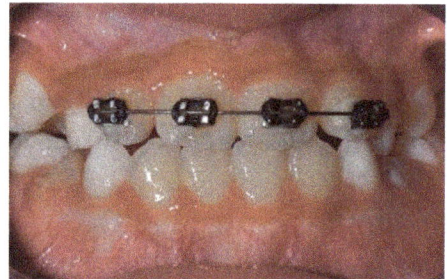

FIGURE 2: Sectional short-span wire-fixed orthodontic appliance in place during treatment.

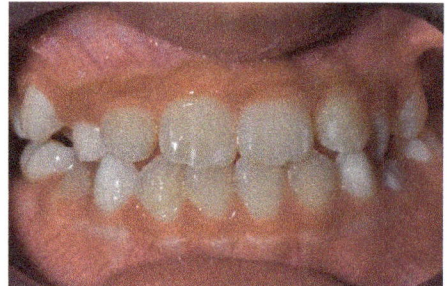

FIGURE 3: Posttreatment photograph at 3-month review after correction of the anterior crossbite.

Intraoral examination showed all primary teeth of the patient missing due to the previous extraction. Both the permanent maxillary and mandibular first molars on either side have erupted into occlusion. Anteriorly, the permanent maxillary right central incisor (tooth 11) was in a crossbite with the permanent mandibular right central incisor (tooth 41). In occlusion, tooth 11 was trapped between tooth 41 and the permanent mandibular right lateral incisor (tooth 42) (Figure 4). Tooth 41 has Class II tooth mobility and gingival recession on its labial aspect.

After discussion with the parents on the treatment options, we decided on using a short-span wire-fixed appliance with two preadjusted edgewise brackets. The patient's bite was raised with 2 mm thickness of GIC placed on the occlusal aspects of the permanent mandibular first molars. GIC placement allowed opening of the anterior bite and released the lock of trapped tooth 11. Two preadjusted edgewise brackets with a 0.022″ slot were bonded to the labial surface of tooth 11 and the permanent maxillary left

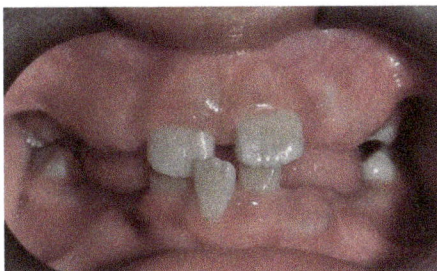

FIGURE 4: Pretreatment photograph of tooth 11 in crossbite.

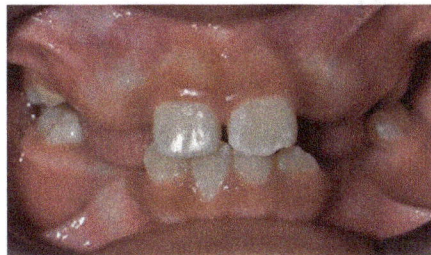

FIGURE 6: Posttreatment photograph at 6 months after correction of the anterior crossbite.

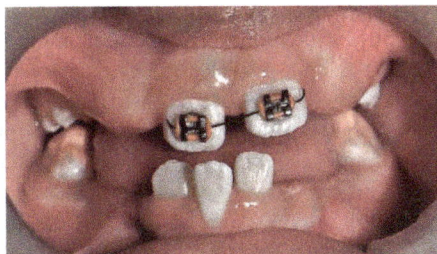

FIGURE 5: Sectional short-span wire-fixed orthodontic appliance in place during treatment.

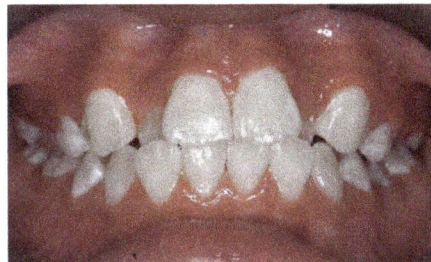

FIGURE 7: Pretreatment photograph of tooth 12 and 22 in crossbite.

central incisor (tooth 21). A short Ni-Ti 0.014″ round archwire was placed into the brackets and held in place with elastic ties (Figure 5).

Two weeks later, the crossbite was corrected. The brackets were debonded, and the GIC on teeth 36 and 46 was removed using an ultrasonic scaler. The occlusion was stable, and the gingival height of tooth 41 showed significant improvement at 6-month review (Figure 6).

2.3. Case 3. An 8-year 2-month old boy presented to the Paediatric Dental Clinic of the Dental Faculty at the National University of Malaysia (UKM) with a chief complaint of trapped upper teeth. He had restorative dental treatment to some of his teeth a year ago, and his medical history was noncontributory.

The intraoral assessment showed that the patient was in his mixed dentition stage and the first permanent molars were in a Class I relationship on either side. The permanent maxillary lateral incisors (teeth 12 and 22) were trapped palatally in an anterior crossbite behind the maxillary deciduous canines (teeth 53 and 63) and the permanent maxillary central incisors (teeth 11 and 21), respectively (Figure 7). He has a Class-I incisor relationship with an overjet and an overbite of 3 mm each. Some evidence of wear facets was noted on the occlusal surfaces of the primary and permanent molars although the patient denied any parafunctional activity. A panoramic radiograph taken a year ago showed the presence of tooth germs of the permanent maxillary canines in a favourable position with no overlapping of the crowns over the roots of teeth 12 and 22 (Figure 8). However, tooth 53 and tooth 63 were relatively big, and limited space was available for teeth 12 and 22 to move anteriorly. Upon consultation with an orthodontist and taking into consideration the patient's molar and incisor

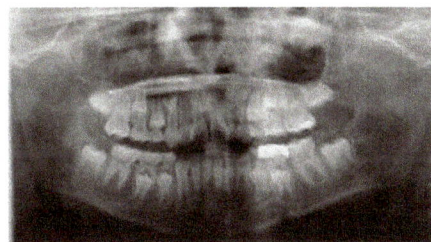

FIGURE 8: Panoramic radiograph view taken 6 months before treatment showing the position of permanent maxillary canines in relation to their primary predecessors and maxillary permanent lateral incisors.

relationship, we decided to extract the primary canines to allow distalization of teeth 12 and 22.

A month later, after observing slight distalization of teeth 12 and 22, a lower removable bite-raising acrylic appliance was made to open up the anterior bite. Then, four preadjusted edgewise brackets were bonded to the labial surfaces of the maxillary incisors, and a short Ni-Ti 0.014″ round archwire was placed into the brackets and held in place with elastic ties (Figure 9). A month later, anterior movement of teeth 12 and 22 was noted. The existing Ni-Ti wire was changed to the Ni-Ti 0.016″ round archwire, and the patient was reviewed monthly. After three months, we were able to correct the anterior crossbite of teeth 12 and 22. At 6-month review, the corrected teeth were still in positive overjet (Figure 10). The patient is currently under review for the monitoring of the permanent canines eruption.

3. Discussion

Anterior crossbite is a common presentation in children during the early mixed dentition stage, and a majority of the

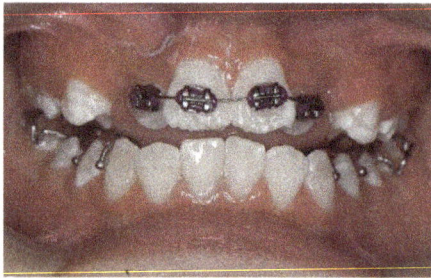

FIGURE 9: Sectional short-span wire-fixed orthodontic appliance in place during treatment.

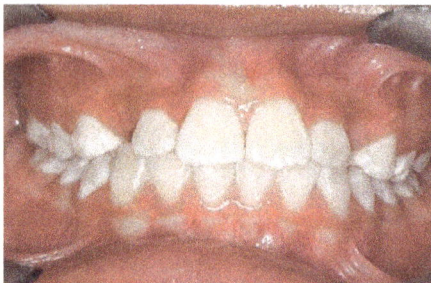

FIGURE 10: Posttreatment photograph at 6 months after correction of the anterior crossbite.

cases are of dental origin [21]. Possible causes of dentally related anterior crossbite are the presence of supernumerary tooth/teeth, odontomas, trauma to the primary predecessor, ectopic position of permanent tooth germ, retained primary predecessor, anomalies in tooth shape and size, arch length inadequacy, and upper lip biting habit [7, 13, 14]. These dentally related factors are responsible for deflection of the normal eruption path of the permanent successor tooth/teeth.

Early treatment to correct the anterior crossbite is often advisable to prevent a much more complicated problem and treatment at a later stage. Early treatment allows harmonisation of the occlusion with time, as the permanent teeth are still erupting during this stage of the dentition [15]. However, provision of early treatment has its own sets of problems such as poor patient compliance and refusal of treatment, and the patient may need another phase of orthodontic treatment later. Nevertheless, early treatment can prevent some of the common detrimental effects of anterior crossbite such as enamel wear, gingival striping and attachment loss, tooth mobility, and jaw deviation [16]. Research has shown that patients' oral health quality of life improves with early treatment [22].

Although the use of the intraoral and extraoral appliances can produce the desired tooth or functional jaw movement, patients' compliance very much dictate the treatment success. Common problems encountered with the use of removable appliances include initial speech difficulty due to palatal coverage of the appliance, progressive loosening of the appliance used, and tendency of the patient to flick the loose appliance in and out with the tongue. Besides that, breakage and loss of appliances also happen due to

patients' carelessness. Other disadvantages of removable appliances include limited tooth movement range, appliance bulkiness, and poor oral hygiene maintenance. Similarly, patients are also not very much in favour of extraoral devices because of their visibility and social stigma attached to its usage. These adverse effects of both the intraoral and extraoral devices often lead to poor patient compliance and failure of treatment [12, 23].

Use of the fixed orthodontic method to correct anterior crossbite during the preadolescent period has not been widely reported in the literature as compared to other methods as described above. Few cases using a simple fixed orthodontic to correct anterior crossbite and alignment of ectopic teeth have shown good clinical outcome [12, 24, 25]. Many of the problems related to the usage of removable appliances can be overcome with the use of a simple fixed orthodontic appliance. One of the described simple fixed orthodontic appliances is the two-by-four (2 × 4) appliance which allows three-dimensional tooth movement that enables correction of not only the crossbite but also the rotated teeth, teeth with incorrect angulation and inclination, and diastema. Besides that, the 2 × 4 appliance is also suitable for mixed dentition patients with a reduced number of teeth, where the retention of the removable appliance used can be a problem [12, 23, 24, 26].

One of the disadvantages of using the 2 × 4 appliance during the early mixed dentition stage is the placement of bands on the maxillary first permanent molars. Placement of the molar band could be a problem if the permanent molar has not fully erupted or it has a short clinical crown height. Sometimes, placement of the band also can cause discomfort, and some children may refuse further treatment. Furthermore, as the brackets are only bonded to the permanent incisors, there will be a long span of a flexible 0.014″ round Ni-Ti archwire extending from the molar bands to the incisors. The dangling wire can be a problem to the young patients especially during eating and tooth brushing as the wire dangles can easily come out from the molar tube. Another disadvantage of the 2 × 4 appliance is plaque retention around the bands and brackets. However, this could be easily overcome with good oral hygiene care.

The cases presented in this article demonstrated the usage of the sectional short-span wire-fixed orthodontic appliance in correcting cases of anterior crossbite. The appliance is as effective as the 2 × 4 appliance but minus the use of orthodontic bands. The short-span wire-fixed orthodontic appliance method is handy for correction of simple anterior crossbite and especially in cases where the first permanent molars are either unavailable or partially erupted for successful placement of orthodontic bands.

Although this is a simple method for anterior crossbite correction, the clinician should perform a thorough clinical assessment of the patient's facial and dental profiles and make an appropriate diagnosis to determine the cause of the crossbite. The sectional short-span wire-fixed orthodontic appliance is very reliable to correct simple labiolingual discrepancies of the dental origin. However, if the labiolingual difference is vast, use of the 2 × 4 appliance is justifiable because it produces a well-controlled movement of teeth. In anterior crossbite of skeletal origin, sole use of the sectional short-span wire-fixed orthodontic appliance may not produce the desired outcome. Similarly, in functional anterior crossbite, the source of the premature contact needs to be eliminated first before commencing with the correction of the crossbite with either the fixed or removable appliance.

4. Conclusion

The highlighted cases showed that it is possible to treat anterior crossbite with the sectional short-span wire-fixed orthodontic appliance, and it offers an alternative treatment option to consider. Early, simple, and tolerable correction of anterior crossbite is beneficial to provide aesthetic and social well-being of the preadolescent children. However, the usage of the sectional short-span wire-fixed orthodontic for treatment of severely rotated teeth, teeth with extreme angulation or inclination, and wide diastema may require further clinical evidence, and consultation with an orthodontist is necessary.

References

[1] American Association of Orthodontists, 2012, https://www.aaoinfo.org/system/files/media/documents/2012 AAO Glossary_0.doc.

[2] M. Shalish, A. Gal, I. Brin, A. Zini, and Y. Ben-Bassat, "Prevalence of dental features that indicate a need for early orthodontic treatment," *European Journal of Orthodontics*, vol. 35, no. 4, pp. 454–459, 2012.

[3] E. R. Reddy, M. Manjula, N. Sreelakshmi, S. T. Rani, R. Aduri, and B. D. Patil, "Prevalence of malocclusion among 6 to 10 year old Nalgonda school children," *Journal of International Oral Health*, vol. 5, no. 6, pp. 49–54, 2013.

[4] H. Kaur, U. S. Pavithra, and R. Abraham, "Prevalence of malocclusion among adolescents in South Indian population," *Journal of Indian Society of Preventive and Community Dentistry*, vol. 3, no. 2, pp. 97–102, 2013.

[5] S. P. Singh, V. Kumar, and P. Narboo, "Prevalence of malocclusion among children and adolescents in various school of Leh Region," *Journal of Orthodontics and Endodontics*, vol. 1, no. 2, pp. 1–6, 2015.

[6] S. N. Vithanaarachchi and L. S. Nawarathna, "Prevalence of anterior cross bite in preadolescent orthodontic patients attending an orthodontic clinic," *Ceylon Medical Journal*, vol. 62, no. 3, pp. 189–192, 2017.

[7] G. Singh, "Management of crossbite," in *Textbook of Orthodontics*, pp. 655–670, Jaypee Publisher, New Delhi, India, 3rd edition, 2015.

[8] K. Ustun, Z. Sari, H. Orucoglu, I. Duran, and S. S. Hakki, "Severe gingival recession caused by traumatic occlusion and mucogingival stress: a case report," *European Journal of Dentistry*, vol. 2, pp. 127–133, 2008.

[9] A. Hanoun, B. Preston, M. Burlingame et al., *Early Diagnosis and Treatment of Anterior Crossbite*, Dental Learning, Manalapan, NJ, USA, 2015, http://www.dentallearning.net/.

[10] A. M. Bollen, "Effects of malocclusions and orthodontics on periodontal health: evidence from a systematic review," *Journal of Dental Education*, vol. 72, no. 8, pp. 912–918, 2008.

[11] V. Wohlberg, C. Schwahn, D. Gesch, G. Meyer, T. Kocher, and O. Bernhardt, "The association between anterior crossbite, deep bite and temporomandibular joint morphology validated by magnetic resonance imaging in an adult non-patient group," *Annals of Anatomy-Anatomischer Anzeiger*, vol. 194, no. 4, pp. 339–344, 2012.

[12] H. F. Mckeown and J. Sandlerd, "The two by four appliance: a versatile appliance," *Dental Update*, vol. 28, no. 10, pp. 496–500, 2001.

[13] P. W. Major and K. Glover, "Treatment of anterior cross-bites in the early mixed dentition," *Journal of Canadian Dental Association*, vol. 58, no. 7, pp. 574–575, 1992.

[14] S. M. Yaseen and R. Acharya, "Hexa helix: modified quad helix appliance to correct anterior and posterior crossbites in mixed dentition," *Case Reports in Dentistry*, vol. 2012, Article ID 860385, 5 pages, 2012.

[15] A. T. Ulusoy and E. H. Bodrumlu, "Management of anterior dental crossbite with removable appliances," *Contemporary Clinical Dentistry*, vol. 4, no. 2, pp. 223–226, 2013.

[16] I. Jirgensone, A. Liepa, and A. Abeltins, "Anterior crossbite correction in primary and mixed dentition with removable inclined plane (Bruckl appliance)," *Stomatologija (Baltic Dental and Maxillofacial Journal)*, vol. 10, no. 4, pp. 140–144, 2008.

[17] S. Bayrak and E. S. Tunc, "Treatment of anterior dental crossbite using bonded resin-composite slopes: case reports," *European Journal of Dentistry*, vol. 2, pp. 303–306, 2008.

[18] P. Prakash Prakash and B. H. Durgesh, "Anterior crossbite correction in early mixed dentition period using catlan's appliance: a case report," *ISRN Dentistry*, vol. 2011, Article ID 298931, 5 pages, 2011.

[19] K. K. Abraham, A. R. James, E. Thenumkal, and T. Emmatty, "Correction of anterior crossbite using modified transparent aligners: an esthetic approach," *Contemporary Clinical Dentistry*, vol. 7, no. 3, pp. 394–397, 2016.

[20] J. A. Dean, "Managing the developing occlusion," in *McDonald and Avery's Dentistry for the Child and Adolescent*, pp. 415–478, Elsevier Publication, St. Louis, Mo, USA, 10th edition, 2016.

[21] G. Vadiakas and A. D. Viazis, "Anterior crossbite correction in the early deciduous dentition," *American Journal of Orthodontics and Dentofacial Orthopedics*, vol. 102, no. 2, pp. 160–162, 1992.

[22] E. Piassi, L. S. Antunes, M. R. T. C. Andrade, and L. A. A. Antunes, "Quality of life following early orthodontic therapy for anterior crossbite: report of cases in twin boys," *Case Reports in Dentistry*, vol. 2016, Article ID 3685693, 5 pages, 2016.

[23] P. Dowsing and J. Sandler, "How to effectively use a 2 × 4 appliance," *Journal of Orthodontics*, vol. 31, no. 3, pp. 248–258, 2004.

[24] R. S. Asher, C. G. Kuster, and L. Erickson, "Anterior dental crossbite correction using a simple fixed appliance: case report," *Pediatric Dentistry*, vol. 8, no. 1, pp. 53–55, 1986.

[25] M. M. Sunil, M. A. Zareena, M. S. Ratheesh, and G. Anjana, "Early orthodontic interception of anterior crossbite in mixed dentition," *Journal of International Oral Health*, vol. 9, no. 2, pp. 88–90, 2017.

[26] R. M. Skeggs and P. J. Sandler, "Rapid correction of anterior crossbite using a fixed appliance: a case report," *Dental Update*, vol. 29, no. 6, pp. 299–302, 2002.

6

Phenotypic Features and Salivary Parameters in Patients with Ectodermal Dysplasia

Mônica Fernandes Gomes ⓘ,[1] Luigi Giovanni Bernardo Sichi,[1]
Lilian Chrystiane Giannasi,[1,2,3] José Benedito Oliveira Amorim,[1]
João Carlos da Rocha,[1] Cristiane Yumi Koga-Ito,[1] and
Miguel Angel Castillo Salgado[1]

[1]Center of Biosciences Applied to Patients with Special Health Care Needs (CEPAPE), Institute of Science and Technology, São Jose dos Campos Campus, São Paulo State University–UNESP, São Paulo, SP, Brazil
[2]Dental School, Metropolitan University of Santos (UNIMES), Santos, SP, Brazil
[3]Sleep Disorders Laboratory, Universitary Center of Anápolis (UniEvangelica), Anápolis, GO, Brazil

Correspondence should be addressed to Mônica Fernandes Gomes; mfgomes@ict.unesp.br

Academic Editor: Luis M. J. Gutierrez

Ectodermal dysplasia (ED) is a rare hereditary disorder affecting the development of ectoderm-derived organs and tissues. The aim of this study was to describe phenotypic features and the therapeutic approach in dentistry among three patients with ED, correlating their data with the literature. Additionally, to investigate the salivary gland disorders and their impacts on oral microbiota, we performed salivary tests, including salivary flow rate, salivary buffering capacity, and concentration levels of mutans streptococci, lactobacilli, and yeasts. All patients presented oligodontia, resulting in a significant masticatory dysfunction and aesthetic impairment. The counts of mutans streptococci ($n = 3$) and yeasts ($n = 2$) were high; on the other hand, the count of lactobacilli ($n = 3$) was low. Therefore, salivary and microbiological tests showed that the patients with ED, particularly the hypohidrotic type, presented a high risk of enamel caries and susceptibility to oral infections, which may be likely triggered by reduction of salivary flow and/or possible immunological disorders.

1. Introduction

Ectodermal dysplasia (ED) is a rare nonprogressive congenital hereditary disorder, characterized by developmental defects of ectoderm-derived organs and tissues, affecting at least two of the following structures: nails, teeth, skin, and secretory organs (eccrine sweat, salivary, lacrimal, and mucous glands of the respiratory and gastrointestinal tracts) [1–3]. The classification of ED is based on genetic findings and phenotypic features, which is divided into two categories: anhidrotic/hypohidrotic (HED; X-linked inheritance) and hidrotic (HidED; autosomal-dominant inheritance) [4–6]. HED is the most frequent form, caused mainly by mutations in the *EDA* gene, located at the long arm of the X-chromosome (Xq12-q13.1), followed by the *EDAR* and *EDARADD* genes

[4,7–10]. These genes regulate specific protein expression, especially the ectodysplasin A, which plays an important role during embryonic development [10, 11]. The HED triad includes sparse hair (hypotrichosis), reduced ability to sweat (hypohidrosis), and the lack of several teeth (hypodontia or oligodontia). Thus, the "classical" clinical characteristics are sparseness or absence of hair, eyebrows, and eyelashes; hypoplasia or agenesis of sweat, submucous, and sebaceous glands leading to episodes of heat intolerance and hyperpyrexia; dry mouth; and dentition abnormalities (incorrect numbers and shape), resulting in impaired mastication, speech disorders, and often affecting the aesthetics [4, 8, 10, 12]. Other relevant symptoms are low tear secretion, poorly functioning mucous membranes, recurrent upper respiratory tract infections, hearing or vision deficits, cleft lip and/or palate, immune

(a)   (b)

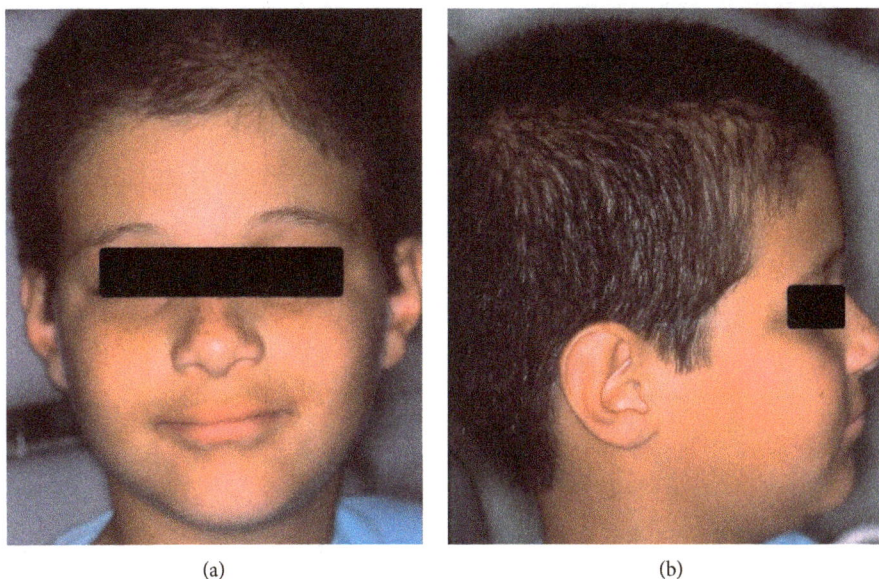

FIGURE 1: Patient 1. Child with hidrotic ED had sparse hair and eyebrows and discrete perioral pigmentation (a and b).

dysfunction, sensitivity to light, and lack of breast development [13, 14]. HidED is caused by mutations in the *GJB6* gene, located on chromosome 13 (locus 13q12), which encodes connexin-30, a component of intercellular gap junctions. The main clinical characteristics are hair loss, palmoplantar keratoderma, dystrophic nails, atrichia or hypotrichosis, and discrete skin hyperpigmentation. Other manifestations may be found, including strabism, conjunctivitis, pterygium, cataracts, sensorineural deafness, polydactyly, and syndactyly [4, 8]. Hypoplastic submandibular glands and abnormal development of minor salivary glands have also been described [7, 13].

Based on this, we describe the phenotypic features and the therapeutic approach in dentistry among three patients with ED, correlating their data with data from literature. We also analyzed their salivary characteristics, such as salivary flow rate, buffering capacity of saliva, and concentration levels of mutans streptococci, lactobacilli, and yeasts, aiming for a better understanding of salivary gland disorders and their impacts on oral microbiota with pathogenic properties. This work was undertaken in accordance with the ethical standards of the Declaration of Helsinki.

2. Case Reports

2.1. Clinical and Radiographic Features

2.1.1. Patient 1. An 11-year-old Caucasian male child complained of oral aesthetic impairment caused by the accentuated diastema. The mother reported delayed eruption of the primary dentition during his childhood. He had good general health; however, episodes of hyperpyrexia were reported, mainly during sports activities. Upon extraoral examination, perioral pigmentation and dry skin were evidenced (Figure 1). Upon intraoral examination, an accentuated diastema between the upper central incisors was observed due to insertion of the labial frenulum into the gum ridge. Fourteen permanent teeth were absent, including the

right left lower central incisors, right left upper and lower lateral incisors, right left upper and lower canines, and right left lower second first premolars (Figure 2). Discrete mild chronic gingivitis due to the presence of supragingival dental biofilm, and no caries were also observed. Thus, an incisional biopsy in the gluteal region was performed to confirm the diagnosis of ectodermal dysplasia, and the histological sections showed few hair follicles and eccrine sweat glands and absence of sebaceous glands (Figure 3). These findings confirmed the diagnosis of HidED. The recommended treatment was dental prophylaxis, topical application of 1.23% fluoride, oral hygiene control, and occlusal adjustment of the preexisting teeth to prevent root resorptions, particularly the deciduous teeth.

2.1.2. Patient 2. A 14-year-old Caucasian adolescent boy with HED had partial anodontia and difficulties in eating, swallowing, and speech, significantly affecting his self-esteem. The medical history reported by the patient was heat intolerance and suffering from hyperpyrexia, frequent colds, and otitis, and recurrent respiratory tract infections were described. Moreover, eye drops and nasal lubricants have been frequently used to relieve eye and nose dryness, respectively. Upon general examination, dry skin and hyperkeratosis, especially in the joints of the upper and lower limbs, were described. Upon extraoral examination, scarce, fine and silky hair, alopecia of the eyelashes and eyebrows, prominent frontal bossing, discrete bilateral deformity and low implantation of the ear, perioral dermatitis and fissures, bilateral angular cheilitis, periorbital pigmentation, and deep nasolabial sulcus were evidenced (Figure 4). Upon intraoral examination, it was verified that almost all permanent teeth were absent, except the right upper permanent canine, resulting in a significant loss of occlusal vertical dimension and an appearance of old age. The upper and lower alveolar ridges were underdeveloped, and the buccal mucosa was found pale and sharply dry. Chronic mouth breathing was also diagnosed.

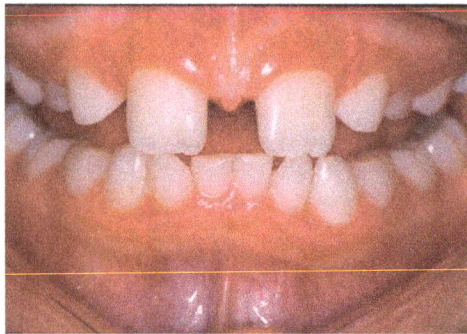

(a)

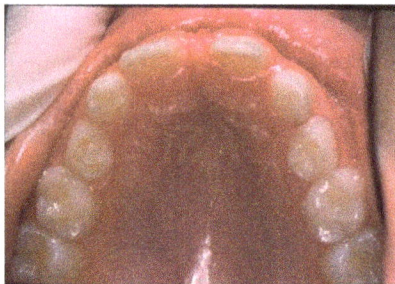

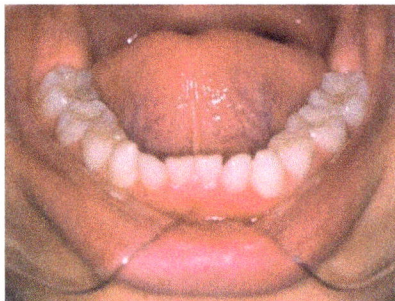

(b)

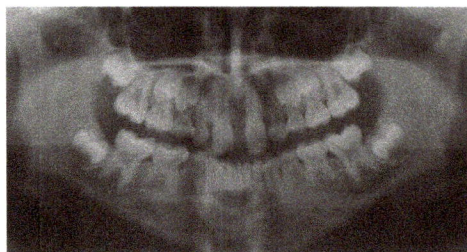

(c)

Figure 2: Patient 1. Accentuated diastema between the upper central incisors due to insertion of the labial frenulum (a), mixed dentition with no caries (b), and absence of the 31, 41, 12, 22, 32, 42, 13, 23, 33, 43, 34, 44, 35, and 45 teeth (c).

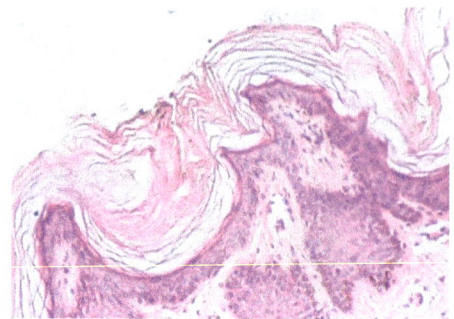

(a)

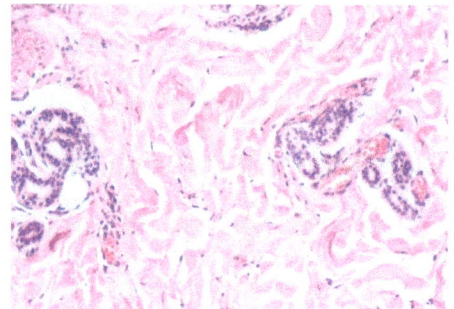

(b)

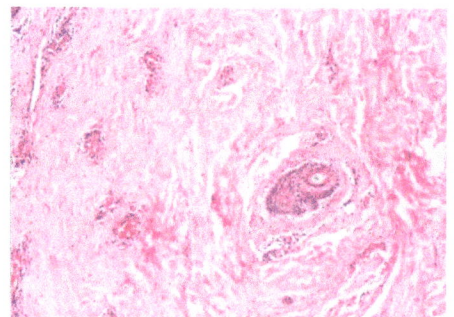

(c)

Figure 3: Patient 1. Histological sections showing hyperkeratosis (a), atresia of sweat glands and absence of sebaceous glands (b), and atrophic hair follicles (c) (original magnification: ×200 and ×100; hematoxylin and eosin).

Initially, the recommended treatment was to make provisional upper and lower dentures (Figure 5), restoring the aesthetics and masticatory functions and, as a consequence, improving the patient's facial appearance and psychological well being. Concomitantly, speech therapy was also accomplished to improve the orofacial motricity after the insertion of the dentures, resulting in rejuvenation with the smoothing of wrinkles and furrows and a balance of orofacial and masticatory muscles. It is important to emphasize that this first phase of treatment was very important to establish the self-esteem of this patient, resulting in his favorable behavior change and, consequently, immediate social inclusion.

After the adaptability of the patient to the provisional dentures, mini dental implants will be inserted into the atrophic alveolar ridges of the edentulous mandible and maxillae in order to effectively retain overdentures and, thus, to promote a better stability for the new removable dentures. This treatment alternative is recommended as the patient's alveolar processes display very thin thickness and reduced height. We believe that this protocol can improve the mastication, comfort, satisfaction, and oral health-related quality of life of this individual.

2.1.3. Patient 3. A 3-year-old afrodescendent male child with HED showed great difficulty eating, swallowing, and

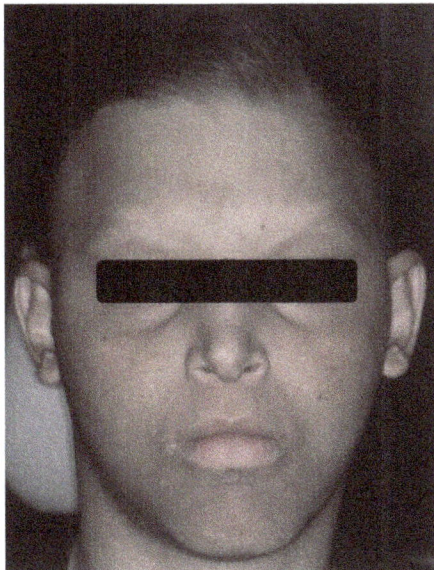

(a)

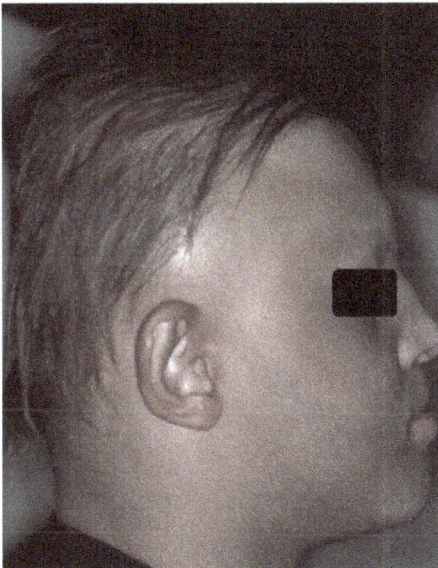

(b)

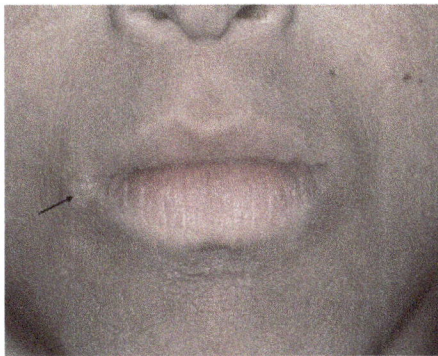

(c)

FIGURE 4: Patient 2. Boy with hypohidrotic ED displaying scarce, fine, and silky hair, alopecia of the eyebrows, prominent frontal bossing, discrete deformity and low implantation of the ear (a and b), angular cheilitis (arrow), dry and scaly skin, and perioral dermatitis and fissures (c).

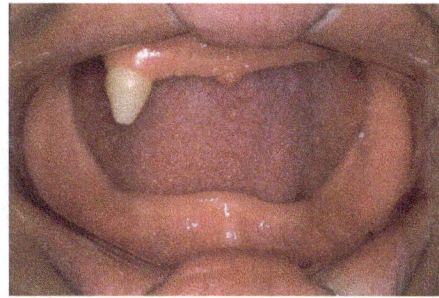

(a)

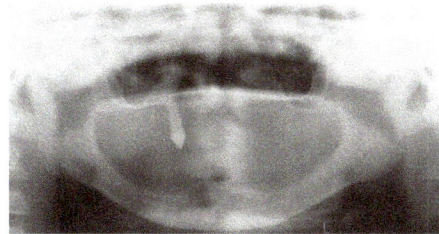

(b)

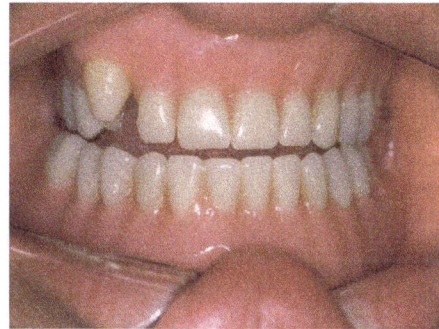

(c)

FIGURE 5: Patient 2. Agenesis of almost all permanent teeth, except the 13th tooth, underdeveloped alveolar ridge with "knife-edge" shape (a and b) and prosthodontic rehabilitation with the use of upper and lower dentures (c).

speech. The medical history reported by the patient was hyperthermic episodes without association with focal infections, reduction of lacrimal secretion, recurrent otitis and colds, and use of antiallergic medication. Upon general examination, the facial skin presented finely wrinkled and dry skin, appearing prematurely aged. Hyperkeratosis was also observed in the elbows, knees, and ankles. Upon extraoral examination, a depressed nasal bridge ("saddle nose"), thin and scanty hair, alopecia of the eyelashes and eyebrows, dry and crusted eyes, periorbital, perioral, and nasal pigmentation, bilateral deformity and low implantation of the ear, perioral fissures, and deep nasolabial sulcus were evidenced (Figure 6). Upon intraoral examination, dry mouth was observed and no deciduous teeth were erupted; however, the radiographic images revealed the presence of the right and left lower and upper deciduous canines and the absence of all permanent dental germs. The upper and lower alveolar ridges were underdeveloped (Figure 7). Firstly, speech therapy was recommended to improve the stomatognathic system functions and to stimulate the growth of the jaw bones. Following

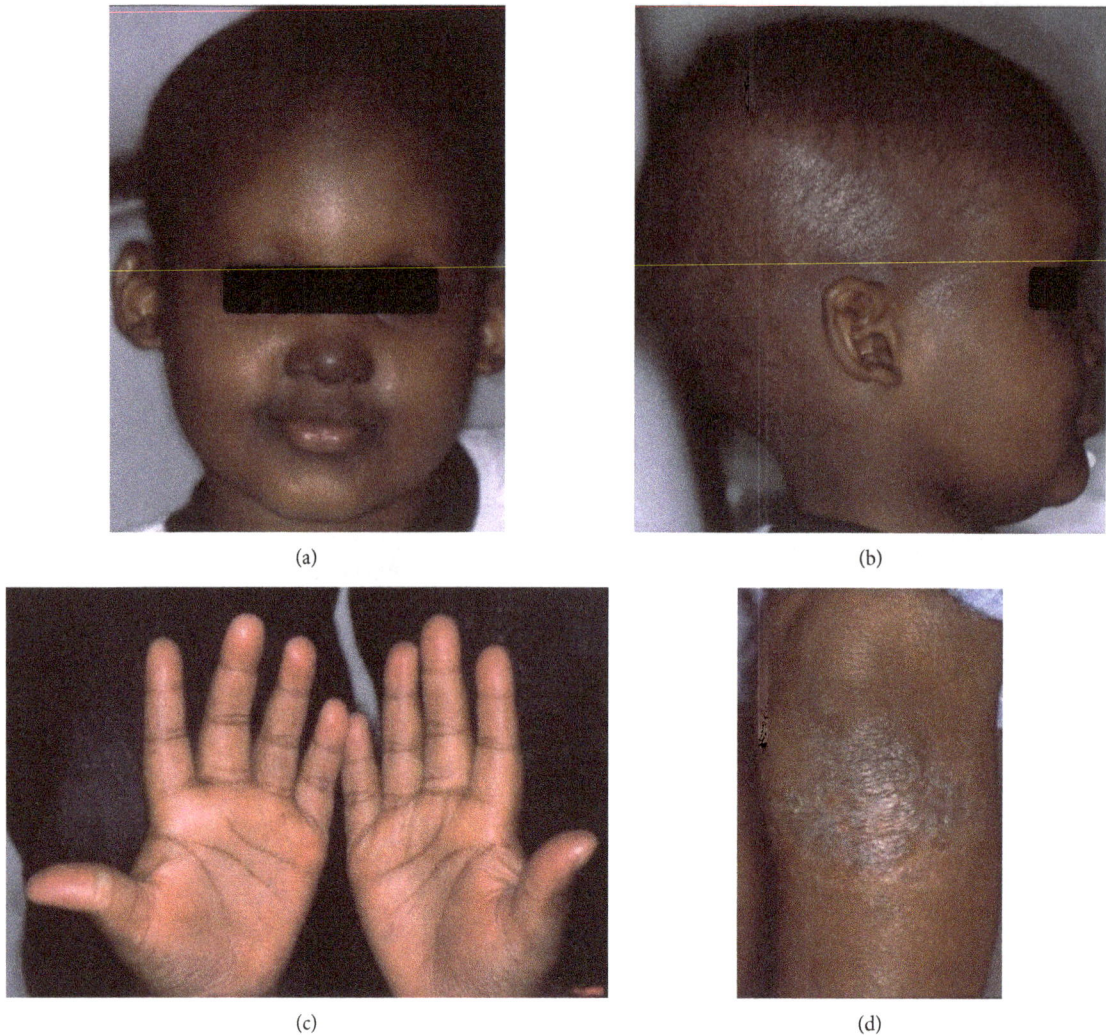

FIGURE 6: Patient 3. Child with hypohidrotic ED presented sparse hair, perioral and nasal pigmentation, ear deformity with pointed shape (a and b), and hyperkeratosis on the palms and knee (c and d).

this, provisional prostheses will continue to be made until the complete development of the mandible and maxilla, after the eruption of the preexisting deciduous teeth.

2.2. Microbiological and Salivary Tests. Initially, saliva was stimulated by using sugarless gum, and then the samples were collected into a sterile cup for 15 min, between 8 and 10 a.m., to prevent circadian rhythm variation. The first saliva sample was discarded to guarantee the fidelity of the results of microbiological analysis. Following this, salivary quantitative and qualitative tests were performed, including salivary flow determination, buffering capacity of saliva, and counts of mutans streptococci (MS), lactobacilli, and yeasts. The methodology applied is described in the study of Koga-Ito et al. [15], and the results obtained are demonstrated in Table 1.

3. Discussion

Due to craniofacial morphological anomalies, the patients with ED often present low self-esteem, psychological pressure, and limited social interactions. The dysmorphic features of

the maxillofacial region and agenesis of salivary and sweat glands can lead to systemic and oral disorders [3]. Among the two types of ED, HED is more prevalent than HidED [5], being in agreement with our studies.

The ability to perspire is reduced due to sweat gland dysfunction, and so patients are predisposed to develop hyperpyrexia due to the misregulation of the body temperature [8, 11, 16, 17]. This clinical symptom was reported by patients 1 and 2, especially during sports activities or high ambient temperatures.

Facial dysmorphy, including a prominent forehead, a depressed nasal bridge, and thick lips, was also noted in patients 2 and 3. All patients have presented congenitally missing dentition since childhood, and consequently, severe oligodontia, leading to masticatory dysfunction and aesthetic impairment. Thus, as a result of several agenesis of permanent and/or deciduous teeth and narrow upper and lower alveolar ridges, the vertical dimension of the face was reduced and the lips became protuberant. These findings were evidenced in patients 2 and 3. Moreover, no dental dysmorphy was found in our patients.

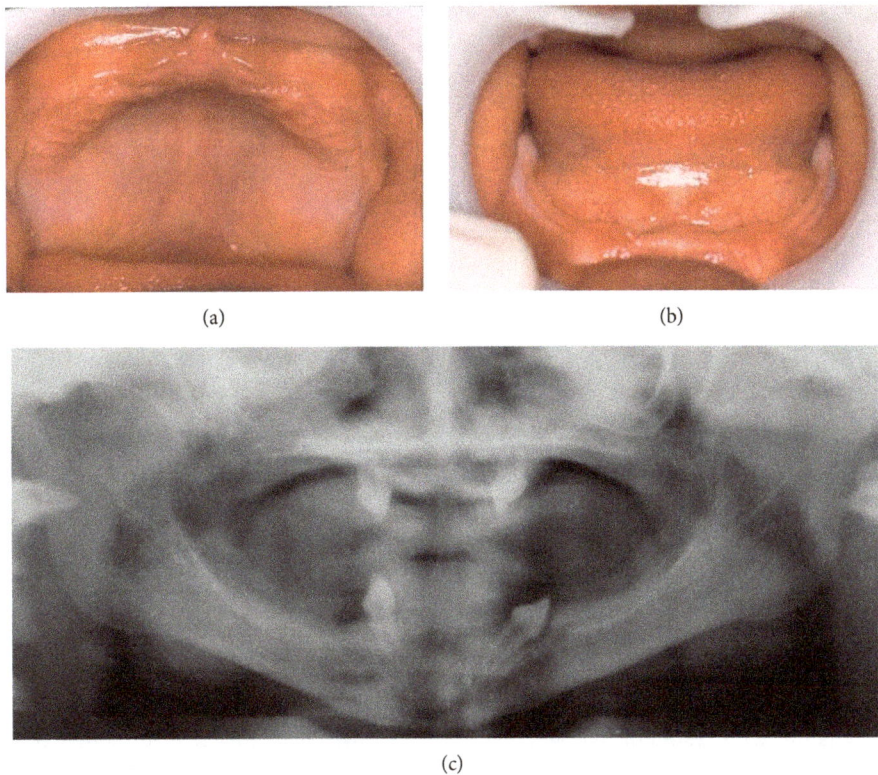

FIGURE 7: Patient 3. (a) Upper and (b) lower alveolar ridges were edentulous and underdeveloped, and (c) radiographic images showing the presence of the 53rd, 63rd, 73rd, and 83rd teeth.

Unfortunately, congenital defects involving oral cavity and facial appearance led to severe masticatory dysfunction and psychosocial disorders negatively influencing the mental health, respectively, especially for the adolescent individuals with ED. Therefore, immediate oral rehabilitation for stabilizing the aesthetics and masticatory functions must be performed, that is, using dental-mini implants due to the extensive bone hypotrophy of the alveolar processes [3]. Some studies report that implant placement in children with ED is highly debatable [3]; on the other hand, others reinforce the use of mini dental implants in children with ED, ensuring better aesthetics and functional and psychosocial development [18]. Thus, treatment strategy should include a comprehensive consideration of patient-specific aspects in order to ensure the best outcomes [3]; however, others reinforce the use of mini dental implants in children with ED, ensuring better aesthetics and functional and psychosocial development [18]. In this study, we can recommend the placement of mini dental implants to better retention of removable dentures only for the adolescent boy (patient 2).

A relevant clinical symptom was a persistent feeling of dry mouth in both patients 2 and 3; however, xerostomia was proved only in patient 3. Probably, this condition caused masticatory, swallowing, and speech difficulties. Our study has some limitations because anatomical and functional abnormalities of salivary glands were not properly investigated, using clinical methods, in particular, sialometry. Some authors described that salivary gland aplasia may lead to variable dysfunctions, including reduction on the salivary flow rate and

alterations on the salivary composition [13, 19]. The oral mucosa becomes dry and atrophic, and the patients can gradually show dysgeusia, dysphagia, and dysarthria, as well as risk of developing ulcerations, caries, gingivitis, periodontitis, candidosis, and bacterial sialadenitis, among others [19]. We suggested that adaptive or assistive technology should be recommended for patients with hyposalivation and dysphagia, as support therapies of gustatory and neuromuscular mechanical stimulation, in order to strengthen the muscular tone, in particular, the masticatory muscles, and to increase the production of saliva.

In this study, our patients were more susceptible to oral infections by bacteria and yeasts. Additionally, risk of malnutrition due to dysphagia and difficulties of mastication and speech may be found, resulting in an important harm to the oral homeostasis and to the quality of life. Another relevant feature is the appearance of rampant caries and severe periodontal disease, resulting in extensive damage of the buffering and antimicrobial properties of saliva [13].

Concerning the immunodeficiency disorder in ED, we consider that patient 2 was immunosuppressed once the diagnosis of angular cheilitis caused by *Candida albicans* was confirmed. Furthermore, recurrent symptoms of colds, otitis, and respiratory tract infections were also reported. Some studies reported that individuals with ED can present abnormalities in the immune system, as protein deficiency of the nuclear factor kappa-β essential modulator (NEMO). This protein is encoded by the *IKBKG* gene. This mutation causes impaired cytotoxicity mediated by natural killer cells

TABLE 1: Amount of salivary flow and buffering capacity of saliva, and counts of mutans streptococci, lactobacilli, and yeast in patients with ED.

Salivary tests	Patient 1 (HidED)	Patient 2 (HED)	Patient 3 (HED)
Salivary flow rate (mL/min)			
Normal flow: >1.0			
Limit value: 1.0	1.0 (limit value)	1.2 (normal)	<0.1 (xerostomia)
Reduced flow: ≤0.7			
Xerostomia: ≤0.1			
Buffering capacity of saliva (pH value)			
Normal: 5.1–7.0			
Limit value: 4.0–5.0	4.0 (limit value)	6.0 (normal)	5.0 (limit value)
Low buffering capacity: <4.0			
Mutans streptococci (log·cfu/mL)			
High caries risk: >5.0	6.2 (high)	5.0 (high)	4.9 (high)
Lactobacilli (log·cfu/mL)			
Low caries risk: 0.0–3.0	0.0 (low)	2.75 (low)	1.70 (low)
Moderate caries risk: 3.0–3.7			
High caries risk: >4.0			
Yeasts (log·cfu/mL)			
No caries risk: 0–1.0			
Moderate caries risk: 2.0–2.6	3.0 (high)	0.0 (no caries risk)	2.78 (high)
High caries risk: >2.6			

HidED, hidrotic ectodermal dysplasia; HED, hypohidrotic ectodermal dysplasia.

and impaired CD40 signaling with resultant hypogammaglobulinemia, decreased antibody response to polysaccharide antigens, and elevated IgM levels. Thus, these factors may impair the patient's defense mechanisms against pathogens, favoring the development of diseases [2, 14]. Although investigations of immune system phenotyping and explorations of NEMO gene mutations were not performed in our patients, we advocate the importance of these specialized biological analyses to confirm the immunodeficiency disorder and to identify its degree of severity, especially in patients with ED.

Regarding the buffering capacity of saliva, no significant alteration was detected in our patients; however, patient 3 was instructed to ingest only basic foods due to xerostomia. According to Chifor et al. [20], the buffering capacity of saliva allows neutralization of plaque acids and remineralization of early enamel caries lesions, leading to a protective effect for potentially pathogenic microorganisms.

Although caries etiology is understood as a polymicrobial and tissue-dependent disease, mutans streptococci are considered one of the most relevant etiologic agents involved in the acidogenic stage [21, 22]. For this reason, counts of mutan streptococci have been used as caries risk indicator or evaluation of anticaries therapy [15, 23]. Besides, counts of lactobacilli are also widely used for caries risk prediction. Lactobacilli are frequently found in low pH areas of caries lesions and exhibit acidogenic ability [24, 25].

It is important to highlight that *Candida* species are associated with caries etiology once they are able to form considerable quantities of acid from carbohydrates, leading to a decrease of the salivary pH [26]. Moreover, *Candida albicans* is also seen as an opportunistic microorganism that may trigger an oral lesion, especially in immunosuppressed individuals [27].

In our study, the counts of mutans streptococci ($n = 3$) and yeasts ($n = 2$) were high; in contrast, the count of lactobacilli

was low. These findings show that our patients presented great predisposition to enamel caries and opportunistic oral infections. It is important to highlight that, although patient 2 has presented no caries risk to yeasts, candidiasis was confirmed bilaterally in the oral commissure. This illness, probably, occurred due to the favorable biological environment promoted by the accentuated loss of vertical dimension, plus the susceptibility of the patient to infections. Therefore, the buccal prophylaxis and orientation of oral hygiene must be indicated as a supportive treatment, especially for the dentulous patient (patient 1) due to predisposition to caries.

Oral cavity is considered a gateway and a reservoir for pathogenic microorganisms, especially in immuno suppressed patients [14]. Considering this, more research related to protein composition of saliva may be performed since the salivary antimicrobial proteins or circulating immune complexes, containing IgA, IgG, and IgM, could be carefully investigated in individuals with ED.

4. Conclusion

Based on these investigations, our patients with ED, particularly the hypohidrotic type, presented a high risk of enamel caries and susceptibility to opportunistic oral infections, which may be likely triggered by reduction of salivary flow and/or possible immunological disorders. However, more investigations must be performed to elucidate the functional behaviors of oral microbiota in these individuals and to explain the appearance of oral lesions caused by biological agents.

Acknowledgments

This work was supported by FAPESP (São Paulo Research Foundation, Grant number: 2017/06835-8). The authors wish to thank the skillful laboratory assistance by Mrs. Clélia Aparecida de Paiva Martins. The authors are also grateful to Danielle Hersey da Silva of the Instituto Cultural Brasil-Estados Unidos (ICBEU), a Brazil-United States Bi-National Center, for the linguistic consultancy.

References

[1] C. F. Salinas, R. J. Jorgenson, J. T. Wright, J. J. DiGiovanna, and M. D. Fete, "2008 International Conference on ectodermal dysplasias classification conference report," *American Journal of Medical Genetics Part A*, vol. 149, no. 9, pp. 1958–1969, 2009.

[2] B. J. Mark, B. A. Becker, D. R. Halloran et al., "Prevalence of atopic disorders and immunodeficiency in patients with ectodermal dysplasia syndromes," *Annals of Allergy, Asthma and Immunology*, vol. 108, no. 6, pp. 435–438, 2012.

[3] Y. Wang, J. He, A. M. Decker, J. C. Hu, and D. Zou, "Clinical outcomes of implant therapy in ectodermal dysplasia patients: a systematic review," *International Journal of Oral and Maxillofacial Surgery*, vol. 45, no. 8, pp. 1035–1043, 2016.

[4] M. Vasconcelos Carvalho, J. Romero Souto de Sousa, F. Paiva Correa de Melo et al., "Hypohidrotic and hidrotic ectodermal dysplasia: a report of two cases," *Dermatology Online Journal*, vol. 19, no. 7, p. 18985, 2013.

[5] M. Mittal, D. Srivastava, A. Kumar, and P. Sharma, "Dental management of hypohidrotic ectodermal dysplasia: a report of two cases," *Contemporary Clinical Dentistry*, vol. 6, no. 3, pp. 414–417, 2015.

[6] R. Yang, Z. Hu, Q. Kong et al., "A known mutation in GJB6 in a large Chinese family with hidrotic ectodermal dysplasia," *Journal of the European Academy of Dermatology and Venereology*, vol. 30, no. 8, pp. 1362–1365, 2016.

[7] M. O. Lexner, A. Bardow, J. M. Hertz, L. Almer, B. Nauntofte, and S. Kreiborg, "Whole saliva in X-linked hypohidrotic ectodermal dysplasia," *International Journal of Paediatric Dentistry*, vol. 17, no. 3, pp. 155–162, 2007.

[8] P. García-Martín, A. Hernández-Martín, and A. Torrelo, "Ectodermal dysplasias: a clinical and molecular review," *Actas Dermo-Sifiliográficas*, vol. 104, no. 6, pp. 451–470, 2013.

[9] D. Li, R. Xu, F. Huang et al., "A novel missense mutation in collagenous domain of EDA gene in a Chinese family with X-linked hypohidrotic ectodermal dysplasia," *Journal of Genetics*, vol. 94, no. 1, pp. 115–119, 2015.

[10] W. H. Trzeciak and R. Koczorowski, "Molecular basis of hypohidrotic ectodermal dysplasia: an update," *Journal of Applied Genetics*, vol. 57, no. 1, pp. 51–61, 2016.

[11] S. Deshmukh and S. Prashanth, "Ectodermal dysplasia: a genetic review," *International Journal of Clinical Pediatric Dentistry*, vol. 5, no. 3, pp. 197–202, 2012.

[12] F. Clauss, N. Chassaing, A. Smahi et al., "X-linked and autosomal recessive hypohidrotic ectodermal dysplasia: genotypic-dental phenotypic findings," *Clinical Genetics*, vol. 78, no. 3, pp. 257–266, 2010.

[13] P. Singh and S. Warnakulasuriya, "Aplasia of submandibular salivary glands associated with ectodermal dysplasia," *Journal of Oral Pathology and Medicine*, vol. 33, no. 10, pp. 634–636, 2004.

[14] T. Fete, "Respiratory problems in patients with ectodermal dysplasia syndromes," *American Journal of Medical Genetics Part A*, vol. 164, no. 10, pp. 2478–2481, 2014.

[15] C. Y. Koga-Ito, C. S. Unterkircher, H. Watanabe, C. A. Martins, V. Vidotto, and A. O. Jorge, "Caries risk tests and salivary levels of immunoglobulins to *Streptococcus mutans* and *Candida albicans* in mouthbreathing syndrome patients," *Caries Research*, vol. 37, no. 1, pp. 38–43, 2003.

[16] S. Joseph, G. J. Cherackal, J. Jacob, and A. K. Varghese, "Multidisciplinary management of hypohydrotic ectodermal dysplasia-a case report," *Clinical Case Reports*, vol. 3, no. 5, pp. 280–286, 2015.

[17] M. Reinholz, G. G. Gauglitz, K. Giehl et al., "Non-invasive diagnosis of sweat gland dysplasia using optical coherence tomography and reflectance confocal microscopy in a family with anhidrotic ectodermal dysplasia (Christ-Siemens-Touraine syndrome)," *Journal of the European Academy of Dermatology and Venereology*, vol. 30, no. 4, pp. 677–682, 2016.

[18] E. Sfeir, N. Nassif, and C. Moukarzel, "Use of mini-dental implants in ectodermal dysplasia children: follow-up of three cases," *European Journal of Paediatric Dentistry*, vol. 15, no. 2, pp. 207–212, 2014.

[19] J. Saleh, M. A. Figueiredo, K. Cherubini, and F. G. Salum, "Salivary hypofunction: an update on aetiology, diagnosis and therapeutics," *Archives of Oral Biology*, vol. 60, no. 2, pp. 242–255, 2015.

[20] I. Chifor, I. Badea, R. Chifor et al., "Saliva characteristics, diet and carioreceptivity in dental students," *Clujul Medical*, vol. 87, no. 1, pp. 34–39, 2014.

[21] N. Takahashi and B. Nyvad, "The role of bacteria in the caries process: ecological perspectives," *Journal of Dental Research*, vol. 90, no. 3, pp. 294–303, 2011.

[22] A. Simón-Soro and A. Mira, "Solving the etiology of dental caries," *Trends in Microbiology*, vol. 23, no. 2, pp. 76–82, 2015.

[23] M. E. Almaz, I. Ş. Sönmez, Z. Ökte, and A. A. Oba, "Efficacy of a sugar-free herbal lollipop for reducing salivary *Streptococcus mutans* levels: a randomized controlled trial," *Clinical Oral Investigations*, vol. 21, no. 3, pp. 839–845, 2017.

[24] T. Klinke, S. Kneist, J. J. de Soet et al., "Acid production by oral strains of *Candida albicans* and lactobacilli," *Caries Research*, vol. 43, no. 2, pp. 83–91, 2009.

[25] N. Kianoush, C. J. Adler, K. A. Nguyen, G. V. Browne, M. Simonian, and N. Hunter, "Bacterial profile of dentine caries and the impact of pH on bacterial population diversity," *PLoS One*, vol. 9, no. 3, article e92940, 2014.

[26] Z. M. Thein, Y. H. Smaranayake, and L. P. Smaranayake, "Dietary sugars, serum and the biocide chlorhexidine digluconate modify the population and structural dynamics of mixed *Candida albicans* and *Escherichia coli* biofilms," *APMIS*, vol. 115, no. 11, pp. 1241–1251, 2007.

[27] S. Shinozaki, M. Moriyama, J. N. Hayashida et al., "Close association between oral *Candida* species and oral mucosal disorders in patients with xerostomia," *Oral Diseases*, vol. 18, no. 7, pp. 667–672, 2012.

7

Large Draining Focal Fibrous Hyperplasia Secondary to Periapical Granuloma

E. I. Ogbureke ⓘ,[1] M. A. Couey,[2] N. Vigneswaran ⓘ,[3] and C. D. Johnson[1]

[1]Department of General Practice and Dental Public Health, School of Dentistry, The University of Texas Health Science Center at Houston, Houston, TX, USA
[2]Department of Oral and Maxillofacial Surgery, School of Dentistry, The University of Texas Health Science Center at Houston, Houston, TX, USA
[3]Department of Diagnostic & Biomedical Science, School of Dentistry, The University of Texas Health Science Center at Houston, Houston, TX, USA

Correspondence should be addressed to E. I. Ogbureke; ezinne.i.ogbureke@uth.tmc.edu

Academic Editor: Gavriel Chaushu

Periapical granuloma is a pathological diagnosis associated clinically and radiographically with a nonvital tooth and a periapical radiolucency, respectively. It is frequently seen as a sequela of long-standing pulpal necrosis. Often times, a draining fistula is observed near the nonvital tooth. We report an unusual case of a large draining focal fibrous hyperplasia in association with a large periapical granuloma treated at our clinic. The diagnosis was made by the clinical presentation, radiologic and histopathologic findings.

1. Introduction

Periapical granuloma, also referred to as chronic apical periodontitis, is a defensive reaction in response to bacterial infection within the pulp chamber which spreads to the root apex [1]. It is a long-standing inflammation of the periodontium that is characterized by the presence of a granulomatous tissue [2]. Radiographically, periapical granulomas are generally indistinguishable from periapical abscesses or cysts. They are often asymptomatic unless the infection spreads to the surrounding tissues.

2. Case Report

A 59-year-old man presented to the urgent care clinic at the School of Dentistry complaining of an upper lip mass for one-year duration. The mass started out as a small bump and had grown steadily since then. 3 months prior to his presentation, a draining parulis developed on the mass. The patient had no history of systemic symptoms such as fever, chills, weight loss, or fatigue. He was aware of a dark-colored "dead tooth" for several decades in the area of concern but denied any previous history of swelling in the area. The patient had recently moved to the United States from Nigeria and had previously been without access to adequate dental care. The patient said that a doctor in Nigeria told him that the lesion was likely cancerous.

On exam, there was a large, painless, fibrous, exophytic mass in the anterior maxillary labial vestibule (Figures 1(a) and 1(b)). The base of the mass approximated the apex of tooth #8. A yellow purulent material was observed draining from the parulis (Figure 1(b)). Tooth #8 was discolored and was confirmed to be nonvital on pulp testing. There was a significant gap between teeth #7 and 8. Tooth #8 was displaced medially and was extruded relative to the adjacent dentition.

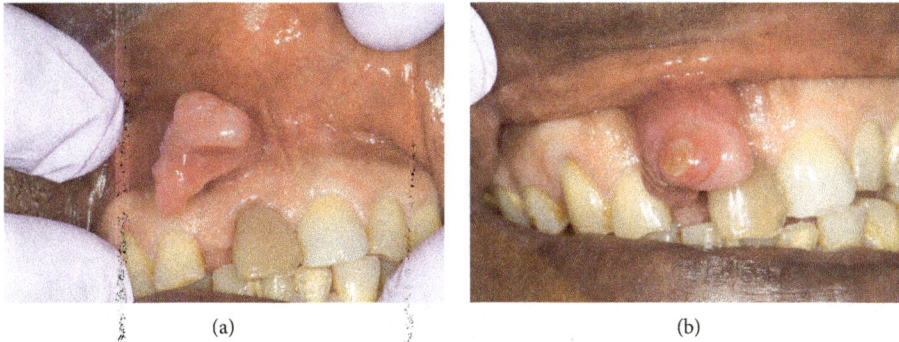

FIGURE 1: (a) Picture of soft tissue exophytic lesion in buccal vestibule. (b) Picture of soft tissue lesion showing purulent exudate.

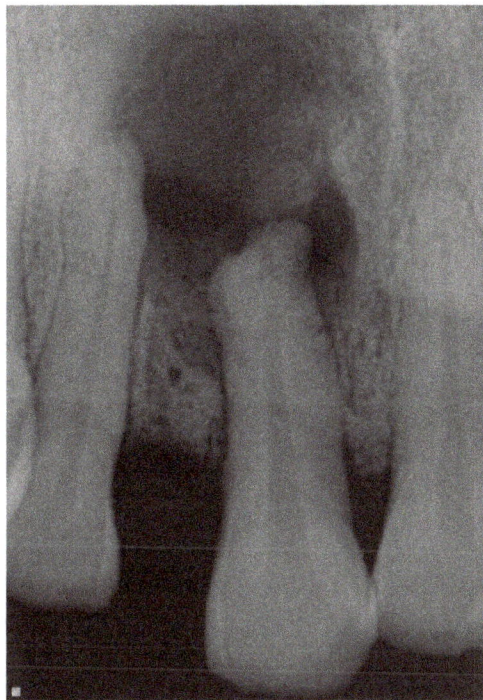

FIGURE 2: Periapical radiograph of large radiolucency associated with necrotic tooth #8.

A periapical radiograph revealed a large unilocular radiolucency associated with the apex of tooth #8 (Figure 2). Cone-beam computed tomography again demonstrated a large cystic-appearing defect in the anterior maxilla with perforation of the buccal and palatal cortices Figure 3. The lesion extended to the nasal floor on the ipsilateral side.

The patient was referred to the oral surgery department for excisional biopsy. After tooth #8 was removed, an incision was made around the base of the stalk that connected the mass to the labial and alveolar mucosa. Sharp dissection was used to free the mass, and the specimen was sent for histopathologic analysis. The mass communicated with a cystic lesion of the maxilla. The cyst was enucleated with a curette and also sent for pathology. Perforation of the cyst through the buccal and palatal cortices was noted during the procedure. Slight undermining of the wound margins allowed for closure with resorbable sutures.

At the patient's one-week follow-up (Figure 4), he was doing very well. He reported minimal pain, no neurosensory disturbances, and no systemic or local symptoms of infection. He and his family were very relieved to learn that the lesion was benign. He was happy with his appearance after having the mass removed.

3. Discussion

A search on PUBMED, google scholar, and google using the terms "focal fibrous hyperplasia" and "draining fibrous hyperplasia" yielded no reported cases of a similar

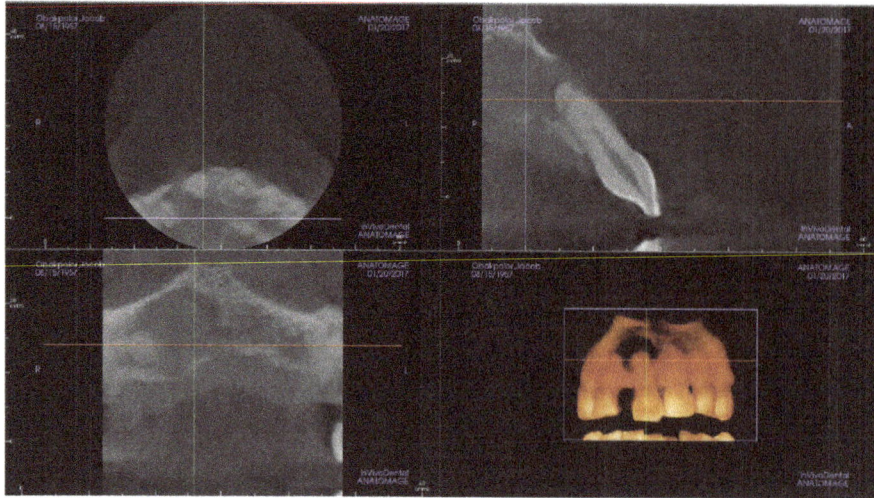

FIGURE 3: CBCT image showing large cystic-appearing defect in the anterior maxilla with perforation of the buccal and palatal cortices.

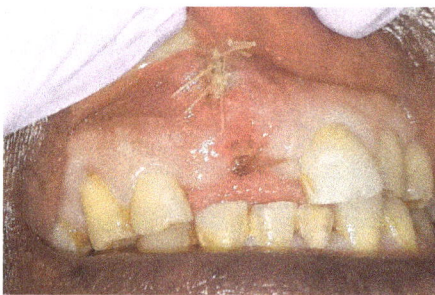

FIGURE 4: Picture at one-week follow-up.

occurrence in the English literature. Focal fibrous hyperplasia (FFH), is a reactive, inflammatory hyperplastic lesion of the connective tissue [3]. It is presumed that mechanical trauma is the primary cause hence it more commonly occurs in the buccal mucosa and tongue [3]. FFH like other reactive soft tissue oral lesions such as pyogenic granuloma (PG), peripheral giant cell granuloma (PGCG), and peripheral ossifying fibroma (POF) are more common in females, and hormones are thought to play a part in its etiology [3, 4]. FFH is distinguishable from the aforementioned lesions by histology. Generally, the teeth associated with FFH and the lesions of PG, PGCG, and POF are vital. The patient in this report is male, and tooth #8 is nonvital and shows a large periapical radiolucency (Figure 2). This leads the authors to postulate that pulpal necrosis of #8 and the subsequent periapical pathology led to a fistula formation in the buccal vestibule adjacent to #8. Trauma and irritation of the fistula opening may have initiated the hyperplastic lesion of FFH.

The location of the periapical lesion is consistent with studies that confirm the anterior maxilla as being the commonest site for periapical granulomas and cysts [4]. This is probably because the anterior maxilla is more prone to trauma than other tooth-bearing areas of the jaws.

4. Histopathological Findings

On gross examination, the growth excised from the gingiva consisted of a yellowish-tan, irregular-shaped fragment of soft tissue measuring $1.5 \times 1.2 \times 0.9$ cm. The intraosseous lesions curated from the cystic lesion of the anterior maxilla composed of multiple tan and irregular-shaped fragments of soft tissue measuring in aggregate $2 \times 2 \times 0.6$ cm.

Microscopic examination of the gingival growth revealed a soft tissue mass surfaced by parakeratinized hyperplastic stratified squamous epithelium (Figure 5). The underlying lamina propria exhibited area of dense fibrous hyperplasia with chronic inflammatory cell infiltrate with increased vascularity. Underneath the hyperplastic, fibrous connective tissue is an abscess consisting of granulation tissue with sheets of neutrophils intermixed with histiocytes and necrotic cellular debris (Figure 5). A sinus tract was present within the middle of the abscess. Biopsy curetted from the accompanying intraosseous lesion revealed dense fibrous connective tissue and granulation tissue with mixed inflammatory cell infiltrate (Figure 5).

5. Conclusion

Few oral lesions are unique or distinctly remarkable in nature. Therefore, it is imperative for oral healthcare providers to follow well-established matrices when encountering atypical oral presentations. The literature strongly suggests high reliability of patients' self-reporting and a thorough account including medical history and the history of the lesion as essential to the diagnostic process. Of secondary importance is delineation of the physical characteristics of the lesion including the size, shape, color,

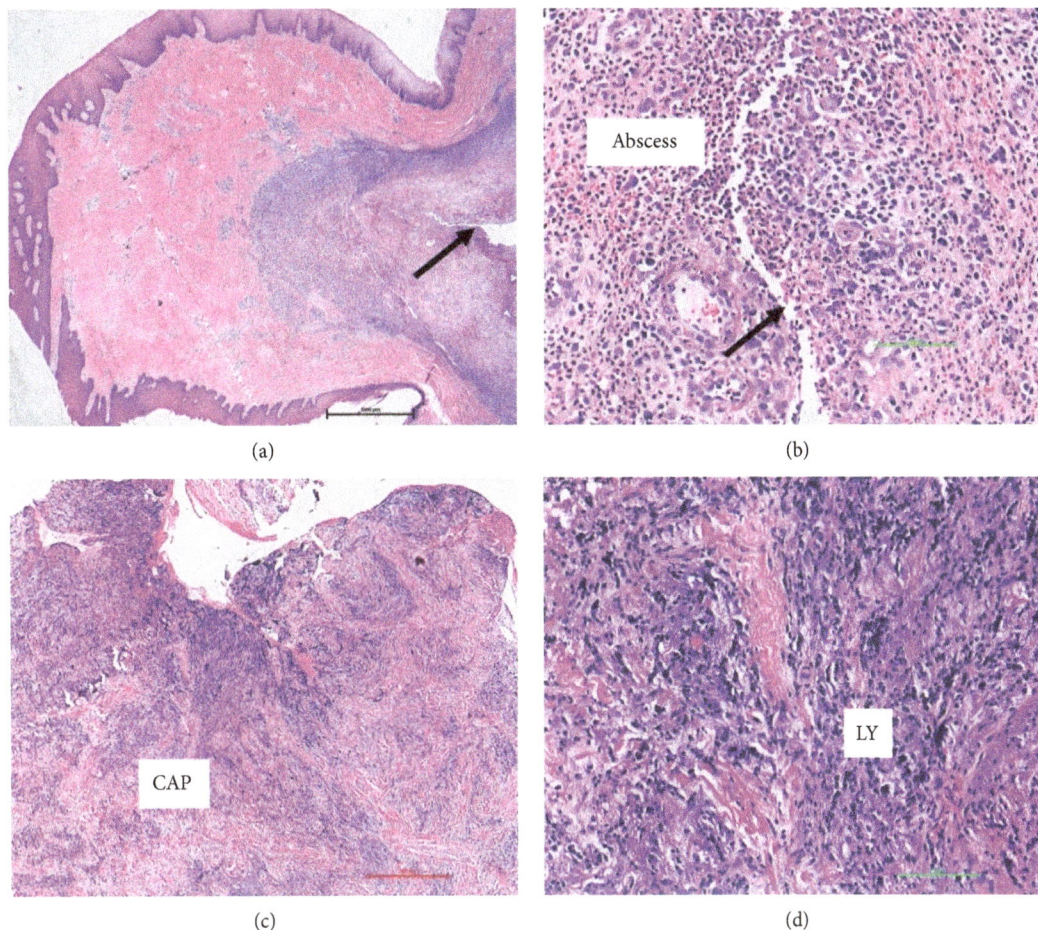

FIGURE 5: Microscopic findings of the gingival growth (a and b) and periapical radiolucent lesion associated with tooth #8 (c and d). Fibrous growth in the gingiva exhibits opening of a sinus tract (arrows) surrounded by an abscess. Periapical radiolucent lesion revealed chronic apical periodontitis (CAP) consisting of mostly lymphocytic infiltrate (LY).

and texture. Radiographic evaluation may assist in narrowing the differential. In our case, despite the atypical appearance, a presumptive differential was limited by the history of the lesion to a fibrous hyperplasia. We, however, advise vigilance in the need for histopathologic evaluation and proper referral when required.

References

[1] B. Neville, D. Damm, C. Allen, and J. Bouquot, *Oral and Maxillofacial Pathology*, W. B. Saunders, Philadelphia, PA, USA, 3rd edition, 2008.

[2] L. Safi, A. Adl, M. R. Azar, and R. Akbary, "A twenty-year survey of pathologic reports of two common types of chronic periapical lesions in Shiraz Dental School," *Journal of Dental Research, Dental Clinics, Dental Prospects*, vol. 2, no. 2, pp. 63–70, 2008.

[3] T. De Santana Santos, P. R. Martins-Filho, M. R. Piva, and E. S. de Souza Andrade, "Focal fibrous hyperplasia: a review of 193 cases," *Journal of Oral & Maxillofacial Pathology*, vol. 18, no. 4, pp. 86–89, 2014.

[4] D. P. Tavares, J. T. Rodrigues, T. dos Santos, L. Armada, and F. R. Pires, "Clinical and radiological analysis of a series of periapical cysts and periapical granulomas diagnosed in a Brazilian population," *Journal of Clinical and Experimental Dentistry*, vol. 9, no. 1, 2017.

8

Diagnosis and Managment of Maxillary Incisor with Vertical Root Fracture: A Clinical Report with Three-Year Follow-Up

Ines Kallel ⓘ,[1,2,3] Eya Moussaoui,[3] Fadwa Chtioui,[1,2,3] and Nabiha Douki[1,2,3]

[1]Department of Dental Medicine, Faculty of Dentistry, Hospital Sahloul, Sousse, Tunisia
[2]Laboratory of Research in Oral Healh and Maxillo Facial Rehabilitation (LR12ES11), Monastir, Tunisia
[3]Faculty of Dental Medicine, University of Monastir, Monastir, Tunisia

Correspondence should be addressed to Ines Kallel; ineskallel@yahoo.fr

Academic Editor: Jiiang H. Jeng

According to the American Association of Endodontists, "a 'true' vertical root fracture is defined as a complete or incomplete fracture initiated from the root at any level, usually directed buccolingually." Vertical root fracture (VRF) usually starts from an internal dentinal crack and develops over time, due to masticatory forces and occlusal loads. When they occur in teeth, those types of fractures can present difficulties in diagnosis, and there are however many clinic and radiographical signs which can guide clinicians to the existence of the fracture. Prognosis, most often, is hopeless, and differential diagnosis from other etiologies may be difficult sometimes. In this paper, we present a case of VRF diagnosed after surgical exploration; the enlarged fracture line was filled with a fluid resin. A 36-month clinical and radiological follow-up showed an asymptomatic tooth, reduction of the periodontal probing depth from 7 mm prior to treatment to 4 mm with no signs of ankylosis. In this work, the diagnosis and treatment alternatives of vertical root fracture were discussed through the presented clinical case.

1. Introduction

A vertical root fracture (VRF) is a root fracture extending along the longitudinal axis of the root; it can be divided into complete and incomplete vertical root fractures based on the separation of the two fragments according to Leubke's classification [1], and it is often observed in endodontically treated teeth. Communly, VRF initiates from the internal root canal wall and extends to the outer root surface, usually in a buccolingual direction. The fracture might involve one surface (buccal or lingual) or both surfaces (buccal and lingual).

These types of fractures can affect either the root or extend coronally towards the cervical periodontal attachment [2, 3]. According to some studies [2–4], they are the third most common cause of tooth loss after dental caries and periodontal disease. VRFs have been reported to occur in both nonendodontically and endodontically treated teeth. The latter represents but the majority of the cases, with or without post insertion.

A retrospective study showed that 94% of teeth with root fractures have a history of endodontic treatment [4]. The prevalence of VRF in endodontically treated teeth (ETT) ranges from 2% to 20% [5]. From a biomechanical standpoint, this condition has been associated with a synergism between chemical and mechanical degradation of the tooth [6].

Patients with VRFs typically present with minimal signs and symptoms during the early stage. Consequently, the entity is generally not noticed until periapical pathology occurs. Under such circumstances, the diagnosis is difficult, as they mimic other conditions [3]. In up to 67% of all root-filled teeth with VRF, symptoms or signs include localized swelling, pain on biting, associated with a fistula or sinus tract, sensitivity to percussion and palpation, and deep localized periodontal probing pocket depth.

Radiographic observation of an angular pattern of apical or lateral bone resorption with a radiolucent halo is considered pathognomonic [7].

Many clinical studies have investigated the different diagnostic and clinical parameters associated with VRF. The use of cone beam computed tomography (CBCT) to identify the presence of VRFs [8, 9] was recommended in many studies. *Their diagnostic accuracy, nevertheless, is still uncertain (but* there is still a considerable uncertainty regarding their diagnosis) [9, 10].

The prognosis of such teeth is generally questionable and the extraction of the tooth being the most common treatment option. However, conservative treatment options such as reconstruction of the fractured fragments with adhesive resin followed by intentional replantation have been recently suggested [11].

The present case report describes the difficulty of diagnosis of an incomplete vertical root fracture in a maxillary right central incisor with a successful management by sealing the fragments with a fluid resin composite. At the three-year follow-up, the tooth was asymptomatic, radiographically sound with probing depth and mobility within normal physiological limits.

2. Case Report Presentation

A 14-year-old male was referred to the Department of Dental Medicine complaining of occasional pain and a mucous fistula which persisted for one year in his upper right central incisor. When history was elicited, the patient revealed that there was a fall two years back in school due to which he sustained fracture of his maxillary permanent central incisors. Both teeth underwent endodontic treatment in a private office. According to his medical history, the patient exhibited no systemic disease.

His extraoral examination was noncontributory. Intraoral examination revealed enamel-dentin fracture involving the incisal edge in tooth #11, in the upper right lateral incisor region (Figure 1). Periodontal probing revealed deep narrow pockets on both facial of tooth 12 and palatal root surfaces of tooth 11 of 5 and 6 millimeters, respectively, while the other teeth showed a nonpathologic probing depth of value of 2-3 mm. Pulp sensibility tests showed a negative response in tooth #12. Radiographic evaluation was performed using a film holder which showed the relationship with tooth #12; both central incisors were endodontically treated (Figure 2). Endodontic treatment of tooth #12 was planned (Figure 3). A 3-month follow-up appointment and coronal restoration of teeth #12 and 11 was scheduled, followed by another appointment 3 months later, but the patient consulted us only 2 years later complaining of the recurrence of the Fistula. A periapical radiograph with film holder has built evidence to show the relation with tooth #12 (Figure 4). A Periapical surgery was carried out and revealed a proliferation of granulation tissue around the apex of the lateral incisor (Figure 5). Periapical curettage followed by a 3 mm root-end resection of tooth #12 (Figure 6) was conducted. After Retrograde root preparation, retrograde filling was performed with glass ionomer cement. The radiological control after root-end filling showed cement excess (Figure 7).

A follow-up appointment was given 3 weeks later. The reappearance of the sinus tract was actually surprising; a periapical radiograph using gutta-percha cones, after fitting them to a gauged apex, showed a relation between both right lateral and central incisors (Figure 8). A second exploratory surgery at routine six-month recall was decided with palatal and buccal full-thickness flaps elevation,

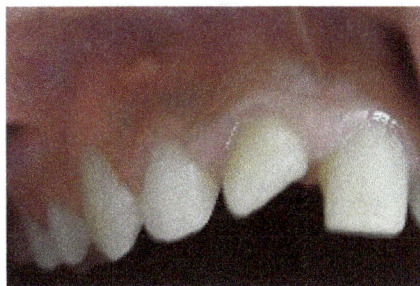

FIGURE 1: Endobuccal examination: mucosa fistula.

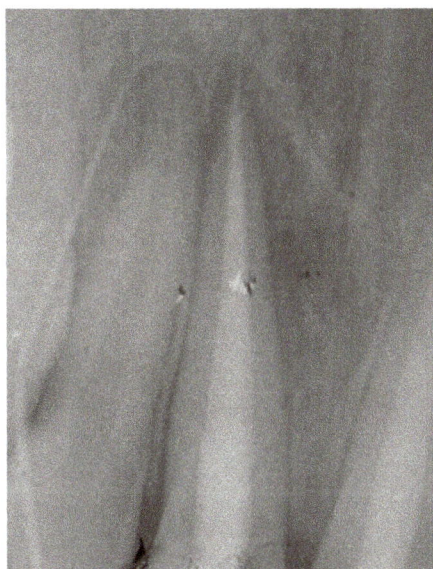

FIGURE 2: Radio using locating cone showing the relationship with tooth 12. Teeth 11 and 21 were both endodontically treated.

revealing the undiagnosed VRF on the palatal side of tooth #11(Figure 9).

We also noted an extended bone loss from the vestibular to palatal side. The alveolar socket was carefully curetted to remove all granulation tissue. The fracture line was sealed using a fluid composite resin (Figure 10).

Clinical and radiographic evaluation was performed after one month (Figure 11), then three months later (Figure 12), and at one-year follow-up (Figure 13). Regular six-month follow-ups were scheduled afterwards.

After three years (Figure 14), the healing of tooth #11 was evident with a probing depth anda mobility ranging within normal physiological limits. No radiographic signs of resorption were observed.

3. Discussion

The retention of microbial dental plaque in these difficult-to-clean areas has been shown to be associated with local periodontal inflammation and periodontal destruction, which is one of the reasons why deep probing pocket against the fracture line is the most common feature of VRF; however, it remains surrounded by normal pocket depths. This may also involve the

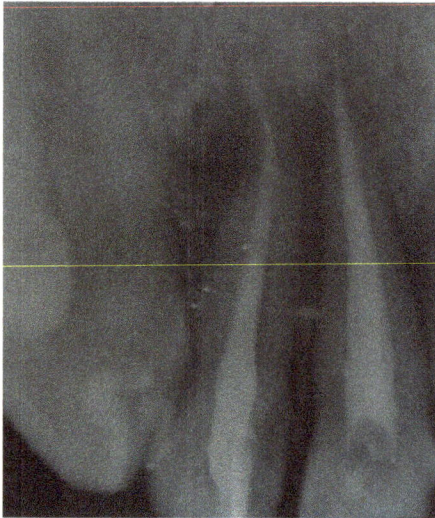

FIGURE 3: Root canal filling of tooth 12.

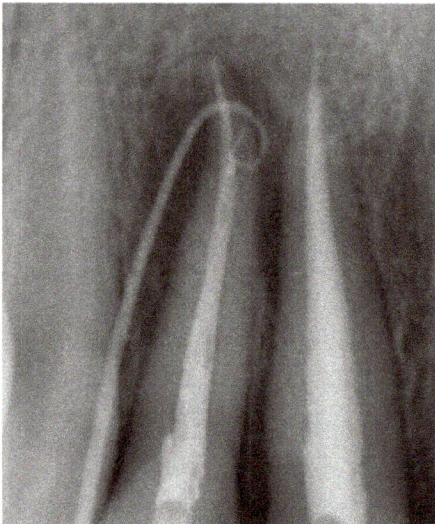

FIGURE 4: Fistula recurrence after 2 years involving tooth 12, persistence of periapical lesion.

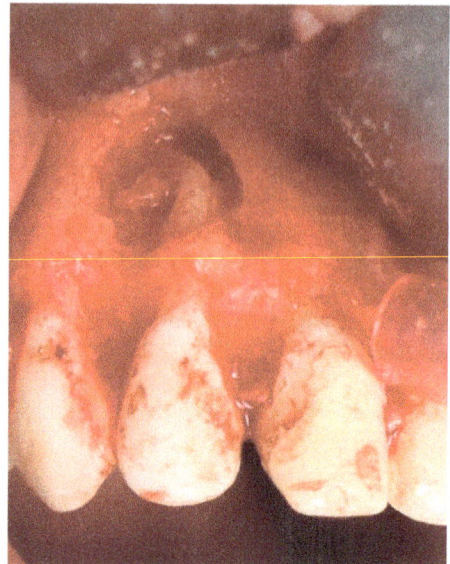

FIGURE 5: Presence of granulation tissue on the periapical side of tooth 12.

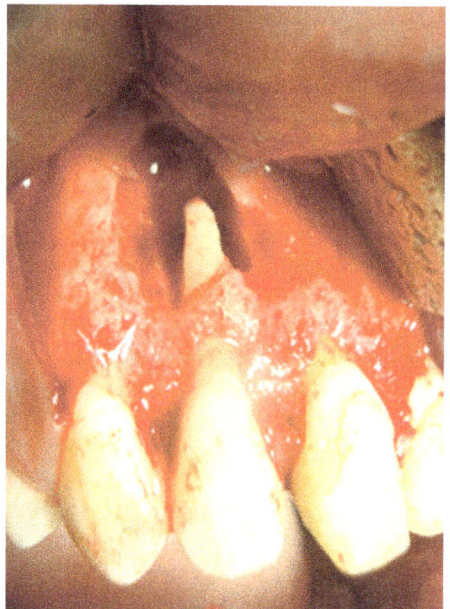

FIGURE 6: Apical root resection.

appearance and recurrence of the fistula, typically located close to the gingival margin, as it was reported in our patient's case. Those characteristics appear because there is bone resorption surrounding the fracture line on the bone plate [12].

Lustig et al. [13] showed after studying 110 vertical fracture cases that the resorption is a consequence of a chronic inflammatory process resulting in a granulation tissue that comes replacing the bone following a bacterial infection. The latter subsequently gains an easy passage through the fracture line bypassing the defense line of the epithelial attachment.

Although one may argue about the viability of the described procedure, and the degradation of the periodontium and osseous architecture during the recall period if the procedure was not successful, periodontal pockets exceeding 6 mm do not necessarily indicate imminent deterioration, and the sites with such deep probing depths may be maintained successfully for a long period by personal plaque control and

professional cleaning. This may explain the successful outcome of the vertically fractured tooth in our case treated by flow resin (ceram x duo DENTSPLY) with residual pockets [14, 15].

This case report presents success even after a period of three years of follow-up as the tooth showed no clinical symptoms, demonstrating periodontal tissue healing/regeneration, and improvements in periodontal probing at the fracture site.

3.1. Difficulty in Diagnosis. Vertical root fractures are most commonly associated with endodontically treated teeth; their presence in a nontreated tooth is rare. There is no single

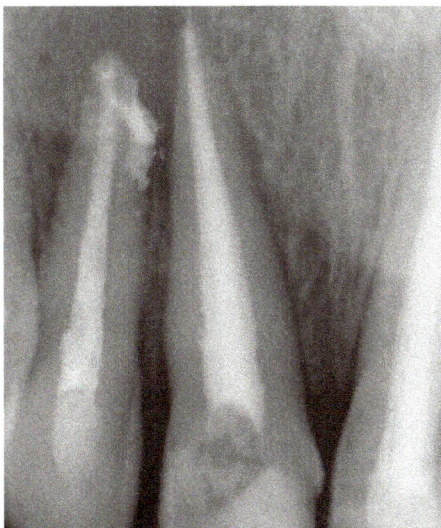

FIGURE 7: Radiological control after root end filling: excess glass ionomer cement.

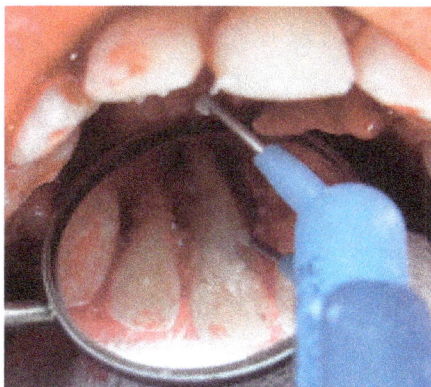

FIGURE 8: Fistula recurrence after 3 weeks. Locating cone showed relation between tooth 12 and tooth 11.

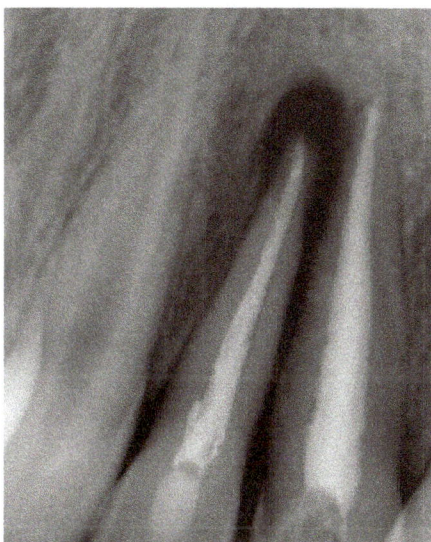

FIGURE 9: Second surgical exploration showing vertical root fracture in the palatal side of tooth 11.

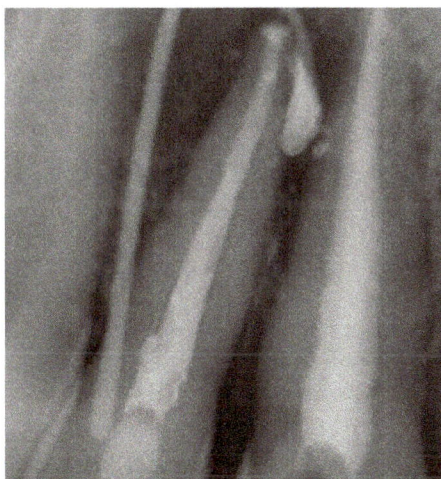

FIGURE 10: Sealing of the vertical root fracture with fluid resin composite.

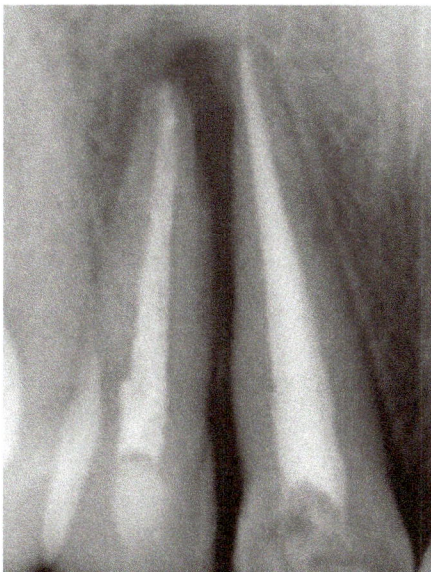

FIGURE 11: Radiograph of control after 1 month.

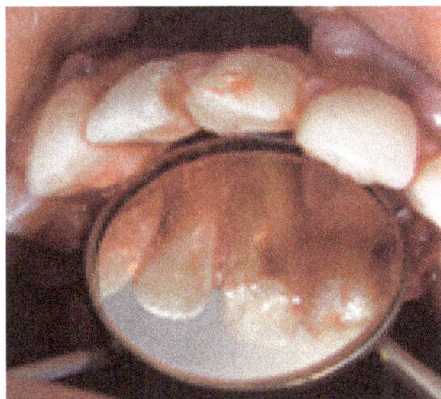

FIGURE 12: Radiograph of control after 3 months.

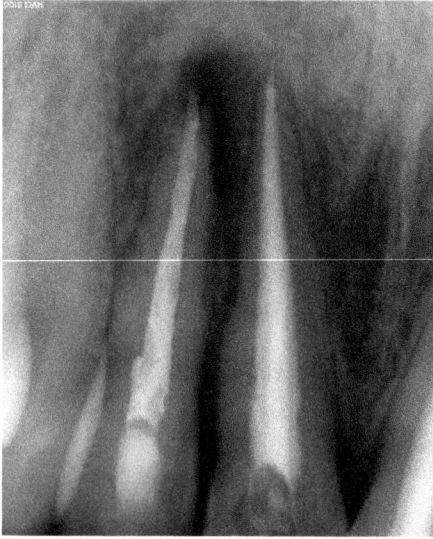

FIGURE 13: Radiograph of control 1 year later.

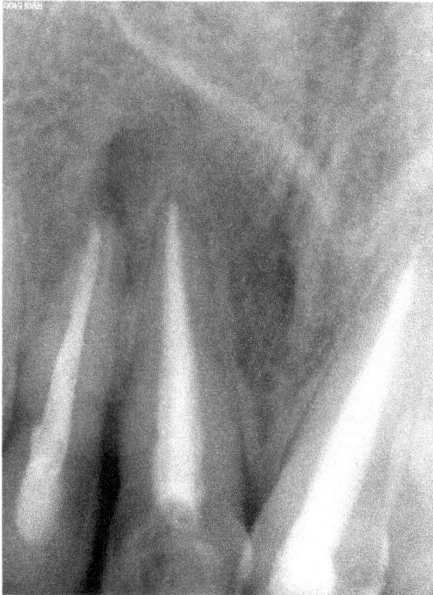

FIGURE 14: Radiograph of control 3 years later.

clinical feature that indicates their presence. They are also difficult to diagnose, as they mimic other conditions. Hence, the diagnosis of vertical root fractures requires more of a predictive rather than a definitive identification. A cumulative assessment of the clinical signs and symptoms and the radiographic features may help us reach a definitive diagnosis [11].

Some clinical tests may guide us towards the right diagnosis of VRF. For instance, periodontal probing may reveal a narrow, isolated, periodontal defect within the gingival attachment.

Tracing the sinus tract using gutta-percha as an endodontic explorer may be used to trace the sinus tract back to its origin, but in our clinical case, we were confused with the periapical lesion of the adjacent tooth.

Bite test, such as biting cotton wool rolls or wood sticks, may be used to reproduce the pain on biting described by the patient. This test is performed tooth-by-tooth or cusp-by-cusp in multirooted teeth. Usually, the patient feels relaxed on biting, and the pain starts while releasing the biting pressure.

Radiographic examination associated with clinical features can lead to a positive diagnosis, and many radiographic features are possible:

(i) Radiolucent lines along the root fillings or posts: appearance of a vertical space adjacent to the root filling material or a space between the edges of a root canal.

(ii) Direct evidence of the fracture line is often difficult to visualize. To be able to see the fracture, the X-ray beam must pass almost directly down the fracture line.

(iii) Fracture line deviating from the long axis of the canal may be radiographically more obvious, as compared to the fracture line running parallel and adjacent to a root filling.

(iv) Double images: when separation of the fragments occurs in a direction other than parallel to the X-ray beam, overlapping of the fragments may result in double images of the external root surface. However, this effect is sometimes seen in normal teeth, for example, in the mesial concavity of maxillary premolar teeth.

(v) Extrusion of cement or filling: extrusion of cement or root filling material may occur into the fracture site or apically when the fracture is present prior to filling. It may also occur during root filling procedure.

(vi) Widening of the periodontal ligament space: along the whole length of the root may indicate VRF. It is different from bone loss seen in a periapical lesion where it occurs apically but without destruction of the lamina dura along the root surface.

(vii) Radiolucent halos: "halo-like" radiolucency running along the whole length of the root surface is a classic sign of VRF.

(viii) Step-like bone defects: oblique fractures often lead to a characteristic step-like bone defect which may mimic endodontic lesions.

(ix) Isolated horizontal bone loss in posterior teeth.

(x) Unexplained bifurcation bone loss: furcation bone loss may occur in molars with root fracture, in the absence of apical pathosis or over a periodontal disease and without any apparent reason like root perforation.

The radiologic signs are highly nonspecific and not detectable during the early stages, in which there are subtle fissures with no separation and those develop late as sequelae of chronic inflammation induced by the fracture. Approximately only one third of the fractures may be visualized directly on conventional dental radiographs. Mesiodistally oriented fractures are not visualized directly in a typical radiographic examination.

Current research has employed cone-beam computed tomography (CBCT) to identify the presence of VRF [8, 9]. Unfortunately, root fractures are difficult to assess, because most of them occur in teeth with RCT. Therefore, the superposition of the fracture line with the filling material decreases the diagnostic accuracy [10].

Currently, there is no evidence supporting the use of CBCT to detect VRF in ETT. Therefore, the diagnosis should be confirmed after surgical flap elevation [3].

An exploratory surgical procedure helps in the definitive diagnosis, if VRF is strongly suspected from the clinical and radiographic signs. Gentle soft tissue retraction may be sufficient to view the fracture line, and a dye material may also be used for a better visualization of the fracture line. As a probe is passed over the fracture line, "clicking" sound may be heard. Reflection of a small full-thickness flap may be required in some cases. This was the case for our patient where diagnosis was made only after a surgical exploration of the side of the vertical fracture, especially that the real cause was hidden by the presence of another periapical lesion of the adjacent tooth which misled us from the correct diagnosis.

3.2. Etiologies.
The etiology of VRFs is multifactorial and can be divided into predisposing and iatrogenic factors.

3.2.1. Predisposing Factors for Endodontically Treated Teeth
(i) Root anatomy: roots with narrow mesiodistal diameter, root curvatures [17, 18], and depressions in the mesial root of mandibular molars as well as in buccal roots of bifurcated maxillary premolars predispose them to fracture, especially at a later stage when additional tooth structure is removed during root canal and dowel space preparations.

(ii) Moisture loss in pulpless teeth [1] was reported to make endodontically treated teeth more brittle. However, this finding was not supported in some studies [19, 20].

(iii) Loss of bone support due to periodontal disease and preendodontic and prosthetic treatment can result in reduced ability of the tooth to withstand functional stresses.

(iv) Preexisting cracks.

(v) Biochemical properties of root dentin: a study on stress-strain response in human dentin showed that the dentin adaptation to functional stress-strain distribution results in a greater mineralization in the buccolingual areas. This may increase the likelihood for a fracture to propagate in this direction, compared with less mineralization and more collagen in the mesiodistal areas [16, 21].

3.2.2. The Iatrogenic Cause of VRF Is Mainly Attributed to Different Phases of Root Canal Treatment
(i) Loss of healthy tooth substance: combined with tooth loss due to caries, the result of intraradicular procedures, the remaining tooth structure is directly related to the ability of endodontically treated tooth to resist fracture [18, 22].

(ii) Change in the architecture of an endodontically treated tooth makes the tooth more prone to fracture and thus requiring a restoration (full cuspal coverage) that will protect the tooth during function.

(iii) Excessive cutting during various phases of root canal treatment.

(iv) Increased stress generated from threaded and tapered posts.

(v) Increased wedging forces with lateral compaction of gutta-percha accounts for 48% to 84% of VRFs. The development of these stresses stands behind crack initiation and propagation, leading eventually to root fracture [17, 23].

Fracture occurring directly during root canal treatment as a result of excessive force application is rare as the required forces for root fractures vary according to the tooth type (approximately 10 to 12 kg) and are well above those that are clinically relevant (1 to 3 kg) during root canal treatment. However, stress caused in dentin may initiate dentinal cracks, which can extend to complete fractures under a functional load. Thus, the multifactorial nature of VRFs has inspired studies in two directions.

Primarily, theoretical research has evaluated the effects of mechanical wear on the dentin in ETT with curved roots and oval channels. Ex vivo studies have associated the presence of isthmus and irregularities in the root canal posterior to mechanical instrumentation with the occurrence of VRF. Whereas in vitro studies have assessed the effects of irrigating solutions, the loss of dentinal moisture after RCT, and the role of tooth restoration and its capacity to respond to masticatory stress on the presence of VRF in ETT.

Secondly, clinical research has investigated factors, such as the type of endodontic treatment and the presence of posts.

A recent study determined that teeth exhibiting dense overfilled root canals significantly increased the odds for VRF by 2.72 times. Another in vitro study of Devale [18] evaluated the effect of instrumentation length and instrumentation systems, and Hand versus Rotary Files on Apical Crack Formation concluded that there was no statistical significance between stainless steel hand and rotary files in terms of crack formation.

Instrumentation length had a significant effect on the formation of cracks when rotary files were used. Using rotary instruments at 1 mm short of the apical foramen caused less crack formation. There was, however, no statistically significant difference in the number of cracks formed with hand files at two instrumentation levels.

Some studies have reported that gender may not play a role in VRFs on endodontically treated teeth; on the contrary, nonendodontically treated teeth VRFs seem to occur more frequently in male patients than females. This may be closely be related to the fact that males often present stronger masticatory muscles and higher bite force values.

Although vertical root fracture (VRF) is mostly found in endodontically treated teeth, it may also occur spontaneously.

If VRF is recognized after endodontic treatment, it is considered to be iatrogenic and can lead to legal trouble. However, legal problems can be averted if the dentist can prove that the VRF existed before endodontic treatment. To determine whether a fracture is iatrogenic or spontaneous, gutta-percha will be found in the fracture line of the transversely sectioned root (after tooth extraction), and it appeared to have penetrated to the fracture line through the generated filling force [21].

Some studies suggest that endodontic treatment procedure, in which some tooth structure is inevitably removed, may weaken the treated tooth, simultaneously increasing the fracture risk even in younger patients [24], which was the case for our patient of only of 14 years of age.

3.3. Treatment and Prognosis. In a multi rooted tooth with VRF, root resection (amputation or hemisection) can save the tooth. However, in single rooted teeth with VRF, the prognosis is unfavorable.

Extraction may be required (because of extensive bone loss and uncertain prognosis).

However, many innovative attempts to treat and retain anterior teeth have been described in various case reports [1, 19, 22].

3.3.1. Extraction and Replantation after Bonding. Studies have reported successfully treating tooth with VRF by atraumatically extracting the fractured tooth, bonding the fragments, and then replanting the tooth either directly or with a 180 degree rotation (especially in cases of anterior teeth). It was advocated that deep and narrow periodontal pockets along the fracture line may remain if teeth with VRF are replanted without rotation as intentional rotational replantation aims to avoid contact with the area where bone and periodontal ligament were lost in the treatment of VRF. The rotation of the tooth was suggested to connect the remnants of the healthy periodontal membrane, remaining on the root, with the connective tissue of the periodontally involved socket wall.

Other treatment options like the use of composite resins, mineral trioxide aggregate, and glass ionomer cements for bonding the fracture line have also been tried [20, 25].

The use of CO2 and Nd:YAG laser to fuse fractured tooth roots was also reported [19].

The Use of dual-cured adhesive resin cement is preferred for bonding the fractured fragments, as it is easy to apply and has a controlled polymerization [26].

In the present case, the extraction of tooth number 11 and its replacement by a removable prosthesis until the age of eighteen was discussed with the patient. However, the patient was reluctant for extraction and an alternative treatment plan was established which included bonding the fragments with a fluid resin cement without extraction and intentional replantation. The use of adhesive resin with intentional replantation has been reported in the literature for complete and incomplete vertical root fractures. Arikan et al. and Dogan et al. reported successful treatment outcome of vertically fractured incisors while adopting this method [27, 28].

The main objective of the treatment adopted was to preserve the natural tooth despite the uncertain prognosis so

that bone support of the tooth is maintained (until the age of 25) along with its normal occlusion. This will genuinely be very useful and important for possible prosthetics or implant treatment needed in the future for this young patient.

However, failure was observed when the same method was used to treat vertically fractured posterior teeth. The possible reasons behind that could include lower occlusal forces applied on the anterior teeth along with a better maintenance of the gingival health in this area. This finding encouraged us to choose the treatment option of bonding and monitoring for the presented case of VRF in the anterior tooth.

Many of the treatment options reported involve extensive procedures often with poor outcomes. Where successful outcomes have been claimed, the long term prognosis has yet to be proven. All the case reports published so far that describe a treatment rationale do not include enough teeth to ascertain the efficacy of any procedure.

Therefore, there is a need for further clinical research on the treatment of teeth with VRF.

References

[1] A. Dhawan, S. Gupta, and R. Mittal, "Vertical root fractures: an update review," *Journal of Restorative Dentistry*, vol. 2, no. 3, p. 107, 2014.

[2] W.-C. Liao, Y.-L. Tsai, C.-Y. Wang et al., "Clinical and Radiographic characteristics of vertical root fracture in endodontically and nonendodontically treated teeth," *Journal of Endodontics*, vol. 43, no. 5, pp. 687–693, 2017.

[3] C. García-Guerrero, C. Parra-Junco, S. Quijano-Guauque, N. Molano, G. A. Pineda, and D. J. Marín-Zuluaga, "Vertical root fractures in endodontically- treated teeth: a retrospective analysis of possible risk factors," *Journal of Investigative and Clinical Dentistry*, 2017, in press.

[4] N. Takeuchi, T. Yamamoto, T. Tomofuji, and C. Murakami, "A retrospective study on the prognosis of teeth with root fracture in patients during the maintenance phase of periodontal therapy," *Dental Traumatology*, vol. 25, no. 3, pp. 332–337, 2009.

[5] E. Chang, E. Lam, P. Shah, and A. Azarpazhooh, "Cone- beam computed tomography for detecting vertical root fractures in endodontically treated teeth: a systematic review," *Journal of Endodontics*, vol. 42, no. 2, pp. 177–185, 2016.

[6] M. Yahyazadehfar, J. Ivancik, H. Majd, B. An, D. Zhang, and D. Arola, "On the mechanics of fatigue and fracture in teeth," *Applied Mechanics Reviews*, vol. 66, no. 3, pp. 0308031–3080319, 2014.

[7] L. Karygianni, M. Krengel, M. Winter, S. Stampf, and K. T. Wrbas, "Comparative assessment of the incidence of vertical root fractures between conven- tional versus surgical endodontic retreatment," *Clinical Oral Investigations*, vol. 18, no. 8, pp. 2015–2021, 2014.

[8] S. Talwar, S. Utneja, R. R. Nawal, A. Kaushik, D. Srivastava, and S. S. Oberoy, "Role of cone- beam computed tomography in diagnosis of verti- cal root fractures: a systematic review and meta- analysis," *Journal of Endodontics*, vol. 42, no. 1, pp. 12–24, 2016.

[9] B. Hassan, M. E. Metska, A. R. Ozok, P. van der Stelt, and P. R. Wesselink, "Detection of vertical root fractures in endodontically treated teeth by a cone beam computed tomography scan," *Journal of Endodontics*, vol. 35, no. 5, pp. 719–722, 2009.

[10] R. F. de Menezes, N. C. de Araújo, J. M. C. S. Rosa et al., "Detection of vertical root fractures in endodontically treated teeth in the absence and in the presence of metal post by cone-beam computed tomography," *BMC Oral Health*, vol. 16, no. 1, p. 48, 2016.

[11] D. Dua and A. Dua, "Reconstruction and intentional replantation of a maxillary central incisor with a complete vertical root fracture: a rare case report with three years follow up," *Journal of Clinical and Diagnostic Research*, vol. 9, no. 9, pp. ZD06–ZD09, 2015.

[12] J. N. R. Martinsa, J. Pedro Canta, A. Coelho, and M. Baharestani, "Vertical root fracture diagnosis of crowned premolars with root canal treatment–Two case reports," *Revista Portuguesa de Estomatologia, Medicina Dentária e Cirurgia Maxilofacial*, vol. 55, no. 1, pp. 60–64, 2014.

[13] J. Lustig, A. Tamse, and Z. Fuss, "Pattern of bone resorption in vertically fractured, endodontically treated teeth," *Oral Surgery, Oral Medicine, Oral Pathology, Oral Radiology, and Endodontology*, vol. 90, no. 2, pp. 224–227, 2000.

[14] T. Sugaya, M. Kawanami, H. Noguchi, H. Kato, and N. Masaka, "Periodontal healing after bonding treatment of vertical root fracture," *Dental Traumatology*, vol. 17, no. 4, pp. 174–179, 2001.

[15] E. J. Nogueira Leal da Silva, G. Romão dos Santos, R. Liess Krebs, and T. de Souza Coutinho-Filho, "Surgical alternative for treatment of vertical root fracture: a case report," *Iranian Endodontic Journal*, vol. 7, no. 1, pp. 40–44, 2012.

[16] A. Kishen, G. V. kumar, and N. N. Chen, "Stress-strain response in human dentine: rethinking fracture predilection in post core restored teeth," *Dental Traumatology*, vol. 20, no. 2, pp. 90–100, 2004.

[17] V. Letchirakam, J. E. Palamara, and H. H. Messer, "Finite element analysis and strain gauge studies of vertical root fracture," *Journal of Endodontics*, vol. 29, no. 8, pp. 529–534, 2003.

[18] M. R. Devale, "Effect of instrumentation length and instrumentation systems: hand versus rotary files on apical crack formation," *Journal of Clinical and Diagnostic Research*, vol. 11, no. 1, pp. ZC15–ZC18, 2017.

[19] S. Arakawa, C. M. Cobb, J. W. Rapley, W. J. Killoy, and P. Spencer, "Treatment of root fracture by CO_2 and ND: YAG lasers: an in vitro study," *Journal of Endodontics*, vol. 22, no. 12, pp. 662–667, 1996.

[20] A. Hasegawa, H. Bando, K. Fukai, T. Vongsurasit, and T. Tsuchida, "Periodontal surgical approach to the vertical fracture of the root: the application of composite resin to the fractured root surface," *Nihon Shishubyo Gakkai Kaishi*, vol. 30, no. 4, pp. 1180–1185, 1988.

[21] M. J. Lim, J. A. Kim, Y. Choi, C. U. Hong, and K. S. Min, "Differentiating spontaneous vertical root fracture in endodontically treated tooth," *European Journal of Dentistry*, vol. 11, no. 1, pp. 122–125, 2017.

[22] R. A. Barkhordar, "Treatment of vertical root fractures: a case report," *Quintessence International*, vol. 22, pp. 707–709, 1991.

[23] A. Tamse, "Iatrogenic vertical root fractures in endodontically treated teeth," *Dental Traumatology*, vol. 4, no. 5, pp. 190–196, 1988.

[24] C. P. Chan, C. P. Lin, S.-C. Tseng, and J.-H. Jeng, "Vertical root fracture in endodontically versus non endodontically treated teeth: a survey of 315 cases in chinese patients," *Oral Surgery, Oral Medicine, Oral Pathology, Oral Radiology, and Endodontology*, vol. 87, no. 4, pp. 504–507, 1999.

[25] R. S. Schwartz, M. Mauger, D. J. Clement, and W. A. Walker III, "Mineral trioxide aggregate: a new material for endodontics," *Journal of the American Dental Association*, vol. 130, no. 7, pp. 967–975, 1999.

[26] M. Oztürk and G. C. Unal, "A successful treatment of vertical root fracture: a case report and 4 year follow-up," *Dental Traumatology*, vol. 24, no. 5, pp. e56–e60, 2008.

[27] F. Arikan, M. Franko, and A. Gurkan, "Replantation of a vertically fractured maxillary central incisor after repair with adhesive resin," *International Endodontic Journal*, vol. 41, no. 2, pp. 173–179, 2008.

[28] M. C. Dogan, E. O. Akgun, and H. O. Yoldas, "Adhesive tooth fragment reattachment with intentional replantation: 36-month follow-up," *Dental Traumatology*, vol. 29, no. 3, pp. 238–242, 2013.

9

Excisional Biopsy of the Pyogenic Granuloma in Very High-Risk Patient

Dirceu Tavares Formiga Nery,[1] **José Ranali,**[2] **Darceny Zanetta Barbosa,**[3] **Helvécio Marangon Júnior,**[4] **Rafael Martins Afonso Pereira,**[4] **and Patrícia Cristine de Oliveira Afonso Pereira**(iD)[4]

[1]*School of Dentistry, Catholic University of Brasília (UCB), Brasília, DF, Brazil*
[2]*Department of Pharmacology, Anesthesiology and Therapeutics, School of Dentistry, University of Campinas (UNICAMP), Piracicaba, SP, Brazil*
[3]*Department of Oral and Maxillofacial Surgery and Traumatology, School of Dentistry, Federal University of Uberlandia (UFU), Uberlândia, MG, Brazil*
[4]*School of Dentistry, University Center of Patos de Minas (UNIPAM), Patos de Minas, MG, Brazil*

Correspondence should be addressed to Patrícia Cristine de Oliveira Afonso Pereira; patriciapereira@unipam.edu.br

Academic Editor: Gavriel Chaushu

Oral surgery to remove pyogenic granuloma in a high-risk patient is reported. A 47-year-old man with gastroesophageal reflux disease, diabetes mellitus II, dyslipidemia, and chronic coronary insufficiency (myocardial infarction within 2 years) with episodes of unstable angina was submitted to an excisional biopsy of hemorrhagic lesion in the lingual right mandibular gingiva. During dental treatment, the arterial blood pressure, oxygen saturation, heart rate, and electrocardiogram were monitored. Local anesthesia was performed with 0.45 ml of 3% prilocaine with 0.03 IU/ml felypressin. The anticoagulant therapy was not interrupted. No local or systemic complications were noticed during or after the surgery.

1. Introduction

Coronary artery disease (CAD) is highly prevalent in industrialized countries, and although prevention, diagnosis, and medication have improved, it is still the main cause of death [1, 2]. When CAD is symptomatic, angina pectoris is the presenting sign. Unstable angina pectoris (UA) and myocardial infarction (MI) are more critical situations and demand prompt medical care [3].

Because of the high prevalence of CAD and the improved preventive measures leading to patients' teeth being preserved into advanced age, the general dental practitioner will more frequently encounter CAD [3, 4]. There are no contraindications to elective dental treatment of patients with stable angina [3]. UA and MI in the period of 6 months after their occurrence were designated by the American Society of Anesthesiologists (ASA) as class IV patients, limiting their dental care to urgency treatment [2, 5–7]. However, in view of the current technological advances in both peri-MI and post-MI treatment and assessment, these guidelines have been revised [5, 6].

If ASA IV patients (UA or IM) with dental pain are given no treatment, this may aggravate the ischemic attacks due to pain and anxiety, thus leading to increased secretion and release of catecholamines [2–7]. On the other hand, the dental treatment itself may endanger the patient's life, if it is not administered and monitored properly [2, 5, 6, 8].

This article reports on the safe management and monitoring of an ASA IV patient during a dental procedure: excisional biopsy of a pyogenic granuloma.

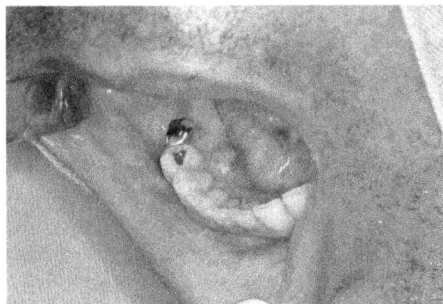

FIGURE 1

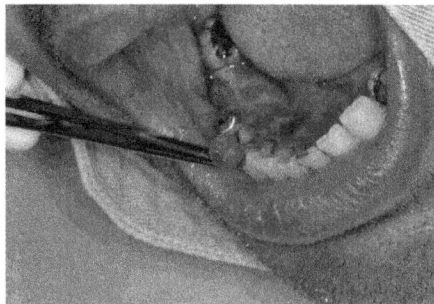

FIGURE 2

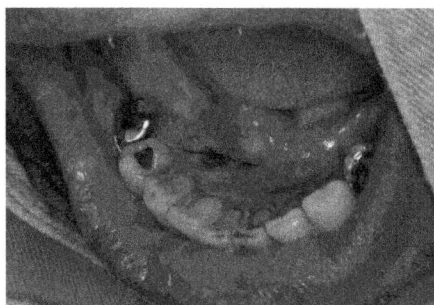

FIGURE 3

2. Clinical Presentation

A 47-year-old man presenting with active CAD and considered to be a very high-risk patient (ASA IV) was referred to the Dentistry School of Uberlândia Federal University exhibiting a solitary nodule, 8 mm in diameter, in the lingual right mandibular gingiva (Figure 1), with spontaneous and intermittent bleeding.

Physical examination revealed a painless lesion, within a well-demarcated violet-colored (hemorrhagic) margin, friable in consistency, and of unknown origin, involving the lingual gingiva in the area of teeth # 43-44. According to the patient, the lesion had been present for approximately two months, exhibiting slow growth. Radiographic examination showed no teeth and/or bone involved. The initial diagnosis was pyogenic granuloma.

The patient's medical history showed gastroesophageal reflux disease, diabetes mellitus II, dyslipidemia, and chronic coronary insufficiency (myocardial infarction within 2 years) with episodes of unstable angina. The patient had been submitted to myocardial revascularization surgery (2 years previously); first, right coronary artery angioplasty (CAA) with stent (within 1 1/2 year); second, CAA (within 1 year), due to intrastent restenosis; third, CAA (about 9 months before) with new restenosis and stent implantation in ACD and previous descending artery (ADA); fourth, stent implantation due to restenosis (within 3 months); and finally, 2 months ago, this patient presented second degree atrium-ventricular block (mobitz II), being submitted to definitive artificial cardiac pacemaker implantation. The patient was receiving anticoagulants, oral nitrates, beta blockers, and calcium channel antagonist. The treatment of choice was an excisional biopsy with curettage (Figure 2), due to the possibility of recurrence. During dental treatment, blood pressure, heart rate, continuous electrocardiogram (ECG), and oxygen saturation were monitored. The emergency service was on stand-by at the ambulatory, and it could be brought into action if necessary. The patient's physician was consulted, and none of the medication being administered to the patient was suspended, including acetylsalicylic and ticlopidine hydrochloride. The patient's international normalized ratio (INR) on the day of the surgery was 2.8.

The surgical appointment started at 9:30 am. No sedation method was used, as the patient was not anxious and the procedure would be performed in a short time. Preoperative vital signs were as follows: blood pressure (BP) 110/86 mmHg,

heart rate (HR) 57 bpm, and 96% oxygen saturation (OS). On that day, the patient complained of chest pain.

After local anesthesia with 0.45 ml of 3% prilocaine with 0.03 IU/ml felypressin, the nodule was excised and sent for histopathologic evaluation. No active bleeding was observed during or after surgery (Figure 3). During dental treatment, the patient did not complain of exacerbation of the symptoms, such as chest pain and dyspnea, or show marked hemodynamic change that necessitated discontinuation or postponement of the surgery, which was completed in 30 minutes. After treatment, the patient was carefully observed for vital signs, cardiac symptoms, pain, and ECG irregularities for 24 hours. Postoperative vital signs were as follows: BP, 111/90 mmHg; HR, 56 bpm; and OS, 95%. Acetaminophen (750 mg each 6 h, for 24 h) was prescribed to control postoperative pain.

Histopathologic examination confirmed the previous diagnosis of pyogenic granuloma (Figure 4). Follow-up examinations have been made every 30 days, to rule out recurrence of the lesion. No local or systemic complications were observed in a period of one month.

3. Discussion

The advances in prevention, diagnosis, and treatment of cardiovascular diseases have led to an increased survival of patients, although this group of diseases continues to be the first cause of death in industrialized countries. For successful dental management of these patients, as with any other disease, a complete medical history and physical examination, including blood pressure, heart rate, and respiratory function, are indispensable. When indicated, medical consultation must be sought [9–11].

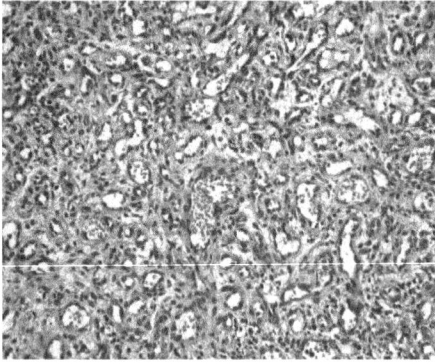

FIGURE 4

Many authors have recommended elective dental treatment only after 6 months of myocardial infarction and with stable angina [7, 9, 12–16]. Therefore, an oral surgery should be postponed in patients with arterial coronary disease, due to the high risk of reinfarction and cardiac arrest [7]. Alexander et al. [17], on the contrary, state that patients with coronary artery disease have a 1.1% perioperative rate of MI after noncardiac surgery, compared with a rate of 0 to 0.7% in the general population.

According to Niwa et al. [6], dental treatment is possible in high-risk patients, but should be limited to procedures of short duration, with good pain control during and after the procedure. In their study, 63 patients received dental treatment after complaints of toothache or masticatory disorder during hospitalization, under local anesthesia with 3% prilocaine with 0.03 IU/ml felypressin, in a maximum period of 30 minutes. The procedures would be stopped if cardiovascular conditions showed signs of deterioration. In some of the cases, sedation (nitrous oxide or diazepam IV) was used. All the procedures were carried out without interruption, and 8 patients had angina in the period of one week after the procedure, 5 of them related to the dental treatment. Of importance is the fact that the incidence of postoperative complications was higher in patients with history of chest pain 2 weeks before the dental treatment and in those who failed to clear the Master Test Single stress test.

In the case presented here, although the patient had a history of unstable angina with complaints of chest pain daily, the procedure was accomplished without postoperative complications. The 24 h ECG monitoring showed no postoperative complications without any new ST depression. Although it is recommended in the literature that patients with cardiovascular disease should be treated under sedation, it is interesting that in the Niwa et al.'s study and in the present case, no relation was observed between the presence of complication and whether or not pharmacological sedation was used. Iatrosedation and the patient's confidence in the dentist are of great importance. In the present case, the medical care is a factor that could also have increased the patient's confidence.

According to Findler et al. [2] and Chapman [7], a prophylactic dose of nitrates a few minutes before the appointment begins is recommended for patients with history of angina. However, this patient presented with continuous chest pain and used isosorbide dinitrate every 4 hours. Due to the risk of hypotension with reflex tachycardia [7], this recommendation was not followed.

As the clinical diagnosis was a pyogenic granuloma, the treatment followed the established protocol, consisting of surgical excision and removal of etiological factors [18–20].

According to Campbell et al. [21], patients can safely undergo routine outpatient oral surgical procedures without alteration of their regular therapeutic anticoagulation regimens [21–26]. It is necessary to establish the prothrombin time/INR on the day of the dental procedure or dental surgery, to ensure that it is in a safe or therapeutic range [23, 27]. Serum level is monitored via the corrected prothrombin time (international normalized ratio—INR). The optimal INR for most conditions is up to 3.018. The case presented here supports this statement, as no excessive bleeding was observed during or after the surgery, with an INR of 2.8 and no anticoagulant withdrawal.

It should be emphasized that in spite of the recommendation that cardiovascular patients should only be treated at least 60 days after myocardial infarction and with clearing the exercise stress testing [5, 6], there are cases such as presence of pain or lesions that must be removed and diagnosis that demands treatment under far from ideal conditions, as in the present case. This shows that it is possible, even in such cases, to offer patients safe treatment.

Dental treatment must therefore be carefully conducted, with proper pain and anxiety management to minimize any elevation in endogenous catecholamine [2, 3, 5, 6] which could cause a number of undesirable effects, such as increased blood pressure and alterations in heart rate.

Therefore, the local anesthetic solution and technique must be those that offer appropriate efficacy and duration without the need for another injection during the procedure to avoid unnecessary pain and stress. In the present case, prilocaine with felypressin was the choice [6], and acetaminophen was prescribed for avoiding postoperative pain.

To avoid additional risks and offer safe treatment in high-risk patients, as in the present case, oral surgery must be performed with cardiovascular monitoring in a medical facility with emergency support.

Acknowledgments

This study was supported by a grant-in-aid from the Brazilian agencies São Paulo Research Foundation (FAPESP (01/13890-7)) and Coordination for the Improvement of Higher Education Personnel (CAPES).

References

[1] W. B. Kammel and T. Y. Tham, "Incidence, prevalence and mortality of cardiovascular disease," in *The Heart*, J. W. Hurst, Ed., p. 627, McGraw-Hill Book Co, New York, NY, USA, 1990.

[2] M. Findler, D. Galili, Z. Meidan, V. Yakirevitch, and A. A. Garfunkel, "Dental treatment in very high risk patients with active ischemic heart disease," *Oral Surgery, Oral Medicine, and Oral Pathology*, vol. 76, no. 3, pp. 298–300, 1993.

[3] R. H. Blanchaert Jr., "Ischemic heart disease," *Oral Surgery, Oral Medicine, Oral Pathology, Oral Radiology, and Endodontics*, vol. 87, no. 3, pp. 281–283, 1999.

[4] N. Jowett and L. Cabot, "Patients with cardiac disease: considerations for the dental practitioner," *British Dental Journal*, vol. 189, no. 6, pp. 297–302, 2000.

[5] H. W. Roberts and E. F. Mitnitsky, "Cardiac risk stratification for postmyocardial infarction dental patients," *Oral Surgery, Oral Medicine, Oral Pathology, Oral Radiology, and Endodontics*, vol. 91, no. 6, pp. 676–681, 2001.

[6] H. Niwa, Y. Sato, and H. Matsuura, "Safety of dental treatment in patients with previously diagnosed acute myocardial infarction or unstable angina pectoris," *Oral Surgery, Oral Medicine, Oral Pathology, Oral Radiology, and Endodontology*, vol. 89, no. 1, pp. 35–41, 2000.

[7] P. J. Chapman, "Chest pain in the dental surgery: a brief review and practical points in diagnosis and management," *Australian Dental Journal*, vol. 47, no. 3, pp. 259–261, 2002.

[8] M. Sugimura, Y. Hirota, T. Shibutani et al., "An echocardiographic study of interactions between pindolol and epinephrine contained in a local anesthetic solution," *Anesthesia Progress*, vol. 42, no. 2, pp. 29–35, 1995.

[9] Research, Science and Therapy Committee, American Academy of Periodontology, "Periodontal management of patients with cardiovascular diseases," *Journal of Periodontology*, vol. 73, no. 8, pp. 954–968, 2002.

[10] W. J. Maloney and M. A. Weinberg, "Implementation of the American Society of Anesthesiologists Physical Status classification system in periodontal practice," *Journal of Periodontology*, vol. 79, no. 7, pp. 1124–1126, 2008.

[11] W. W. Herman, J. L. Konzelman, and L. M. Prisant, "New national guidelines on hypertension: a summary for dentistry," *The Journal of the American Dental Association*, vol. 135, no. 5, pp. 576–584, 2004.

[12] J.-P. Goulet, R.'n. Pe'russe, and J.-Y. Turcotte, "Contraindications to vasoconstrictors in dentistry: part III: pharmacologic interactions," *Oral Surgery, Oral Medicine, Oral Pathology*, vol. 74, no. 5, pp. 692–697, 1992.

[13] R.'n. Pe'russe, J. P. Goulet, and J. Y. Turcotte, "Contraindications to vasoconstrictors in dentistry: part I: cardiovascular diseases," *Oral Surgery, Oral Medicine, Oral Pathology*, vol. 74, no. 5, pp. 679–686, 1992.

[14] F. J. Silvestre, L. Miralles-Jorda, C. Tamarit, and R. Gascon, "Dental management of the patient with ischemic heart disease: an update," *Medicina Oral*, vol. 7, no. 3, pp. 222–230, 2002.

[15] L. F. Rose, B. Mealey, L. Minsk, and D. W. Cohen, "Oral care for patients with cardiovascular disease and stroke," *The Journal of the American Dental Association*, vol. 133, pp. 37S–44S, 2002.

[16] J. R. Hupp, "Ischemic heart disease: dental management considerations," *Dental Clinics of North America*, vol. 50, no. 4, pp. 483–491, 2006.

[17] R. W. Alexander, R. C. Schlant, and V. Fuster, Eds., *Hurst's the Heart*, McGraw-Hill, New York, NY, USA, 1998.

[18] J. A. Regezi, J. J. Sciubba, and R. C. K. Jordan, Eds., *Patologia bucal: correlações clínicopatológicas*, Elsevier, Rio de Janeiro, Brazil, 2017.

[19] T. Al-Khateeb and K. Ababneh, "Oral pyogenic granuloma in Jordanians: a retrospective analysis of 108 cases," *Journal of Oral and Maxillofacial Surgery*, vol. 61, no. 11, pp. 1285–1288, 2003.

[20] J. Bakshi, R. S. Virk, and M. Verma, "Pyogenic granuloma of the hard palate: a case report and review of the literature," *Ear, Nose, & Throat Journal*, vol. 88, no. 9, pp. E4–E5, 2009.

[21] J. H. Campbell, F. Alvarado, and R. A. Murray, "Anticoagulation and minor oral surgery: should the anticoagulation regimen be altered?," *Journal of Oral and Maxillofacial Surgery*, vol. 58, no. 2, pp. 131–135, 2000.

[22] R. L. Campbell and W. G. Langston, "A comparison of cardiac rate-pressure product and pressure-rate quotient in healthy and medically compromised patients," *Oral Surgery, Oral Medicine, Oral Pathology, Oral Radiology, and Endodontology*, vol. 80, no. 2, pp. 145–152, 1995.

[23] R. Alexander, A. C. Ferretti, and J. R. Sorensen, "Stop the nonsense not the anticoagulants: a matter of life and death," *The New York State Dental Journal*, vol. 68, no. 9, pp. 24–26, 2002.

[24] D. E. van Diermen, J. Hoogstraten, and I. van der Waal, "Dental procedures for patients using oral anticoagulation: new insights," *Nederlands Tijdschrift voor Tandheelkunde*, vol. 115, no. 4, pp. 225–229, 2008.

[25] M. Caliskan, H. C. Tukel, E. Benlidayi, and A. Deniz, "Is it necessary to alter anticoagulation therapy for tooth extraction in patients taking direct oral anticoagulants?," *Medicina Oral Patología Oral y Cirugia Bucal*, vol. 22, no. 6, pp. e767–e773, 2017.

[26] T. Yagyuu, M. Kawakami, Y. Ueyama et al., "Risks of postextraction bleeding after receiving direct oral anticoagulants or warfarin: a retrospective cohort study," *BMJ Open*, vol. 7, no. 8, article e015952, 2017.

[27] T. Badoual, N. Lellouche, M. Bourraindeloup et al., "Pathology and dental care in the context of cardiovascular conditions: myths beliefs and realities," *Archives des maladies du coeur et des vaisseaux*, vol. 96, no. 6, pp. 637–644, 2003.

10

Unexpected Complication Ten Years after Initial Treatment: Long-Term Report and Fate of a Maxillary Premolar Rehabilitation

Davide Augusti and **Gabriele Augusti**

DDS, Private Dental Practice, Cosmetic and Restorative Dentistry, Via Papa Giovanni XXIII 37, 20091 Bresso Milan, Italy

Correspondence should be addressed to Gabriele Augusti; g.augusti@libero.it

Academic Editor: Jiiang H. Jeng

Full-coverage restorations represent a well-known rehabilitation strategy for compromised posterior teeth; in the last years, new ceramic materials like zirconia have been introduced and widely adopted for the prosthetic management of molar and premolar areas. A long-term follow-up of a maxillary premolar rehabilitation using a veneered zirconia crown is presented; after ten years of uneventful clinical service of the tooth-restoration complex, a serious complication—namely, a vertical root fracture (VRF)—occurred. An extended time lapse (9 years) between the end of restorative procedures and development of symptoms due to VRF has been observed. On the other hand, a complete functional and esthetic integrity of the zirconia crown (without chippings or crack development) is documented along the follow-up period. Due to periodontal breakdown and severity of fracture, the premolar was extracted. The illustrations of our late failure, aetiological factors, and available data on the literature regarding VRF are addressed. Patients and clinicians should be aware of potential occurrences of some long-term, serious complications when dealing with previously treated and/or structurally weakened teeth. The development of a VRF might be unexpected and might occur many years after the end of tooth rehabilitation, despite adoption of contemporary restorative protocols and techniques.

1. Introduction

The prosthetic crown placement on posterior, endodontically treated teeth has been suggested in the literature to improve their long-term prognosis [1–4]. According to Aquilino and Caplan, endodontically treated teeth without a crown restoration after filling of the canals were lost at a 6.0 times greater rate than teeth with full coverage after obturation [1]. An old study investigated a large number of extracted root-canal-treated (RCT) teeth [5]: the author found significant differences in the longevity between crowned teeth and those without cuspal protection, in favor of the former (average time before extraction of 87 and 50 months, respectively). In particular, RCT teeth restored with indirect prosthetic restorations (i.e., crown, bridge, and gold partial crown, with or without prefabricated posts) demonstrated a significantly lower mean fracture rate (14-year survival before fracture) than non-vital teeth provided with just a composite filling (10-year survival before fracture) [6].

New all-ceramic prosthetic materials, like yttrium tetragonal zirconia polycrystal (Y-TZP), represent a clinical alternative to the metal frameworks of single crowns, bridges, and also for minimally invasive, adhesively luted resin-bonded fixed partial dentures [7, 8]. This material offers high resistance to masticatory stresses and effectively reproduces the appearance of a natural dentition [9].

The reported contemporary survival rate for all-ceramic, single restorations is generally high: according to Ozer et al., more than 90% of posterior porcelain fused-to-zirconia crowns survived after a mean period of 7.4 years [10]. A meta-analysis of Sailer et al. demonstrated a 96% survival rate for densely sintered zirconia fixed dental prostheses at a 5-year follow-up; a statistically similar value (94.7%) was also found for metal-ceramic restorations [11]. A recent

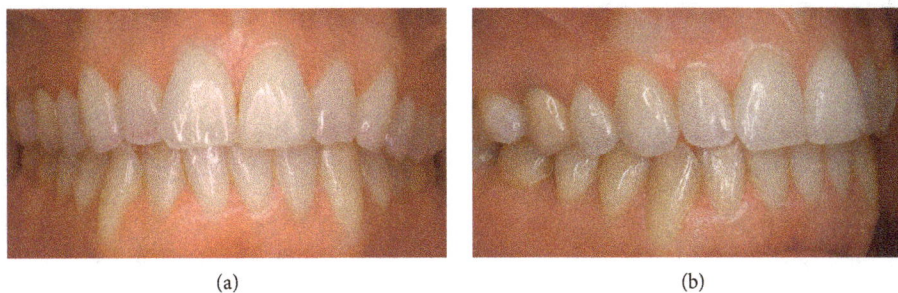

(a)   (b)

FIGURE 1: Preoperative intraoral frontal (a) and lateral (b) views showing the preexisting upper second premolar crown (tooth 1.5).

systematic review set the success (absence of any kind of technical or biological complications) of single crowns on RCT teeth at 92%, after 6 years of service [12].

However, extensive operative procedures might be required on compromised teeth before they receive a full occlusal coverage. The long-term prognosis of multidisciplinary treated teeth (endodontic, periodontal, prerestorative, and prosthetic steps) might decrease substantially. For example, Moghaddam et al. have found a survival rate of 83% and of 51% for multidisciplinary treated teeth at 10- and 13-year recalls, respectively [13]. In other words, potential complications should be expected on severely damaged teeth when they are restored with multidisciplinary procedures and followed up for a long time.

Vertical root fractures (VRF) are defined as longitudinally oriented cracks confined to the root [14]: they are included among the potential reasons for failures of crowned teeth [15], leaving the clinician with few or limited treatment options. According to their 3-dimensional direction and extension, VRF can be classified as partial or complete [16]: a full separation and displacement of root fragments might eventually lead to tooth extraction [17, 18]. VRF are encountered more frequently on specific tooth types due to biomechanical factors: first lower molars (mesial root) and upper/lower premolars are predominantly affected, mainly due to a reduced mesio-distal diameter of the roots [19]. The reasons for extraction of a group of RCT teeth were analysed in a prospective study: the authors showed that 13.4% of the specimens were affected by a vertical root fracture [20]. An overall prevalence of 3 to 5% has been reported for that kind of complication; however, an underestimation of the problem might exist and be related to unrecognized cracks after extraction and/or other diagnostic difficulties [21].

The purpose of this paper is to report a long term, 10-year follow-up case of a maxillary premolar restored by contemporary endodontic and prosthetic procedures: after several years of uneventful service of the tooth-restoration complex, a serious complication—vertical root fracture—occurred. About 18% of VRFs are developed within 1 year from endodontic procedures [22]; in another study, the failure of teeth (i.e., extraction) associated to longitudinal fracture was established 1–5 years postoperatively [19]. In our case, an extended time lapse (9 years) between the end of restorative procedures and development of symptoms due to VRF has been observed. At the same time, a complete functional and esthetic integrity of the zirconia crown (without

chippings or crack development) is documented along the entire follow-up period. After case illustration, potential causes of the failure and analysis of available data in the literature related to VRF will be addressed.

2. Case: Report Presentation

2.1. Patient Presentation and Preliminary Care. A healthy female Caucasian patient (M.M, 46 years old) with an overall good oral hygiene attitude presented at our private dental practice in 2008; following a preliminary full-mouth dental bleaching and direct conservative therapies (i.e., restorations at elements 1.6–1.7) at the right maxillary quadrant, a decision was made to replace an old metal-ceramic prosthetic crown of tooth 1.5. Lateral and occlusal views of the preexisitng restoration are shown in Figures 1(a) and 1(b). Esthetic reasons guided the replacement, in order to achieve a new optimal integration with adjacent bleached teeth. At start of the new restorative cycle, informed consent was obtained.

2.2. Treatment Plan for Upper Premolar. The previously treated abutment (>10 years ago, by other colleagues) was originally restored with a metal cast post-and-core extending up to the coronal third of the root; the intraoral periapical X-ray revealed a partially treated and/or filled root canal space, accompanied by a slight radiolucency at the mesial side of the apex (Figure 2). Periodontal clinical parameters were all within normal limits.

After a complete clinical and radiographic evaluation, preprosthetic treatments were deemed necessary for the second maxillary premolar: our efforts were addressed towards delivering an all-ceramic restoration, in order to satisfy high patient's expectations and esthetic needs.

2.3. Disassembly and Endodontic Retreatment. Previous metal-based reconstructions would have been replaced by resin-based materials, in association with the adoption of adhesive techniques.

The preexisting crown was sectioned and gently removed. The abutment disassembly was accomplished with the aid of ultrasonic inserts until mobilization of cast post was obtained; then, a nonsurgical root canal retreatment (NSRCR) was planned. Standardized endodontic procedures included the use of stainless steel manual files and rotary Ni-Ti instruments (ProTaper® Universal Series, Dentsply

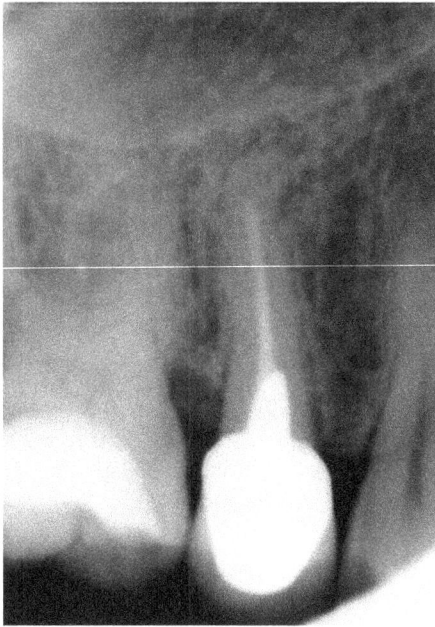

FIGURE 2: Periapical radiograph showing previous endodontic and prosthetic treatments on upper second premolar.

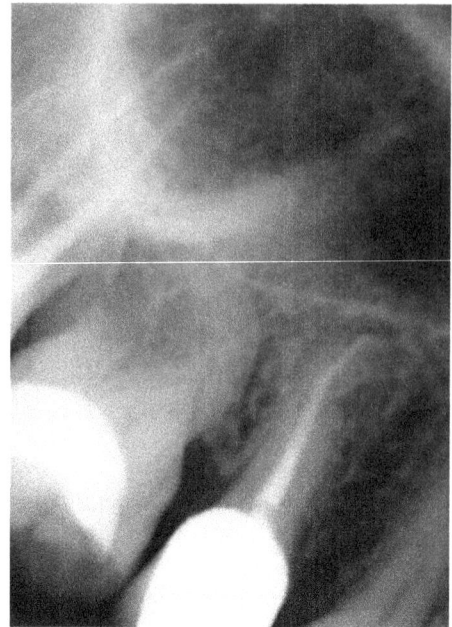

FIGURE 3: Periapical radiograph showing immediate outcome of nonsurgical endodontic retreatment performed at our dental office.

Maillefer), along with NaOCl and EDTA irrigations; the single-cone gutta-percha technique was chosen for final obturation (Figure 3) of the root canal (finishing file instrument and gutta-percha point: size *F1*, ProTaper® Universal, Dentsply Maillefer).

2.4. Core Build-Up, Prosthetic Preparation, and Crown Delivery. The abutment was finally restored using a tapered translucent glass-fiber post (D.T. Light-Post®, Bisco Inc.) luted with dual-polymerizing resin cement (Clearfil® SA, Kuraray Medical Ltd.); core build-up was completed with universal nanohybrid composite (Clearfil Majesty™, Kuraray Medical Ltd.) applications. A full-crown prosthetic preparation with a chamfer finishing line was accomplished: axial (1.0 to 1.5 mm) and occlusal reductions (1.5 to 2.0 mm) were carried out according to all-ceramic restoration's guidelines [23]; the cervical margin width was approximately 0.8 mm.

Medium-grit followed by fine-grit diamond burs provided a smooth preparation; due to its high precision and physical performances [24], a VPS material was chosen for a one-step impression technique, in association with retraction cords for gingival displacement (Elite HD+ putty soft; Elite HD+ light body, Zhermack SpA, Badia Polesine, Italy).

The porcelain-zirconia restoration was CAD/CAM fabricated starting from a presintered zirconia blank (Zirkonzhan, GmbH), milled with a dedicated machine (5 + 1 axis milling unit, M5, Zirkonzhan GmbH); the framework was refined, completely sintered (Zirkonofen 600, Zirkonzahn GmbH), and veneered. The definitive crown was adhesively luted as previously reported [25]: briefly, the inner surface of zirconia framework was pretreated with low-pressure (1 bar) 50 µm alumina sandblasting and ultrasonically cleaned; an MDP-based, dual polymerizing luting agent (Clearfil® SA, Kuraray Medical Ltd.) was subsequently applied for final cementation (Figures 4(a) and 4(b)). After luting, the occlusion was verified to avoid both interferences during excursive (protrusive and lateral) jaw movements and prematurities at maximum intercuspation.

2.5. Regular Check-Ups and Development of Symptoms. The premolar rehabilitation was completed within the same year (2008), and the tooth entirely recovered its function in the mouth; regular check-ups (approximately every 6 months) were carried out during subsequent years. Marginal integrity, signs of wear and visible cracks of the artificial crown, shade matching, and development of secondary caries at the interface with the tooth were assessed during the check-ups [26, 27]: the clinical examinations included periodontal probing and were accompanied by radiographic analyses. While the patient received other dental therapies in the meantime, no further problems or complications related to the premolar treatment were detected at follow-ups. About seven years later, in 2015, some modifications of the soft tissues were noted, as multiple gingival recession developed on upper posterior teeth: however, the margin at the premolar restoration was just slightly affected (0.5 mm recession, Figures 5(a) and 5(b)). High compliance was shown by the patient throughout the treatment, as demonstrated by strict attendance at check-ups, adequate biofilm control, and copings with discontinuous pain/symptoms during later stages.

Development of symptoms started about nine years later, in March 2017: at physical examination, a vestibular draining sinus tract on attached gingiva was discovered, with a mild positive response of the tooth to palpation (Miller class I score, for mobility test) and percussion tests. Diffuse widening of the periodontal ligament (in comparison with X-ray at time of root canal filling) and lamina dura modifications near the apex were observed from radiographic analysis,

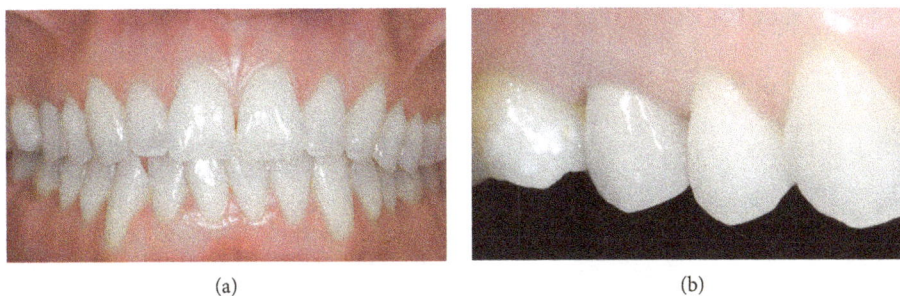

(a)   (b)

FIGURE 4: Postoperative intraoral frontal (a) and lateral (b) views showing good integration of the new veneered-zirconia crown on tooth 1.5.

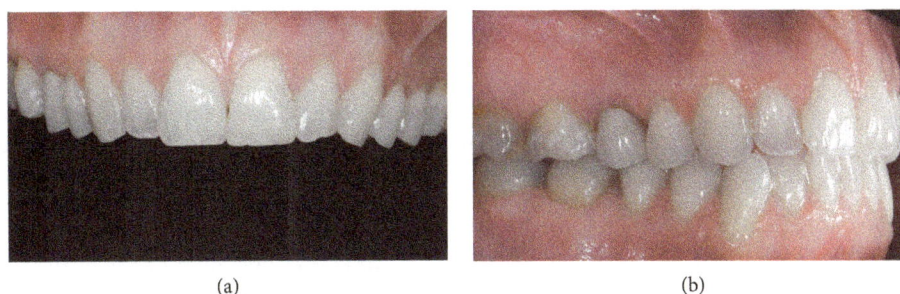

(a)   (b)

FIGURE 5: Frontal (a) and lateral (b) views 7 years after crown delivery: an overall dental deterioration is visible associated with soft tissue modifications.

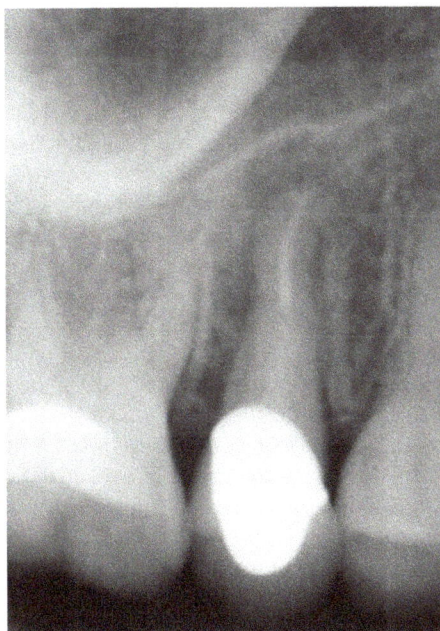

FIGURE 6: Development of clinical symptoms 9 years after crown delivery: the radiograph revealed a periapical radiolucency, with widening of periodontal ligament/lamina dura modifications.

occlusal status was checked, in order to identify potential trauma or overloads to the tooth: the patient presented a class I interarch relationship, with lateral canine guidance and absence of interferences during jaw movements. Minor signs of wear were identified at some locations (slight indentations at incisal margins of left central incisor, left lateral incisor, and canine: Figure 5(a)); the zirconia-porcelain crown, however, was free from chippings and visible cracks.

Following a pharmacologic treatment for acute phase management and resolution of the sinus tract, a surgical intervention was planned for several reasons: (1) direct inspection of potential fracture lines that were not visible on 2D radiographic images; (2) to assess the status of periradicular tissues and bone; and (3) to investigate the presence of accessory lateral canals, especially along the body (middle third) or at the apical mesial curvature of the root (last 3-4 mm). Patient and clinician's shared efforts were all addressed towards achieving a definite diagnosis and, possibly, tooth preservation: from this perspective, the open-flap surgical intervention was well accepted by the patient.

2.6. Surgical Procedure. During May 2017, a papilla-sparing, trapezoidal, full-thickness flap was reflected and extensive cortical bone loss was confirmed at the vestibular side of the root. Under magnification and fiber-optic illumination, however, the exposed area of the root appeared free of cracking lines. Interproximal bone peaks were still preserved. A root-end resection was performed to ensure the removal of apical ramifications and/or residual bacterial contamination as potential aetiologic factors (Figure 7). The periapical granulation tissue was carefully removed with the aid of curettes and hand excavators; the residual cleaned cavity

despite the apparently well-performed root canal therapy (Figure 6). At this time point, a deep vestibular pocket was also detected by the periodontal exam (manual probing depth > 10 mm). Due to clear alterations of the attachment system, the analyses of tooth mobility and pain on biting were also carried out at subsequent examinations. The

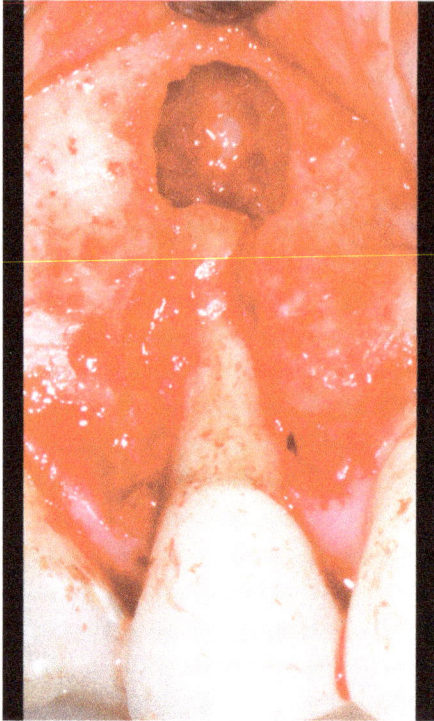

FIGURE 7: Apical resection of premolar root showing vertical bone resorption at the cortical vestibular side.

was finally irrigated with saline solution. The flap was repositioned and sutured.

The clinical scenario did not improve after apical surgery: during subsequent months (July and September 2017), the radiographic follow-up revealed a progressive radiolucency also involving the distal areas of the tooth and proximal peaks (Figures 8(a) and 8(b)). Increased horizontal tooth mobility (Miller class II score) and pain on biting at the premolar tooth were present in September 2017.

2.7. Vertical Root Fracture. On December 2017, a vertical fracture associated with separation of root fragments came to light both clinically and radiographically (Figures 9(a) and 9(b)). The vestibular view showed a clear, 1 mm wide gap between the two root halves, running up to gingival margin of the prosthetic crown. Considering the extensive periodontal breakdown, type of fracture, and apical splitting, the second upper premolar was scheduled for extraction. Despite some emerging treatments are available for VRF, like fragment reattachment and tooth replantation, they still need long-term validation [28]; in order to prevent further bone loss and achieve rapid resolution of symptoms, the extraction treatment was proposed and accepted by the patient. Two main tooth fragments were retrieved from the extraction procedure: a larger one, formed by the crown, post and gutta-percha obturation and a smaller slice with unoccupied root canal space, detached from all the other restorative materials (Figures 10(a) and 10(b)). The fracture was running for the entire bucco-lingual root length: it was considered "complete" in the horizontal extent or type "A" according to the classification of von Arx and Bosshardt [16], being visible

from both the vestibular and palatal sides (Figures 11(a) and 11(b)). On the longitudinal plane, the cracking line was also complete, extending from the prosthetic margin to the root-end resection. The fracture was off-centered in the axial plane (i.e., asymmetric involvement of the root), locating itself mainly outside the root canal space in the apical third (Figure 11(c)). A detailed analysis of the fragments shows a close adaptation between post/endodontic filling and the dentinal walls, which also appeared of adequate thickness; in addition, an incomplete cracking line was visible on the coronal third of the small fragment (Figure 12).

3. Discussion

3.1. Type of Complications for Single-Tooth Restorations. Biological and technical complications are currently reported in the literature for zirconia-based, tooth-supported single crowns. The predominant recorded failures during the first 5–7 years of service were technical, related to the prosthesis: according to Monaco et al. [26], delamination of the veneering ceramic, also known as chipping, was frequently associated with parafunctional habits of the patients. Rinke et al. also reported fractures of the veneering material (12.4% of the considered crowns, observation time: 7 years), along with crown decementations (10% of the considered crowns) [15]. That kind of technical complications might require a minimally invasive intervention. In fact, loss of retention is usually managed with adhesive reluting; polishing/composite repair or crown replacement might be selected for minor and major chipping, respectively. In our study, the premolar crown was not affected by any technical problems during the entire study period: the postextraction analysis also showed optimal marginal accuracy and fitting of the restoration. In other words, survival and success (no occurrence of postcementation complications, up to the extraction procedure) related exclusively to the restoration itself were demonstrated.

Biological failures, on the other hand, are less frequently encountered and strictly related to the supporting tooth: they include secondary caries, periodontal disease, or structural problems such as fractures [15].

In our study, the occurrence of a complete VRF was relatively unexpected in relation to the time elapsed from initial operative procedures (about 9 years). In fact, according to the study of Fuss et al. [22], 50% of the extractions due to VRF were recorded between 1 year and 5 years after root canal treatment or retreatment, while 18% of teeth failed within 1 year from endodontic procedures. Pradeep Kumar et al. also reported that pulpless teeth covered with crowns are more likely to develop VRFs within 5 years postoperatively (mean time of 4.35 ± 1.95 years) [19]. Among restored teeth, premolars could be particularly affected by fractures due to anatomical reasons: (1) their crowns are bulkier than anterior teeth (incisors and canines) but they show reduced mesio-distal diameters of the roots: second maxillary premolars, in addition, are usually single-rooted; (2) premolars are characterized by crowns with steep cuspal inclination and are located midway (between molars and anteriors) along the occlusal arch: in this way, they are subjected to significant lateral

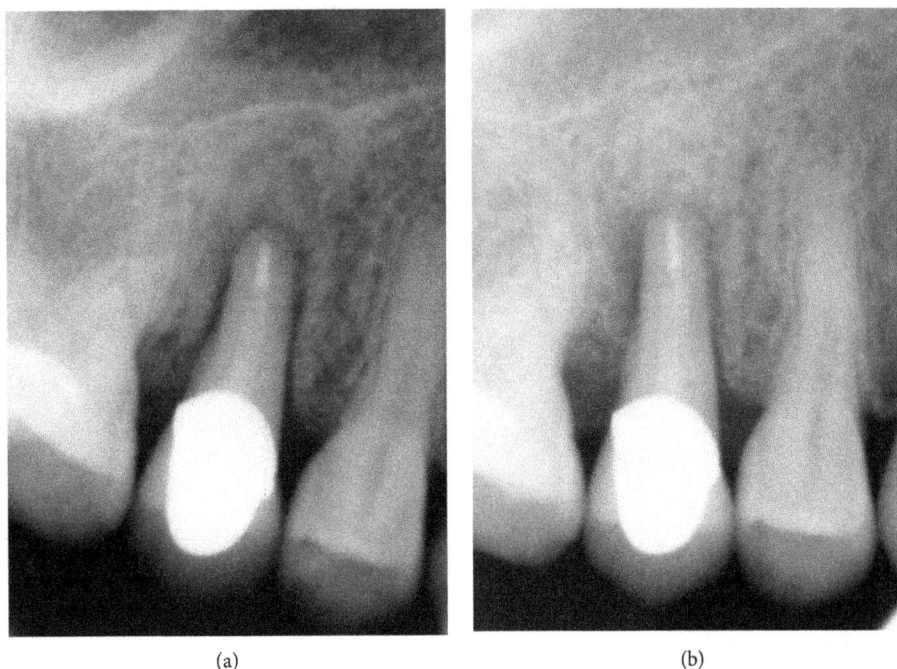

(a)   (b)

FIGURE 8: Three (a) and five (b) months after endodontic surgery, the clinical scenario did not improve: a progressive radiolucency involved the distal areas of the tooth and proximal peaks.

forces during functional and parafunctional activities. Ferrari et al. [29] carried out a cornerstone randomized controlled trial on endodontically treated and restored/crowned premolars, showing the importance of coronal tissue preservation: they found the highest number of root fractures on compromised teeth with one or two residual coronal walls; on the other hand, no failures (cracks) were recorded on elements with 3 and 4 preserved walls.

3.2. Aetiological Factors Related to VRF.
Recovery of compromised teeth might include a number of preprosthetic steps that have been identified as risk factors for development of VRF: from a chronological perspective, aetiological variables usually described in the literature play a role before the placement of a full-occlusal coverage. The impact of endodontic procedures on structural integrity of teeth and retreatments, in particular, have been investigated [19, 21, 22]: canal shaping appears to cause stresses in dentin along with apical microcracks, regardless the type of rotary instrument motion [30, 31]; further propagation and extension of that partial fractures might be sustained by functional occlusal loads, despite the existence of a full-crown restoration. The use of chemical agents (i.e., irrigants) has been associated with a deterioration of dentinal properties of nonvital teeth [32, 33]. With endodontic retreatments, both mechanical and chemical agents are applied once again on inner root surfaces, producing a relative enlargement of the canal walls and increased loss of radicular dentin: in fact, endodontically retreated teeth have shown a reduced resistance to fracture when compared to first-time treated elements [34]. According to the above data, we may speculate that microcrack development or propagation, in our study, may have been facilitated by the endodontic retreatment procedures and/or

by the removal of preexisting cast post. Among filling techniques, however, the adopted single-cone obturation is considered relatively safe regarding the development of lateral condensation forces [30].

An increased risk of fractures could be associated with repetitive restorative cycles: they lead to a progressive removal of dental tissues and should be avoided [35]. During a patient's life, multiple replacements of artificial crowns may be required for a wide number of reasons: aging and wear, loss of marginal integrity, fractures, caries at the interface, and endodontic problems [36]. In addition, previous indirect restorations might become damaged, inaccurate, and in need of replacement when performing disassembly and/or adequate access for root canal retreatments. In our case, a new restorative cycle was started mainly for esthetic and endodontic reasons. Delivering state-of-the-art first-time treatments along with adoption of durable prosthetic materials might reduce the need for new restorative cycles [35].

3.3. Diagnostic Challenges.
Despite technological improvements, a clear detection of VRFs is still a clinical challenge: early signs are similar to those of other conditions such as periodontal disease, apical periodontitis, or combined endo-perio lesions [21, 37]. According to the results of Yoshino et al. [37], a definite diagnosis of longitudinal fracture was established about 18 months after the initial onset of clinical symptoms, on upper second premolars; diagnostic rate for VRF was just nearly 50% at 12 months and 79.5% at 24 months.

In the present study, the time span from initial symptoms to final diagnosis was 9 months (from March to December 2017): no dislodgment of the crown/build-up restoration and absence of cracking lines during first months were the

(a)

(b)

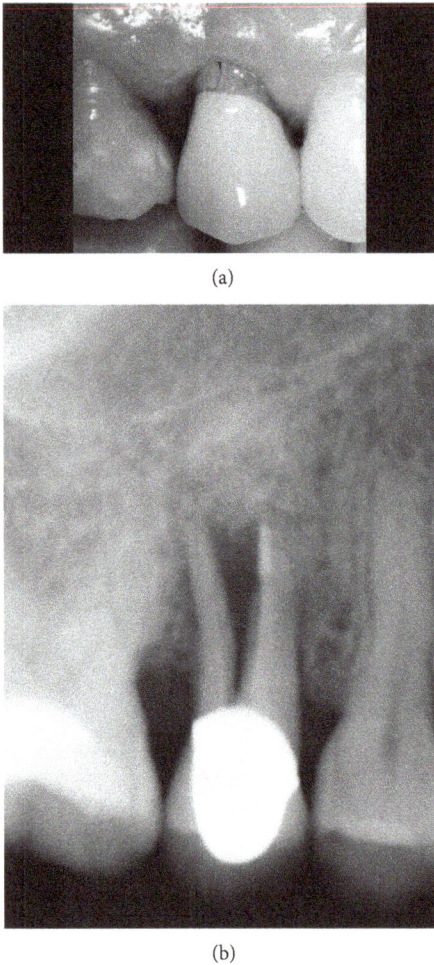

FIGURE 9: Clinical (a) and radiological (b) presentation of the vertical root fracture: splitting of the premolar root into two halves is clearly visible.

main misguiding factors. On the other hand, mild symptoms, positive periodontal probing, and progressive enlargement of lamina dura (radiolucent halo) were typical features of root fracture's presentation [21, 38]. The challenges related to identification of a VRF were also explained to the patient: after proper communication, she was confident and allowed the clinician adequate time for follow-ups and reevaluations, in order to reach a final diagnosis.

While a CBCT exam was not performed, the diagnostic capabilities of that radiological instrument have not been fully explored: the in vivo accuracy of fracture detection, for crack width in the range of 50–330 μm, was low [39]; in addition, filling materials and posts in the canal may also impair clear visualization of VRF.

3.4. Limitations of the Study and Future Directions. A careful evaluation and control of patient-based or tooth-related variables, along with specific identification of VRF's origin, are not possible with a case report study design. The description of our clinical event, on the other hand, might be helpful to understand features, timing, and presentation's mode of a serious long-term complication. The mechanical behavior

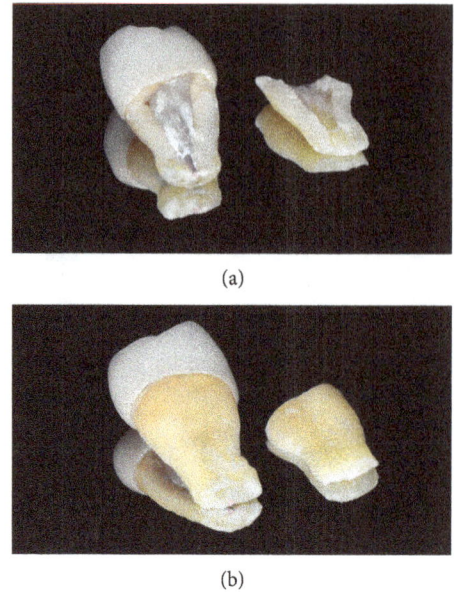

(a)

(b)

FIGURE 10: Inner (a) and outer (b) views of the two fragments produced by the longitudinal fracture, retrieved after tooth extraction.

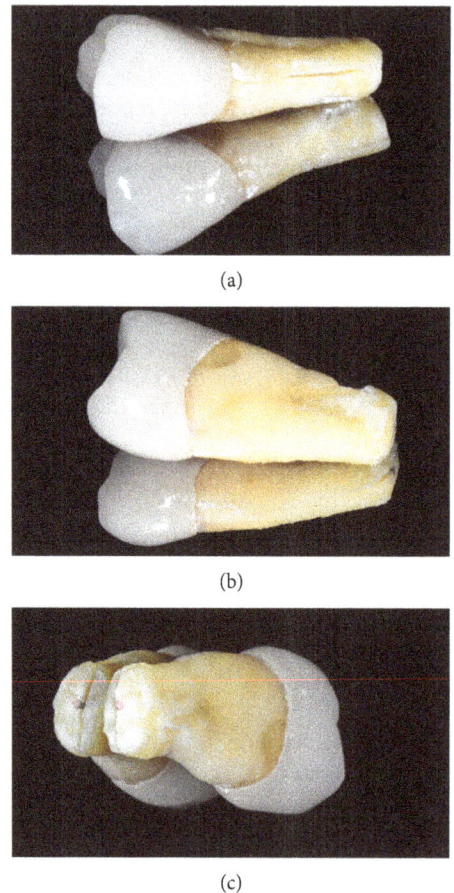

(a)

(b)

(c)

FIGURE 11: Extraoral close readaptation of fragments: the fracture runs for the entire bucco-lingual length of the tooth, as shown by separation on the vestibular (a) and palatal (b) sides. The fracture line was off-centered from the canal when observed on the axial plane (c).

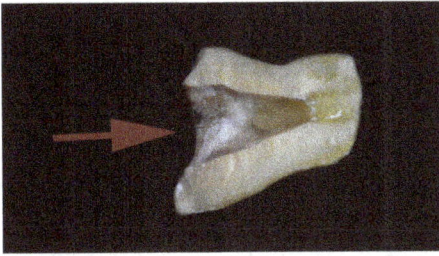

FIGURE 12: An incomplete cracking line (arrow) involved the coronal area of the small fragment.

of the tooth-restoration unit, when high-strength ceramic frameworks are chosen, should be further explored. In particular, future research should be performed to evaluate force transmission or dissipation from all-ceramic coronal restorations to the roots of endodontically treated teeth.

3.5. Final Remarks. Potential long-term complications should be taken into account when dealing with previously treated and/or structurally weakened teeth. The development of a vertical root fracture might be unexpected and might occur many years after the end of a tooth rehabilitation.

Patients should always be aware and well informed about risks associated with recovery of compromised teeth and their prosthetic rehabilitations.

References

[1] S. A. Aquilino and D. J. Caplan, "Relationship between crown placement and the survival of endodontically treated teeth," *Journal of Prosthetic Dentistry*, vol. 87, no. 3, pp. 256–263, 2002.

[2] R. Nagasiri and S. Chitmongkolsuk, "Long-term survival of endodontically treated molars without crown coverage: a retrospective cohort study," *The Journal of Prosthetic Dentistry*, vol. 93, no. 2, pp. 164–170, 2005.

[3] Y. L. Ng, V. Mann, and K. Gulabivala, "Tooth survival following non-surgical root canal treatment: a systematic review of the literature," *International Endodontic Journal*, vol. 43, no. 3, pp. 171–189, 2010.

[4] A. F. Stavropoulou and P. T. Koidis, "A systematic review of single crowns on endodontically treated teeth," *Journal of Dentistry*, vol. 35, no. 10, pp. 761–767, 2007.

[5] D. E. Vire, "Failure of endodontically treated teeth: classification and evaluation," *Journal of Endodontics*, vol. 17, no. 7, pp. 338–342, 1991.

[6] T. Dammaschke, K. Nykiel, D. Sagheri, and E. Schafer, "Influence of coronal restorations on the fracture resistance of root canal-treated premolar and molar teeth: a retrospective study," *Australian Endodontic Journal*, vol. 39, no. 2, pp. 48–56, 2013.

[7] Y. Zhang and B. R. Lawn, "Novel zirconia materials in dentistry," *Journal of Dental Research*, vol. 97, no. 2, pp. 140–147, 2018.

[8] D. Augusti, G. Augusti, A. Borgonovo, M. Amato, and D. Re, "Inlay-retained fixed dental prosthesis: a clinical option using monolithic zirconia," *Case Reports in Dentistry*, vol. 2014, Article ID 629786, 7 pages, 2014.

[9] R. Shahmiri, O. C. Standard, J. N. Hart, and C. C. Sorrell, "Optical properties of zirconia ceramics for esthetic dental restorations: a systematic review," *Journal of Prosthetic Dentistry*, vol. 119, no. 1, pp. 36–46, 2018.

[10] F. Ozer, F. K. Mante, G. Chiche, N. Saleh, T. Takeichi, and M. B. Blatz, "A retrospective survey on long-term survival of posterior zirconia and porcelain-fused-to-metal crowns in private practice," *Quintessence International*, vol. 45, no. 1, pp. 31–38, 2014.

[11] I. Sailer, N. A. Makarov, D. S. Thoma, M. Zwahlen, and B. E. Pjetursson, "All-ceramic or metal-ceramic tooth-supported fixed dental prostheses (FDPs)? A systematic review of the survival and complication rates. Part I: single crowns (SCs)," *Dental Materials*, vol. 31, no. 6, pp. 603–623, 2015.

[12] A. Ploumaki, A. Bilkhair, T. Tuna, S. Stampf, and J. R. Strub, "Success rates of prosthetic restorations on endodontically treated teeth; a systematic review after 6 years," *Journal of Oral Rehabilitation*, vol. 40, no. 8, pp. 618–630, 2013.

[13] A. S. Moghaddam, G. Radafshar, M. Taramsari, and F. Darabi, "Long-term survival rate of teeth receiving multidisciplinary endodontic, periodontal and prosthodontic treatments," *Journal of Oral Rehabilitation*, vol. 41, no. 3, pp. 236–242, 2014.

[14] E. Chang, E. Lam, P. Shah, and A. Azarpazhooh, "Cone-beam computed tomography for detecting vertical root fractures in endodontically treated teeth: a systematic review," *Journal of Endodontics*, vol. 42, no. 2, pp. 177–185, 2016.

[15] S. Rinke, K. Lange, M. Roediger, and N. Gersdorff, "Risk factors for technical and biological complications with zirconia single crowns," *Clinical Oral Investigations*, vol. 19, no. 8, pp. 1999–2006, 2015.

[16] T. von Arx and D. Bosshardt, "Vertical root fractures of endodontically treated posterior teeth: a histologic analysis with clinical and radiographic correlates," *Swiss Dental Journal*, vol. 127, no. 1, pp. 14–23, 2017.

[17] K. Yoshino, K. Ito, M. Kuroda, and N. Sugihara, "Prevalence of vertical root fracture as the reason for tooth extraction in dental clinics," *Clinical Oral Investigations*, vol. 19, no. 6, pp. 1405–1409, 2015.

[18] S. Schwarz, U. Lohbauer, A. Petschelt, and M. Pelka, "Vertical root fractures in crowned teeth: a report of 32 cases," *Quintessence International*, vol. 43, no. 1, pp. 37–43, 2012.

[19] A. R. Pradeep Kumar, H. Shemesh, S. Jothilatha, R. Vijayabharathi, S. Jayalakshmi, and A. Kishen, "Diagnosis of vertical root fractures in restored endodontically treated teeth: a time-dependent retrospective cohort study," *Journal of Endodontics*, vol. 42, no. 8, pp. 1175–1180, 2016.

[20] B. Toure, B. Faye, A. W. Kane, C. M. Lo, B. Niang, and Y. Boucher, "Analysis of reasons for extraction of endodontically treated teeth: a prospective study," *Journal of Endodontics*, vol. 37, no. 11, pp. 1512–1515, 2011.

[21] H. Haueisen, K. Gartner, L. Kaiser, D. Trohorsch, and D. Heidemann, "Vertical root fracture: prevalence, etiology and diagnosis," *Quintessence International*, vol. 44, no. 7, pp. 467–474, 2013.

[22] Z. Fuss, J. Lustig, A. Katz, and A. Tamse, "An evaluation of endodontically treated vertical root fractured teeth: impact of operative procedures," *Journal of Endodontics*, vol. 27, no. 1, pp. 46–48, 2001.

[23] D. Re, F. Cerutti, G. Augusti, A. Cerutti, and D. Augusti, "Comparison of marginal fit of Lava CAD/CAM crown-copings with two finish lines," *The International Journal of*

Esthetic Dentistry, vol. 9, no. 3, pp. 426–435, 2014.

[24] D. Re, F. De Angelis, G. Augusti et al., "Mechanical properties of elastomeric impression materials: an in vitro comparison," *International Journal of Dentistry*, vol. 2015, Article ID 428286, 8 pages, 2015.

[25] D. Re, D. Augusti, G. Augusti, and A. Giovannetti, "Early bond strength to low-pressure sandblasted zirconia: evaluation of a self-adhesive cement," *The European Journal of Esthetic Dentistry*, vol. 7, no. 2, pp. 164–175, 2012.

[26] C. Monaco, M. Caldari, R. Scotti, and AIOP Clinical Research Group, "Clinical evaluation of 1,132 zirconia-based single crowns: a retrospective cohort study from the AIOP clinical research group," *The International Journal of Prosthodontics*, vol. 26, no. 5, pp. 435–442, 2013.

[27] U. S. Beier, I. Kapferer, and H. Dumfahrt, "Clinical long-term evaluation and failure characteristics of 1,335 all-ceramic restorations," *International Journal of Prosthodontics*, vol. 25, no. 1, pp. 70–78, 2012.

[28] N. Nizam, M. E. Kaval, O. Gurlek, A. Atila, and M. K. Caliskan, "Intentional replantation of adhesively reattached vertically fractured maxillary single-rooted teeth," *International Endodontic Journal*, vol. 49, no. 3, pp. 227–236, 2016.

[29] M. Ferrari, A. Vichi, G. M. Fadda et al., "A randomized controlled trial of endodontically treated and restored premolars," *Journal of Dental Research*, vol. 91, no. 7, pp. S72–S78, 2012.

[30] I. D. Capar, G. Saygili, H. Ergun, T. Gok, H. Arslan, and H. Ertas, "Effects of root canal preparation, various filling techniques and retreatment after filling on vertical root fracture and crack formation," *Dental Traumatology*, vol. 31, no. 4, pp. 302–307, 2015.

[31] A. Jamleh, T. Komabayashi, A. Ebihara et al., "Root surface strain during canal shaping and its influence on apical microcrack development: a preliminary investigation," *International Endodontic Journal*, vol. 48, no. 12, pp. 1103–1111, 2015.

[32] L. S. Gu, X. Q. Huang, B. Griffin et al., "Primum non nocere – the effects of sodium hypochlorite on dentin as used in endodontics," *Acta Biomaterialia*, vol. 61, pp. 144–156, 2017.

[33] F. M. Pascon, K. R. Kantovitz, P. A. Sacramento, M. Nobre-dos-Santos, and R. M. Puppin-Rontani, "Effect of sodium hypochlorite on dentine mechanical properties. A review," *Journal of Dentistry*, vol. 37, no. 12, pp. 903–908, 2009.

[34] A. Ganesh, N. Venkateshbabu, A. John, G. Deenadhayalan, and D. Kandaswamy, "A comparative assessment of fracture resistance of endodontically treated and re-treated teeth: an *in vitro* study," *Journal of Conservative Dentistry*, vol. 17, no. 1, pp. 61–64, 2014.

[35] D. B. Henry, "The consequences of restorative cycles," *Operative Dentistry*, vol. 34, no. 6, pp. 759–760, 2009.

[36] R. Uzgur, Z. Uzgur, H. Colak, E. Ercan, M. Dalli, and M. Ozcan, "A cross-sectional survey on reasons for initial placement and replacement of single crowns," *European Journal of Prosthodontics & Restorative Dentistry*, vol. 25, no. 1, pp. 42–48, 2017.

[37] K. Yoshino, K. Ito, M. Kuroda, and N. Sugihara, "Duration from initial symptoms to diagnosis of vertical root fracture in dental offices," *The Bulletin of Tokyo Dental College*, vol. 59, no. 1, pp. 59–61, 2018.

[38] W. C. Liao, Y. L. Tsai, C. Y. Wang et al., "Clinical and radiographic characteristics of vertical root fractures in endodontically and nonendodontically treated teeth," *Journal of Endodontics*, vol. 43, no. 5, pp. 687–693, 2017.

[39] I. M. Makeeva, S. F. Byakova, N. E. Novozhilova et al., "Detection of artificially induced vertical root fractures of different widths by cone beam computed tomography in vitro and in vivo," *International Endodontic Journal*, vol. 49, no. 10, pp. 980–989, 2016.

11

Regenerative Endodontic Treatment of a Maxillary Mature Premolar

Qingan Xu [1,2] and Zhou Li [3]

[1]School of Nursing and Medical Technology, Jianghan University, Wuhan, China
[2]Wuhan First Stomatology Hospital, Wuhan, China
[3]Department of Pediatric Dentistry, Stomatology Hospital of Guangzhou Medical University, Guanghzou, China

Correspondence should be addressed to Qingan Xu; xu.qa@wuhankq.com

Academic Editor: Jiiang H. Jeng

Regenerative endodontic treatment was performed on a mature maxillary premolar diagnosed as chronic pulpitis. The root canals were chemomechanically prepared and placed intracanal medicaments at the first appointment. Then 2 weeks later, a blood clot was created in the canals, over which mineral trioxide aggregate was placed. At 6-month follow-up, cementum-like tissue seemed to be formed in the root canal along with nearly recovered pulp vitality. At 12-month recall, the radiographic results revealed evidence of root wall thickening. At 30-month recall, no periapical lesion was found. This case report indicates that regenerative endodontic treatment for the mature premolar is feasible. More cases are needed for further validation.

1. Introduction

Regenerative endodontics is the use of biologically based procedures designed to replace damaged structures, including dentin and root structures, as well as cells of the pulp-dentin complex [1]. It shows a broad prospect in both tissue engineering and clinical application, which was adopted as a procedure code by the American Dental Association in January 2011 [2].

Traditionally, for pulpitis or apical periodontitis, root canal treatment (RCT) is the most common treatment method. However, RCT results in complete removal of pulp tissues, which means loss of a warning system, immunoresponse and formation of dentin as active defense mechanisms against invading toxins and bacteria, and cease of root development in the cases of young patients. Moreover, in some special cases, the absence of an apical constriction makes RCT problematic. Apexification also has some disadvantages such as variability of treatment time, patient compliance, and increased risk of tooth fracture, which may do not promote the continued development of the root and just "closed" the open apex by a calcific barrier. In contrast, the goal of regenerative endodontics is to induce biologic replacement of dental tissues and regenerate a functional and healthy pulp-dentin complex. So, regenerative endodontic treatment may be a good alternative to conventional endodontic therapies, especially for immature permanent teeth.

To date, more and more case reports and case series showed the feasibility of regenerative endodontic treatment [3–5]; however, most of these cases were performed on immature teeth. Recently, cases on mature teeth with closed apex were occasionally reported [6, 7]. In the present report, we described the treatment of a mature tooth with pulpitis by using regenerative endodontic therapy, and the follow-up period lasted for 30 months.

2. Case Report

A 15-year-old girl in good health presented to the Department of Endodontics, Wuhan University Hospital of Stomatology, in November, 2014, with a chief complaint of cold water pain on her left upper posterior tooth for the last 5 days. Three months earlier, she had caries filled in the same region. Intraoral examination revealed that tooth #13 had an existing distal occlusal composite restoration. Tooth #13 showed sensitivity to pulp test and no sensitivity to palpation and percussion. Radiographic examination showed a filling shadow close to the pulp and a fully developed root and closed apex (Figure 1). On the basis of the results of the clinical and radiographic examinations, the diagnosis for tooth #13 was chronic pulpitis.

An informed consent was obtained from the patient and her parent for regenerative endodontic treatment. An access cavity preparation was performed after local anesthesia with 2% lidocaine and rubber dam isolation. The canal was irrigated copiously with 5.25% sodium hypochlorite and 17% EDTA. The canal was partially dried with sterile paper points and then dusted with a mixture powder of ciprofloxacin and metronidazole. The tooth was then temporized with zinc oxide eugenol cement.

At 2-week follow-up, the patient was asymptomatic. The tooth was not sensitive to percussion and palpation. After local anesthesia by using 2% lidocaine and rubber dam isolation, the temporary restoration was removed. The antibiotic mixture was completely removed with 5.25% sodium hypochlorite. The apical foramen was enlarged up to 0.6 mm with a size #60 hand file (K-file). Seventeen percent EDTA was used as a final irrigating agent and left in the canal for about 1 minute. Then, the canal was dried with sterile paper points. A size #25 K-file was introduced into the root canal to irritate the periapical tissue and to create some bleeding into the root canal. The mineral trioxide aggregate (MTA) was placed approximately 2 mm below the cementoenamel junction. The tooth was restored with glass ionomer cement (Figure 2).

At 3-month recall, the patient was asymptomatic. The tooth was not sensitive to percussion or palpation and not responsive to pulp testing. The radiograph showed nearly a normal periodontal ligament space (Figure 3). The tooth was restored with composite resin after removal of the glass ionomer cement.

At 6-month follow-up, tooth #13 regained pulp sensibility and responded positively to the electric pulp tester (EPT) and Endo-Ice at a similar extent as the control tooth. The radiographic results showed narrowing of the canal space with radiopaque shadows (Figure 4).

At 12-month recall, there was no pain on percussion and palpation. Tooth #13 was normally responsive to Endo-Ice and EPT. The radiographic results revealed evidence of root wall thickening (Figure 5).

At 30-month recall, tooth #13 still showed normal pulp vitality compared to the control tooth, and no periapical lesion was found on the X-ray film (Figure 6). The recovery of pulp vitality at different follow-up time points was summarized in Table 1.

3. Discussion

Age of thirteen to fifteen years is the period of a premolar maturation, during which the apex is gradually closed. In this case, the patient was 15 years old. The X-ray showed that the apex was fully developed. Furthermore, during the regenerative endodontic treatment, a #15 K-file was used to probe the apical foramen and an obvious sense of friction was found, so we judged the tooth in this case belongs to

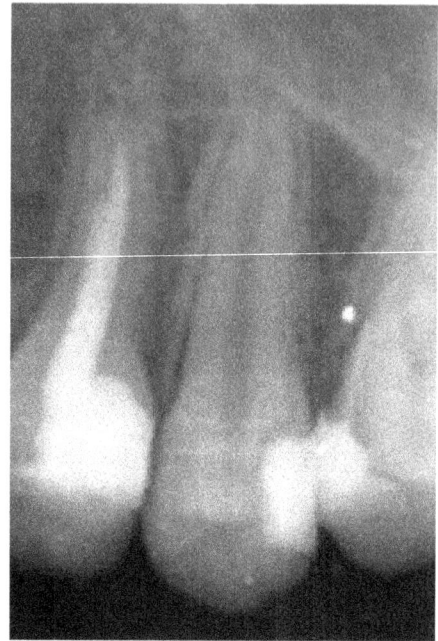

FIGURE 1: Preoperative radiograph showing a filling shadow close to the pulp and a fully developed root and closed apex of tooth #13.

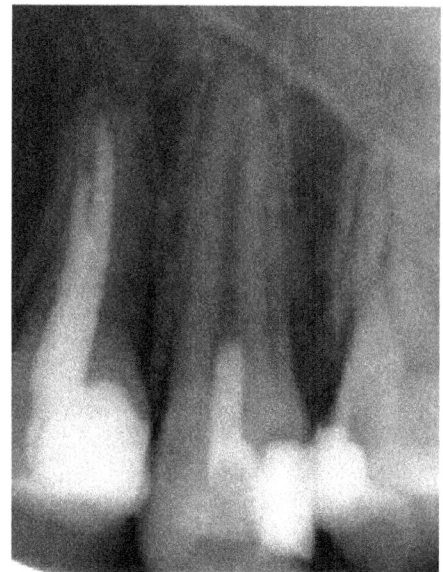

FIGURE 2: Postoperative radiograph presenting placement of the MTA and glass ionomer cement.

mature permanent tooth. Apical bleeding was induced into the root canal, leading to a suitable environment for pulp regeneration with an enrichment of host endogenous stem cells and growth factors in a bioactive scaffold. The new-grown tissue was not a pulp tissue revealed by the calcified shadows in the root canal. Instead, it might be a newly generated cementum-like tissue termed herein "intracanal cementum" as reported in relevant literature [8].

The concept of regenerating pulpal tissue was promulgated by the classic studies of Nygaard-Ostby in 1961.

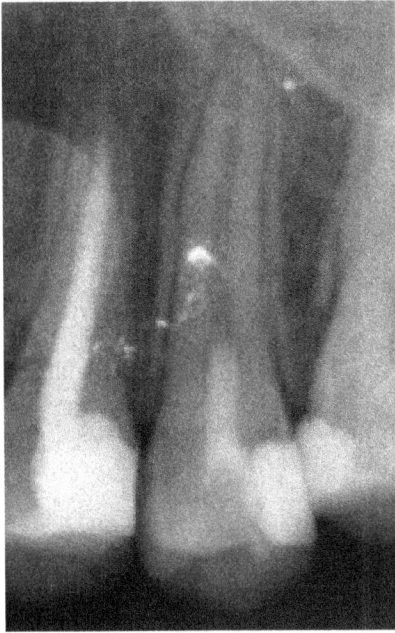

FIGURE 3: Three-month follow-up radiograph showing a normal periodontal ligament space.

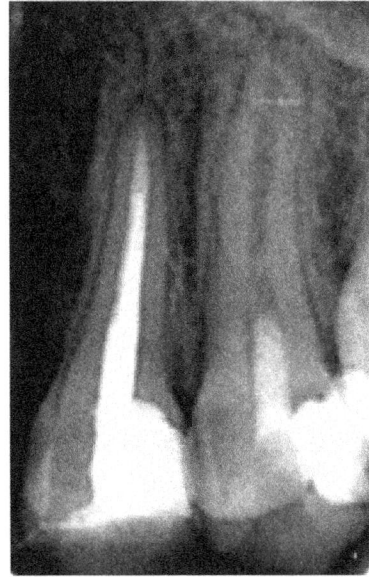

FIGURE 5: Twelve-month follow-up radiograph showing root wall thickening.

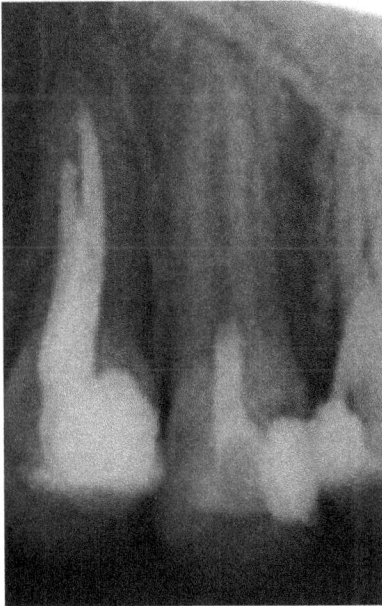

FIGURE 4: Six-month follow-up radiograph showing narrowing of the canal space with radiopaque shadows.

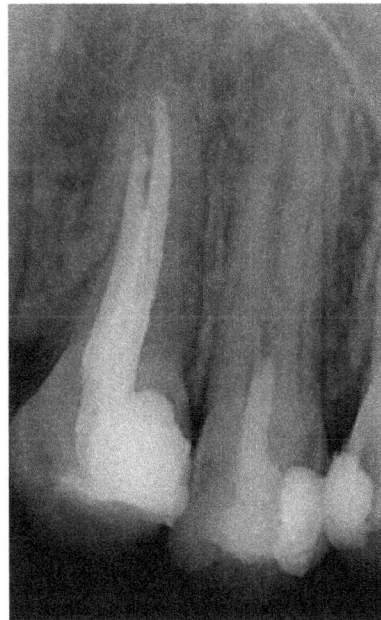

FIGURE 6: Thirty-month follow-up radiograph showing a normal periapical image.

His early research revealed tissue repair (fibroblasts, collagen, and sparse vascularity) without histologic evidence of regeneration of the pulp-dentin complex, while a newly mineralized tissue appeared to be cementum was evident on some dentinal walls. The second case series 10 years later showed histologic evidence of an ingrowth of vascularized fibrous connective tissue in the most of the teeth. Wang et al. [8] analyzed the histologic characterization of regenerated tissues in the canal space after the revitalization/revascularization procedure of immature dog teeth with apical periodontitis. It is found that the canal dentinal walls were thickened by the apposition of a newly generated cementum-like tissue which was similar to cellular cementum. One of the cases showed partial survival of pulp tissue juxtaposed with fibrous connective tissue that formed intracanal cementum on canal dentin walls. Bone or bone-like tissue, the so-called intracanal bone, and connective tissue similar to periodontal ligament were also present in the canal space surrounding the intracanal cementum and/or intracanal bone. In the

TABLE 1: Recovery of pulp vitality at different follow-up time points.

Follow-up time points	Response to pulp testing
3 months	Not responsive
6 months	Nearly normal
12 months	Normal
30 months	Normal

present case, the intracanal cementum may be able to explain the imaging manifestations well, including the radiopaque shadows and root wall thickening. But further studies are still needed to prove whether the recovery of pulp vitality means there is regeneration of nerve fibers and whether there are blood vessels, fibroblast, newly formed dentin, etc.

It is believed that stem cells play an important role in histogenesis as well as pulp regeneration. To our knowledge, at least five types of postnatal mesenchymal stem cells can differentiate into odontoblast-like cells based upon the studies of recent years, including dental pulp stem cells (DPSCs), stem cells of human exfoliated deciduous teeth (SHED), dental follicle progenitor cells (DFPCs), stem cells of the apical papilla (SCAP), and bone marrow-derived mesenchymal stem cells (BMMSCs). Promisingly, studies in vivo have shown that transplantation of stem cells can yield ectopic dental pulp-like tissues in tooth slices or fragments. However, no clinical trials of stem cell transplantation have been reported to date. It has been adopted by the American Dental Association (ADA) to induce apical bleeding into the root canal in immature permanent teeth with necrotic pulps which have been extirpated in January 2011 [9]. The evoked bleeding during endodontic regenerative procedures conducted on immature teeth reveals a massive influx of mesenchymal stem cells into the root canal space. In contrast to cell-based approaches of stem cell transplantation and/or tissue engineering, this "induced bleeding" technique was named "cell-free approach" [10], which was applied in our present case as well.

Scaffold is thought of as an indispensable element for pulp/dentin regeneration. In this report, sterile blood clot induced into the root canal also acted as the 3-dimensional scaffold [11] for tissue ingrowth which supplied potent chemoattractants and growth factors simultaneously to induce cell migration, proliferation, and differentiation. Therefore, no other scaffold materials or growth factors were used in this case while considering noninvasion and avoiding rejection. But they may be the substitution when ideal blood clot is absent. For instance, after dressing with the antibiotic mixture to resist inflammatory reaction, or if the root apex of the upper posterior tooth is adjacent to maxillary sinus, it may be more difficult to induce enough blood.

Clinical regenerative endodontics has been focused on immature teeth because they have a greater chance of pulp tissue regeneration. It is believed that immature teeth with open apices allow more stem cells to migrate into root canals, and more stem cells found near immature root apices have been shown to possess a great regeneration potential in

pulp regeneration [12]. Moreover, there are narrower apical pathways for cell migration in mature teeth, and sufficient disinfection is more challenging than that in immature teeth.

In conclusion, the present case demonstrates the resolution of clinical signs and symptoms with cementum-like tissue formed in the root canal and pulp vitality nearly recovered in the mature permanent premolar with pulpitis after regenerative endodontic treatment. Current regenerative procedures successfully produce root development, but still no evidence is there to reestablish a real pulp tissue. Higher level of evidence with large-scale investigations and randomized controlled clinical trials is still needed. Anyway, it might be possible that regenerative endodontic treatment could be widely used on mature teeth in the future and become an alternative to conventional endodontic therapies.

Acknowledgments

This case report was financially supported by grants (nos. 81570968 and 81570972) from the National Natural Science Foundation of China.

References

[1] K. M. Hargreaves and S. Cohen, *Pathways of the Pulp*, Mosby Elsevier, St. Louis, MO, USA, 10th edition, 2011.

[2] American Dental Association, *CDT 2011-2012: The ADA Practical Guide to Dental Procedure Codes*, American Dental Association, Chicago, IL, USA, 2010.

[3] R. Y. Ding, G. S. Cheung, J. Chen, X. Z. Yin, Q. Q. Wang, and C. F. Zhang, "Pulp revascularization of immature teeth with apical periodontitis: a clinical study," *Journal of Endodontics*, vol. 35, no. 5, pp. 745–749, 2009.

[4] A. Nosrat, A. Seifi, and S. Asgary, "Regenerative endodontic treatment (revascularization) for necrotic immature permanent molars: a review and report of two cases with a new biomaterial," *Journal of Endodontics*, vol. 37, no. 4, pp. 562–567, 2011.

[5] S. Y. Shin, J. S. Albert, and R. E. Mortman, "One step pulp revascularization treatment of an immature permanent tooth with chronic apical abscess: a case report," *International Endodontic Journal*, vol. 42, no. 12, pp. 1118–1126, 2009.

[6] K. Paryani and S. G. Kim, "Regenerative endodontic treatment of permanent teeth after completion of root development: a report of 2 cases," *Journal of Endodontics*, vol. 39, no. 7, pp. 929–934, 2013.

[7] T. M. Saoud, G. Martin, Y. H. Chen et al., "Treatment of mature permanent teeth with necrotic pulps and apical periodontitis using regenerative endodontic procedures: a case series," *Journal of Endodontics*, vol. 42, no. 1, pp. 57–65, 2016.

[8] X. Wang, B. Thibodeau, M. Trope, L. M. Lin, and G. T.-J. Huang, "Histologic characterization of regenerated tissues in canal space after the revitalization/revascularization procedure of immature dog teeth with apical periodontitis," *Journal of Endodontics*, vol. 36, no. 1, pp. 56–63, 2010.

[9] American Dental Association, *Changes to the Code 2011–2012. Current Dental Terminology*, American Dental Association, Chicago, IL, USA, 2010.

[10] K. M. Galler, A. Eidt, and G. Schmalz, "Cell-free approaches for dental pulp tissue engineering," *Journal of Endodontics*, vol. 40, no. 4, pp. S41–S45, 2014.

Change of TGF-β1 Gene Expression and TGF-β1 Protein Level in Gingival Crevicular Fluid and Identification of Plaque Bacteria in a Patient with Recurrent Localized Gingival Enlargement before and after Gingivectomy

Lilies Anggarwati Astuti,[1] **Mochammad Hatta** (ID),[2] **Sri Oktawati,**[3] **Rosdiana Natzir,**[4] **and Ressy Dwiyanti**[1,5]

[1]*Post-Graduate Program of Medical Sciences, Faculty of Medicine, University of Hasanuddin, Makassar, Indonesia*
[2]*Molecular Biology and Immunology Laboratory, Faculty of Medicine, University of Hasanuddin, Makassar, Indonesia*
[3]*Department of Periodontology, Faculty of Dentistry, University of Hasanuddin, Makassar, Indonesia*
[4]*Department of Biochemistry, Faculty of Medicine, University of Hasanuddin, Makassar, Indonesia*
[5]*Department of Medical Microbiology, Faculty of Medicine, Tadulako University, Palu, Indonesia*

Correspondence should be addressed to Mochammad Hatta; hattaram@yahoo.com

Academic Editor: Sukumaran Anil

This case report highlights the change of TGF-β1 gene expressions and TGF-β1 protein level in gingival crevicular fluid (GCF) and identification of plaque bacteria in a patient with recurrent localized gingival enlargement before and after *gingivectomy* treatment. A 26-year-old woman came to AG Dental Care Clinic, South Sulawesi, Indonesia, in October 2015 with a chief complaint that her gingiva often bled spontaneously and she felt pain on her gingiva and felt less comfortable and no self-confidence with her anterior and posterior gingival condition on the right maxilla region which is slightly larger than normal. She often felt that her gingiva could bleed spontaneously when she was talking or remains silent though. The patient is disturbed by the malodor she felt. At that moment, the patient sought for gingivectomy treatment. Three years afterward, the patient came back with the same complaint. Gingival crevicular fluid has been taken from the gingival sulcus before and after gingivectomy. Clinical and GCF follow-up examination was performed one week and three weeks after gingivectomy, and successful results on biological, functional, and aesthetic parameters were observed.

1. Introduction

The gingival disease has common features such as an increase in the size of the gingiva. This condition nowadays is known as gingival enlargement or gingival overgrowth [1]. This term has replaced gingival hyperplasia (increase in cell number) and gingival hypertrophy (increase in cell size) as these are histological diagnosis and do not accurately describe the varied pathological processes seen within the tissues [2].

Gingival enlargement or gingival overgrowth is a common finding in clinical practice. This condition affects the patient's oral hygiene practice and aesthetics and hampers speech, mastication, and natural self-confidence [3]. Many

types of gingival enlargement can be classified according to etiologic factors and pathologic changes such as inflammation, drug-induced enlargement, systemic diseases or conditions, neoplasms, and false enlargement. Gingival enlargement can be designated using the criteria of location and distribution along with the degree [1].

Based on distribution, gingival enlargement may be described as localized or generalized [2, 4]. Localized gingival enlargements are limited to the gingiva adjacent to a single tooth or a group of teeth that started as ballooning papillae and then progressed to involve the marginal gingiva and in more severe cases can cover occlusal aspects of dentition [1, 2]. Historically, this condition termed as epulis refers to

TABLE 1: Change of TGF-β1 gene expression and TGF-β1 protein level in gingival crevicular fluid (GCF).

	Before gingivectomy (day 1)	After gingivectomy (day 7)	After gingivectomy (day 21)
Change of TGF-β1 gene expression	9.72121	4.10328	9.7010
Change of TGF-β1 protein level	1129.736 pg/dl	662.242 pg/dl	1079.391 pg/dl

any solitary/discrete, pedunculated, or sessile masses of the gingiva with no histologic characterization of a particular lesion. The precise term "reactive lesion of the gingiva" seems to be more appropriate for these swelling conditions [2, 4].

Gingival enlargement commonly was an inflammatory process related to plaque accumulation and trauma. This condition has the clinical appearance such as soft, edematous, hyperemic or cyanotic, and usually painful or at least sensitive. These gingivae bleed quickly when probed and have smooth and distended appearance; the normal stippling has usually been lost clinically as well [2, 5].

The appropriate treatment for gingival enlargement depends on precisely diagnosing the cause of enlargement. Gingival enlargement caused by plaque (inflammatory enlargement) should be resolved with nonsurgical treatment including debridement of plaque and calculus (scaling and root planing), improved oral hygiene (oral hygiene instruction), and administration of antibiotics, usually amoxicillin and metronidazole, along with anti-inflammatory (ibuprofen) and analgesic (paracetamol) drugs and the use of chlorhexidine mouth rinse [5, 6].

If the resolution of enlargement did not occur, resulting in the persistence of periodontal pocket such as in fibrotic gingival tissues, this condition may require more detailed assessment and a longer-term management plan. Surgical management to remove enlarged tissue such as the use of laser/electrosurgery excision and internal/external bevel gingivectomy can be provided to improve access for the patient's oral hygiene [5, 6]. Removal must be thorough and based on the understanding of the lesion type. This removal usually includes complete excision of the lesion after the elevation of full-thickness mucoperiosteal flaps and thorough curettage of the area to its origin from the periosteum and periodontal ligament cells to prevent recurrence. Sutures were then given after achieving proper hemostasis [7–9].

Hence, plaque control is an essential aspect of management in all patients. An excisional/incisional biopsy and/or hematologic/histologic examination may be needed occasionally to precisely diagnose the uncommon cases of gingival enlargement. Every effort should be made to obtain primary closure of the surgical site to facilitate healing and so discourage the proliferation of granulation tissue which heralds early recurrence. A follow-up is required to ensure that any recurrence is detected early and dealt with and that the postsurgical gingival contour is maintained as close as possible to its preoperative state [4, 7].

2. Case Presentation

A 26-year-old woman came to AG Dental Care Clinic, South Sulawesi, Indonesia, in October 2015 with a chief complaint that her gingiva often bled spontaneously and she felt pain on her gingiva and felt less comfortable and no self-confidence with her anterior and posterior gingival condition on the right maxilla region which is slightly larger than normal. She often felt that her gingiva could bleed spontaneously when she was talking or remains silent though. The patient is disturbed by the malodor she felt. At that moment, the patient sought for gingivectomy treatment. Three years afterward, the patient came back with the same complaint. Gingival crevicular fluid has been taken from the gingival sulcus before and after gingivectomy. Clinical and GCF follow-up examination was performed one week and three weeks after gingivectomy, and successful results on biological, functional, and aesthetic parameters were observed.

The expected results with the gingivectomy treatment are that patients should not perceive any more complaint such as spontaneously gingival bleeding, pain on the gingiva, and malodor. Besides, after the gingivectomy treatment, the patient already felt comfortable and had her self-confidence back with her anterior and posterior gingival condition on the right maxilla region not having the appearance that is slightly larger than normal. Besides, the expected results after gingivectomy and scaling and root planing treatment such as localized gingival enlargement on the anterior and posterior of the right maxilla region do not recur.

Gingival crevicular fluid (GCF) was taken from the gingival area with enlargement using a paper point. The paper point was inserted into the gingival sulcus to absorb the gingival fluid. Then, the paper point was inserted to medium fluid L6. GCF was then checked using real-time polymerase chain reaction (RT-PCR) to find TGF-β1 gene expression and examined using enzyme-linked immunosorbent assay (ELISA) to find TGF-β1 protein level (Table 1). On the other hand, smear plaque was taken from the tooth surface both supragingival and subgingival and then inserted to medium transport.

Furthermore, the transport medium containing plaque and calculus was taken to the microbiology laboratory for bacterial culture examination, and the bacterial culture was cultured using Brain-Heart Infusion Broth (BHIB) medium (Figure 1). Then, the observation of swabs of dental plaque samples incubated for 1×24 hours in the incubator at a certain temperature was conducted. Identification of bacteria under a microscope was performed to determine bacterial species based on bacterial morphology before and after gingivectomy treatment (Table 2). On excised gingival tissue, biopsy was performed to find tissue morphology and tumour subtype and to grade gingival cells.

3. Discussion

Periodontal disease is multifactorial, including the case with recurrent localized gingival enlargement. When microbial

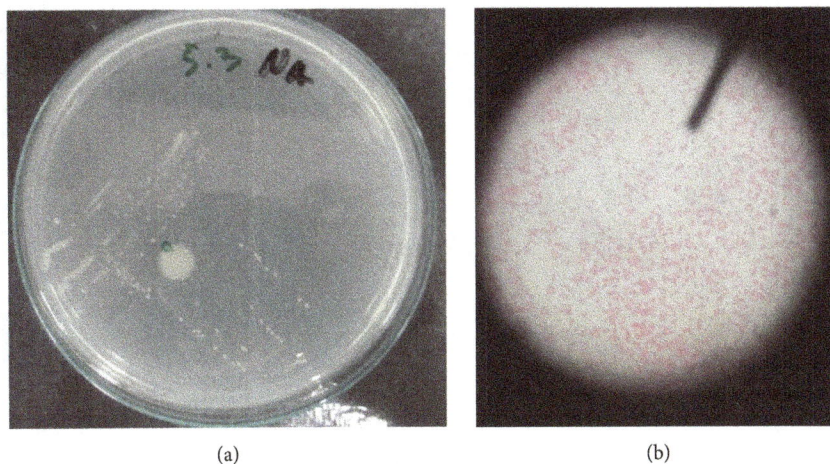

(a)   (b)

FIGURE 1: The smear of dental plaque on the medium to show the growth of *Streptococcus* sp. bacteria on the control at day 21 (a). Under a microscope with 1000x magnification, the growth of *Klebsiella* sp. bacteria was visible at the time before gingivectomy and at the time of the first control at day 7 (b).

TABLE 2: Identification of plaque bacteria.

Before gingivectomy (day 1)	After gingivectomy (day 7)	After gingivectomy (day 21)
Klebsiella sp.	*Streptococcus* sp.	*Streptococcus* sp.

(bacterial biofilm) and other environmental factors such as gender were believed to initiate and modulate periodontal disease development, now there has been powerful supporting data explaining that genetic and environmental factor risk plays a role in the trend for recurrence and severity development of periodontal disease. The enlargement could be due to a reduction of collagen degradation by collagenase or the outcome of overproduction of extracellular ground substance. Some literature has reported the synergistic effect of proinflammatory cytokines on the possible factors involved in this enlargement [10]. Genetic and technology information applied for prediction, diagnosis, and periodontal condition treatment conceptually is very interesting at this moment. Some features such as cytokines, cell surface receptors, chemokines, and enzymes, related to the recognition of antigen, immune system, and host response, among the other things, are determined by a polymorphism genetic component that possibly increases the individual's vulnerability to periodontal disease. Growth factors and cytokines play an important role in the regulation of the gingival extracellular matrix turnover. Tumour necrosis factor-α (TNF-α) and interleukins induce the expression of MMPs while transforming growth factor-β (TGF-β) downregulates their synthesis and secretion and promotes the production of their natural tissue inhibitors, TIMPs [11]. Gene and polymorphism identification could result in a new diagnostic for risk examination, early detection of disease, and individual treatment approach. Thus, genetic epidemiology includes knowledge about polymorphism genetic, which is promising as one of the tools that can contribute to the understanding of the periodontal disease. Gingival crevicular fluid could be a diagnostic tool for analysis of oral diseases. GCF, as a biomonitoring fluid, plays a constructive role in the diagnosis of oral diseases, especially for periodontitis and gingivitis. Its limited amount compromises biochemical and proteomic analysis, and the severity of inflammation in the periodontium affects its collection [12].

Gingival crevicular fluid is a serum exudate that originates from the periodontal sulcus or pocket and is regarded as a promising biological fluid for the detection of periodontal disease. Its composition resembles normal serum, but its volume fluctuates in certain conditions such as those of gingivitis, caries, external root resorption, and chronic periodontitis, as well as during orthodontic movement. GCF is composed of variable substances that include immunoglobulin, enzymes, local mediators, toxin cells, protein peptides, tissue breakdown products, and microorganisms [12].

The TGF-β superfamily consists of several multifunctional structurally related growth and differentiation factors associated with the inflammatory response. Five distinct isoforms of TGF-β have now been described, and three of these—TGF-β1, TGF-β2, and TGF-β3—are found in all mammalian species [11, 13]. TGF-β1 is expressed in epithelial, hematopoietic, and connective tissue cells. It is predominantly produced by T regulatory (Treg) cells and macrophages and could also induce a wide range of essential functions. Because TGF-β1 exhibits both proinflammatory and anti-inflammatory properties besides its ability to stimulate migration and synthesis of ECM molecules and to inhibit the breakdown of ECM, it has been intensively evaluated in relation to all types of gingival enlargement [11, 14].

Real-time polymerase chain reaction (RT-PCR) examination was conducted using TGF-β1 primary Macrogen to find TGF-β1 gene expression with results before gingivectomy and SRP treatment of 9.72121. A week after, gingivectomy and SRP treatment decreased to 4.10328, and three weeks after, gingivectomy and SRP treatment rebound to 9.7010. The expression of the TGF-β1 gene decreased on the seventh day after gingivectomy and SRP treatment and increased

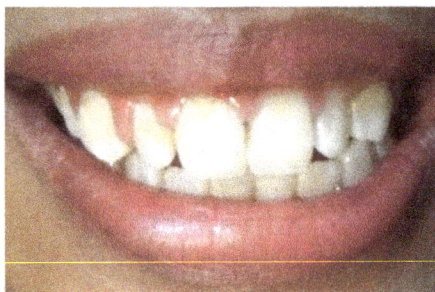

Figure 2: Clinical examination. An enlarged gingiva appears on the anterior and posterior teeth of the right maxilla region.

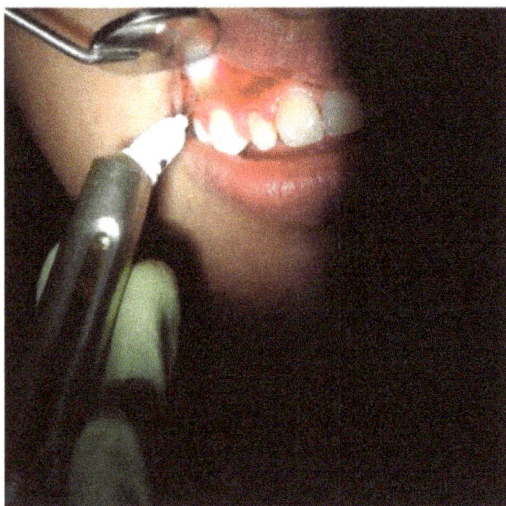

Figure 3: After disinfection, a local anesthetic was injected using 2% lidocaine norepinephrine.

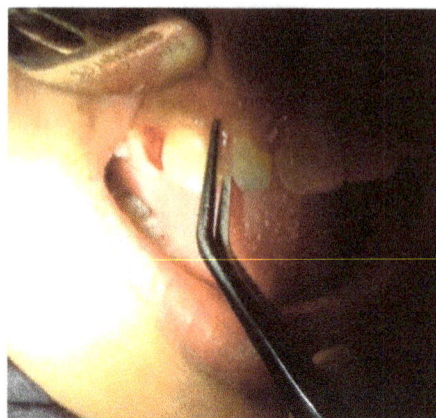

Figure 4: Determining the baseline pocket using an Ossung® pocket marker that will result in a bleeding point.

again on the 1st day, and the TGF-β1 gene here acted as an anti-inflammatory. Babel et al. who conducted a study involving patients with chronic periodontitis discovered that high TGF-β1 production might be a protective factor for periodontitis. Although TGF-β1 levels are elevated in moderate disease, they declined in fluid samples obtained from the pockets in more advanced experimental periodontitis [15].

Enzyme-linked immunosorbent assay (ELISA) examination was conducted to find TGF-β1 protein level using the Human TGF-β1 ELISA kit LSBio (Lifespan Biosciences Inc.) with results before gingivectomy and SRP treatment of 1129.736 pg/dl. A week after, gingivectomy and SRP treatment decreased to 662.242 pg/dl, and three weeks after, gingivectomy and SRP treatment rebound to 1079.391 pg/dl. These results were similar to those of the study conducted by Sattari et al. who found a significant decrease in TGF-β1 level from phase 1 (baseline or before surgery) to phase 3 (12 weeks after surgery). However, they did not assess the changes in TGF-β1 concentration between phase 1 and phase 2 (4 weeks after surgery) [14]. A study involving 60 patients by Mutlak et al. reported insignificant differences for the chronic periodontitis group in comparison with the control group, even though TGF-β1 depicted the highest correlation

of the biochemical and immunohistological expression only in the chronic periodontitis group [16].

Gram staining has been done with bacteria in BHIB bacterial suspension, and gram-negative bacteria is obtained in the form of bacil composed of monobacil. The BHIB media are turbid indicating bacterial growth in the media. The bacteria are bacil and streptobacil. Bacteria in red are bacteria fading with alcohol but are able to bind to the dye comparator safranin. Positive results were found in all the sugars used (glucose, maltose, lactose, sucrose, and mannitol). Positive results are indicated by the color change indicator (from blue to yellow) contained in this medium.

The color change is caused by the bacteria that grow in it and are able to ferment all the confectionery products in the form of acid products. Positive results were obtained using Simmons' citrate agar because the color in the media is changed from green to blue. This is because the Klebsiella bacteria is one of the species that use citrate as a carbon source for metabolism by producing an alkaline atmosphere. In one series of urease biochemical tests, the results obtained are positive because the color of the media turns to pink.

Indole reaction can only be seen when this medium with growing bacteria is added with Covac's reagent. Indole is positive when it has a red ring on its surface. The red color is produced from the residual which results from the reaction of the amino acid tryptophan to indole with the addition of Covac's reagent. Bacteria capable of producing indole signify that the bacteria use the tryptophan amino acid as a carbon source. In the observation results obtained, indole was negative, so it can be concluded that the growing bacteria do not use tryptophan amino acids as the carbon source. From the result of identification and isolation that have been done (staining, breeding, differential test, biochemical test, and sugar) on the dental plaque sample, Klebsiella sp. bacteria were found before gingivectomy and SRP treatment.

The results of the identification of bacteria contained on plaque and calculus preparation through bacterial culture examination before gingivectomy and SRP treatment found the existence of Klebsiella sp.; then, on the first control, we did not find any Klebsiella sp. a week after gingivectomy and SRP treatment, but we found Streptococcus sp., and on

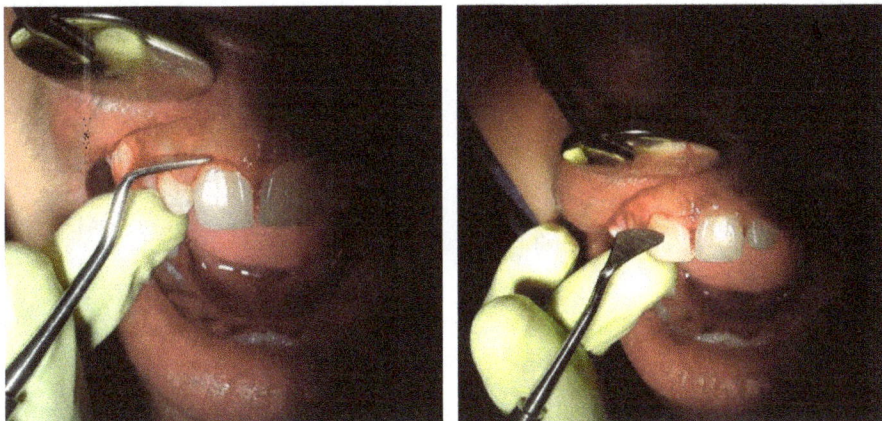

FIGURE 5: Incision and excision conducted on the buccal region of the gingiva using an Ossung Kirkland knife.

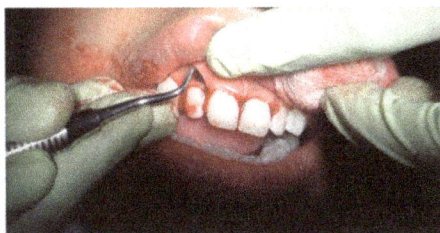

FIGURE 6: Incision and excision conducted on the interdental gingival area using an Ossung Orban knife.

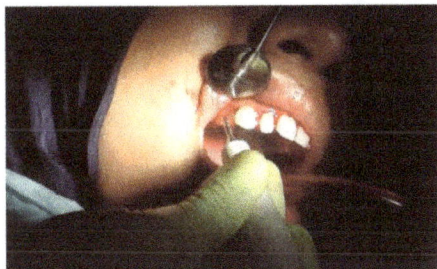

FIGURE 7: Scaling and root planing (SRP) performed with an electric scaler (Satelec P5 Newtron).

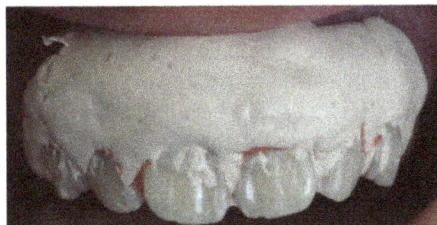

FIGURE 8: The periodontal pack being fixed after gingivectomy (Coe Pack®).

the second control, three weeks after gingivectomy and SRP treatment, we still found *Streptococcus* sp.

A study conducted by Uzel et al. stated that *A. gerencseriae*, *A. israelii*, *A. odontolyticus*, *C. sputigena*, *E. nodatum*, *F. nucleatum* subsp. *polymorphum*, *F. nucleatum* subsp.

vincentii, *F. periodonticum*, *P. nigrescens*, *T. denticola*, and *T. socranskii* were found in periodontally healthy subjects on day 1 observation. On the other hand, *C. rectus*, *E. nodatum*, *P. intermedia*, and *S. constellatus* were found in the periodontitis group. But *Veilonella parvula*, *Neisseria mucosa*, and *A. oris* were found in both groups. In this study, they compared the shift of microbes taken from the supragingival and subgingival plaque sample in healthy and periodontitis subjects before and after tooth cleaning. They also concluded that the hypothesis that biofilm redevelopment would be more rapid in periodontitis than in periodontally healthy subjects was rejected for supragingival biofilms but could not be rejected for subgingival biofilm redevelopment [17].

The result of anatomical pathology examination on gingival tissue macroscopically was that the tissue has a size of ±1 cm in diameter with red bright color while microscopically showed biopsy tissue was coated by epithelium squamosum complex which some seem hyperplastic but the nuclei within normal size, subephithelial composed of stroma of edematous fibrocollagenous tissues which was pounding with massive lymphosites, PMNs, and hystiocytes and were accompanied by vascular proliferation and hemorrhage, but there wasn't sign of malignancy. We concluded that this case was nonspecific gingival enlargement.

On clinical examination (Figure 2), there are swollen gingivae in the anterior and posterior (labial, buccal) region of the right maxilla. The gingiva was seen to have edema and hyperemia on interdental 11, 12, 13, and 14. Bleeding occurred when the pocket depth (probing) was examined. The depth of the gingival pocket was approximately 4 mm in region 11, 12, 13, and 14. Besides, a plaque on the tooth surface and subgingival calculus was evident. There was no traumatic occlusion in the maxillary anterior teeth and mandibular anterior teeth. On the other hand, there is no tooth mobility found. Povidone iodine was used for disinfection; then, local anesthetic infiltration was performed using 2% lidocaine mixed with norepinephrine in the labial and buccal part of the tooth 11, 12, 13, and 14 region (Figure 3). Furthermore, the pocket base was marked using a pocket marker to obtain the bleeding point on each enlarged gingiva. This procedure was performed to obtain the pocket base as a reference for gingivectomy (Figure 4). Gingival incision was

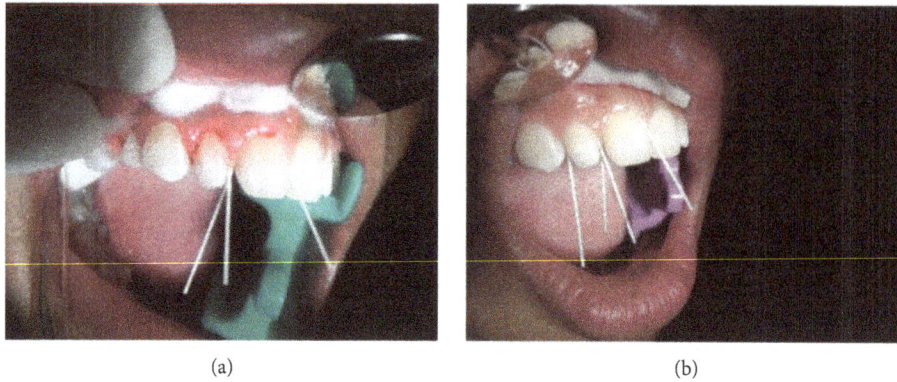

FIGURE 9: Gingival crevicular fluid (GCF) taken before gingivectomy (a) and after gingivectomy (b).

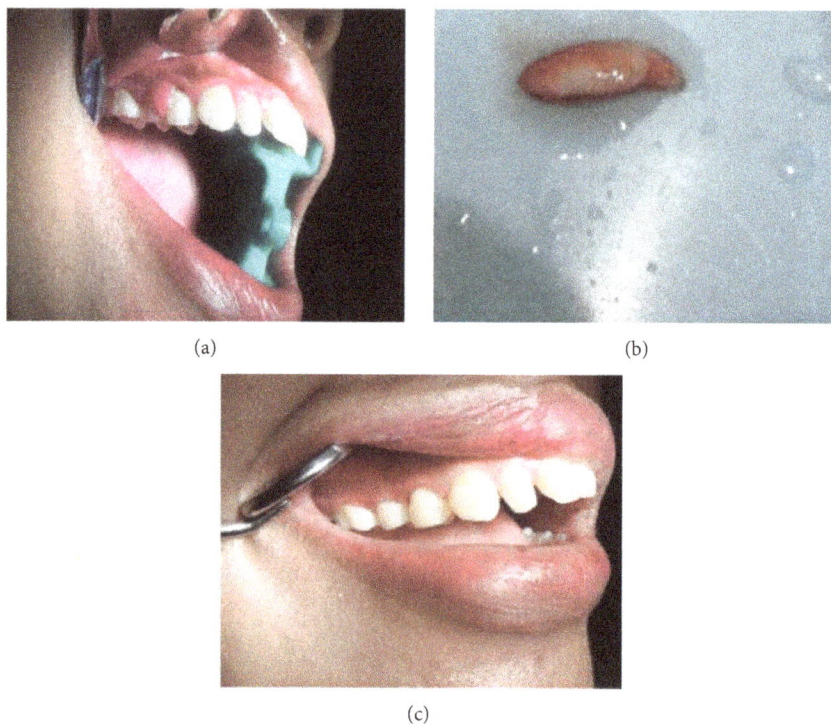

FIGURE 10: Appearance before gingivectomy (a), gingival tissue that has been excised (b), and appearance after gingivectomy (c).

performed on the bleeding point at the buccal region using a Kirkland knife. It was placed on the enlarged interdental area of the gingiva of the enlarged teeth. The Kirkland knife was placed at 45° to the gingiva to obtain a bevel on the gingival surface (Figure 5). Gingival excision on the interdental part of the pocket base was performed to take the gingival tissue that has been enlarged due to inflammation using an Orban knife. Furthermore, scaling and root planing was performed. Gingival tissue removal can be done after the previous incision (Figure 6). Scaling and root planing is performed to eliminate plaque and calculus, especially in subgingival areas using an electric scaler. Irrigation was performed using a 0.12 chlorhexidine solution in areas where gingivectomy and scaling have been performed. This is to make sure that the area is clean from plaque and calculus (Figure 7). The final procedure is the fastening of periodontal dressing using periodontal pack that covers all gingival areas where gingivectomy has been performed. The utilization of periodontal dressing is to ease the healing process. Placement of periodontal dressing does not cover the entire surface of the tooth for aesthetic reason (Figure 8). GCF has been taken from the gingival sulcus before the gingivectomy procedure using size 15 paper points (Figure 9(a)). They are placed on the interdental and buccal areas of teeth 11 and 12 (Figure 9(b)). The clinical features before gingivectomy are shown in Figure 10(a). The gingival tissue that has undergone gingivectomy is shown in Figure 10(b). As shown in Figure 10(c), a change of contour on the gingival surface was observed 3 weeks after gingivectomy, no reenlargement and no bleeding were observed, and edema, hyperemia, and attached gingiva formed well on the tooth surface.

Acknowledgments

This research work was supported by Lembaga Pengelola Dana Pendidikan (LPDP), and the authors would like to thank all the staff of Molecular Biology and Immunology Laboratory, Faculty of Medicine, Hasanuddin University, Makassar, South Sulawesi, Indonesia, for their help.

References

[1] F. A. Carranza and E. L. Hogan, "Gingival enlargement," in *Carranza's Clinical Periodontology*, M. G. Newman, H. H. Takei, and P. R. Klokkevold, Eds., Elsevier Saunders, Missouri, USA, 11th edition, 2012.

[2] J. Beaumont, J. Chesterman, M. Kellett, and K. Durey, "Gingival overgrowth: part 1: aetiology and clinical diagnosis," *British Dental Journal*, vol. 222, no. 2, pp. 85–91, 2017.

[3] C. G. Devaraj, A. Yadav, S. Sharma, M. Meena, and K. Goyal, "Diagnosis and management of chronic gingival overgrowth," *Journal of Mahatma Gandhi University of Medical Sciences and Technology*, vol. 2, no. 1, pp. 47–50, 2017.

[4] A. A. Agrawal, "Gingival enlargements: differential diagnosis and review of literature," *World Journal of Clinical Case*, vol. 3, no. 9, pp. 779–788, 2015.

[5] N. Tomar, M. Vidhi, and K. Mayur, "Inflammatory gingival enlargement – a case report," *Journal of Advanced Medical and Dental Sciences*, vol. 2, no. 1, pp. 109–113, 2014.

[6] K. Gawron, K. Łazarz-Bartyzel, J. Potempa, and M. Chomyszyn-Gajewska, "Gingival fibromatosis: clinical, molecular, and therapeutic issues," *Orphanet Journal of Rare Diseases*, vol. 11, no. 1, pp. 9–14, 2016.

[7] N. W. Savage and C. G. Daly, "Gingival enlargements and localized gingival overgrowths," *Australian Dental Journal*, vol. 55, Supplement 1, pp. 55–60, 2010.

[8] B. R. Rajanikanth, S. Moogla, G. Suragimath, B. S. J. Pai, A. Walvekar, and R. Kumar, "Localized gingival enlargement – a diagnostic dilemma," *Indian Journal of Dentistry*, vol. 3, no. 1, pp. 44–48, 2012.

[9] S. Banerjee and T. K. Pal, Localized gingival overgrowths: a report of six cases," *Contemporary Clinical Dentistry*, vol. 8, no. 4, pp. 667–671, 2017.

[10] R. Livada and J. Shiloah, "Gingival enlargement and medication use," *Dimensions of Dental Hygiene*, vol. 11, no. 9, pp. 51–55, 2013.

[11] C. Pisoschi, C. Stanciulescu, and M. Banita, "Growth factors and connective tissue homeostasis," in *Periodontal Disease, Pathogenesis and Treatment of Periodontitis*, N. Buduneli, Ed., INTECH, Rijenka, Kroasia, 2012.

[12] Z. Khurshid, M. Mali, M. Naseem, S. Najeeb, and M. Zafar, "Human gingival crevicular fluids (GCF) proteomics: an overview," *Dentistry Journal*, vol. 5, no. 1, pp. 1–8, 2017.

[13] A. B. Roberts, B. K. McCune, and M. B. Sporn, "TGF-β: regulation of extracellular matrix," *Kidney International*, vol. 41, no. 3, pp. 557–559, 1992.

[14] M. Sattari, A. Fathiyeh, F. Gholami, H. Darbandi Tamijani, and M. Ghatreh Samani, "Effect of surgical flap on IL-1β and TGF-β concentrations in the gingival crevicular fluid of patients with moderate to severe chronic periodontitis," *Iranian Journal of Immunology*, vol. 8, no. 1, pp. 20–26, 2011.

[15] N. Babel, G. Cherepnev, D. Babel et al., "Analysis of tumor necrosis factor-α, transforming growth factor-β, interleukin-10, IL-6, and interferon-γ gene polymorphisms in patients with chronic periodontitis," *Journal of Periodontology*, vol. 77, no. 12, pp. 1978–1983, 2006.

[16] S. S. Mutlak, N. A. RazzakHasan, and A. Y. Al-Hijazi, "Biochemical and immunohistochemical evaluation of transforming growth factor-β1 and tumor necrosis factor-α in dental diseases," *International Journal of Research Pharmacy and Chemistry*, vol. 5, no. 4, pp. 736–752, 2015.

[17] N. G. Uzel, F. R. Teles, R. P. Teles et al., "Microbial shifts during dental biofilm re-development in the absence of oral hygiene in periodontal health and disease," *Journal of Clinical Periodontology*, vol. 38, no. 7, pp. 612–620, 2011.

13

Alteration of Occlusal Plane in Orthognathic Surgery: Clinical Features to Help Treatment Planning on Class III Patients

Daniel Amaral Alves Marlière◉,[1] **Tony Eduardo Costa**,[2] **Saulo de Matos Barbosa**,[3] **Rodrigo Alvitos Pereira**,[4] **and Henrique Duque de Miranda Chaves Netto**[5]

[1]*Division of Oral and Maxillofacial Surgery, Piracicaba Dental School, State University of Campinas, 13414-903 Piracicaba, SP, Brazil*
[2]*Division of Dentistry, Faculty of Medical Science and Health – SUPREMA, 36033-003 Juiz de Fora, MG, Brazil*
[3]*Division of Dentistry, Faculty São Leolpoldo Mandic – SLM, 13045-755 Campinas, SP, Brazil*
[4]*Department of Oral and Maxillofacial Surgery, Pedro Ernesto University Hospital, State University of Rio de Janeiro, 20551-030 Rio de Janeiro, RJ, Brazil*
[5]*Department of Clinical Dentistry, Juiz de Fora Dental School, Federal University of Juiz de Fora, 36036-300 Juiz de Fora, MG, Brazil*

Correspondence should be addressed to Daniel Amaral Alves Marlière; ctbmf.marliere@gmail.com

Academic Editor: Daniel Torrés-Lagares

Dentofacial deformities (DFD) presenting mainly as Class III malocclusions that require orthognathic surgery as a part of definitive treatment. Class III patients can have obvious signs such as increasing the chin projection and chin throat length, nasolabial folds, reverse overjet, and lack of upper lip support. However, Class III patients can present different facial patterns depending on the angulation of occlusal plane (OP), and only bite correction does not always lead to the improvement of the facial esthetic. We described two Class III patients with different clinical features and inclination of OP and had undergone different treatment planning based on 6 clinical features: (I) facial type; (II) upper incisor display at rest; (III) dental and gingival display on smile; (IV) soft tissue support; (V) chin projection; and (VI) lower lip projection. These patients were submitted to orthognathic surgery with different treatment plannings: a clockwise rotation and counterclockwise rotation of OP according to their facial features. The clinical features and OP inclination helped to define treatment planning by clockwise and counterclockwise rotations of the maxillomandibular complex, and two patients undergone to bimaxillary orthognathic surgery showed harmonic outcomes and stables after 2 years of follow-up.

1. Introduction

The exact prevalence of significant dentofacial deformities (DFD) that requires orthognathic surgery as a part of definitive treatment is not quite clear [1]. However, it was estimated that about 5% of the UK or USA population present with DFD that had needed orthognathic surgery as a part of their definitive treatment [2, 3]. Among the DFD, the most prevalent was Class III malocclusion [1], who had been shown in similar studies by findings of several samples in Brazil [4], Saudi Arabia [5], Hong Kong [6], UK [6, 7], Norway [8], and the USA [9].

An index of orthognathic functional treatment needs (IOFTN) had been developed to objectively identify patients that seemed to need orthognathic surgery with low- or high-priority treatments. This index has 5 categories, from a very great need (score 5) through to no need for treatment (score 1), there being patients with scores 4 or 5 had more priority treatment [10]. Borzabadi-Farahani et al. [11] assessed retrospectively the functional needs using the index in DFD patients who had undergone orthognathic surgery. The most Class III patients had presented score 5 of the index that was higher percentages than other malocclusion indicating a functional need for orthognathic surgery.

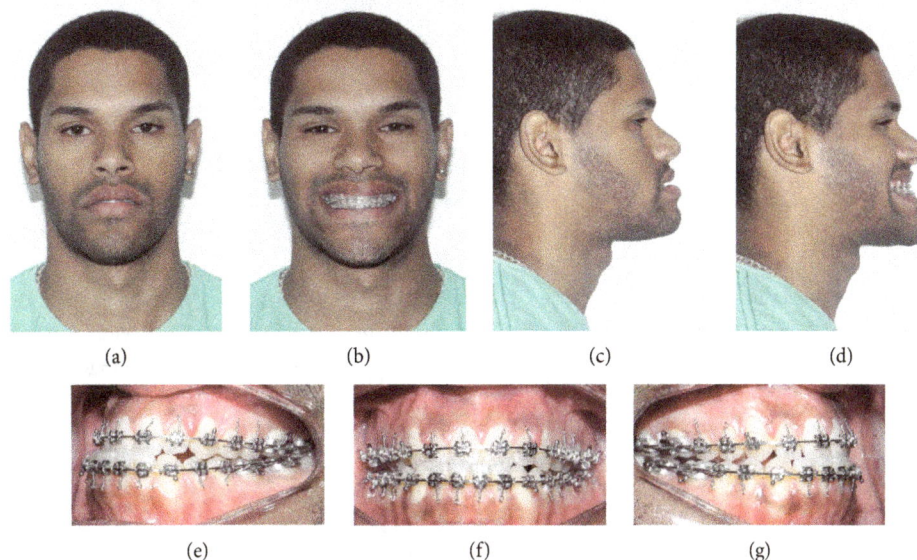

FIGURE 1: (a–d) Preoperative evaluation at rest and smiling. (e–g) Intraoral images.

Regardless of the malocclusion classification, prevalence or priority treatment, Class III patients can present different facials features that will be correlated with cephalometric aspects, one of them is the occlusal plane (OP) angulation [12]. The OP angle is defined as the angle formed by the Frankfort horizontal plane and the line tangent to the canine tips of the lower premolars and the buccal groove of the second molars. The normal value for adults is $8°$ ($\pm4°$). DFD are often related to an abnormal OP angulation, and surgical alteration of this angle may have a substantial impact on the functional and esthetic outcomes for patients [12].

Class III patients may present two facial types correlated to the angulation of the OP and can be highlighted brachycephalic with low OP ($<4°$) and dolichocephalic with high OP ($>12°$). The low OP facial type presents with the following characteristics: decreased OP angle; low mandibular plane angle; prominent mandibular gonial angles; strong chin relative to the mandibular dental alveolus; and Class I, Class II, or occasionally, Class III malocclusion. The HOP facial type presents with the following basic characteristics: increased OP angulation; anterior vertical maxillary hyperplasia and/or posterior vertical maxillary hypoplasia; anteroposterior mandibular hypoplasia; high mandibular plane angulation; and Class I, Class II, or Class III malocclusion with or without an anterior open bite [12].

One of the ways to benefit Class III patients such aesthetically as functionality is performed bimaxillary orthognathic surgery by means of treatment plannings based on alterations of the OP [13, 14]. Thus, Class III patients with different angulations of the OP can benefit from rotations of counterclockwise and clockwise of the maxillomandibular complex (MMC) [13]. In this sense, Marlière et al. [13] and Parente et al. [14] showed three clinical cases in Class III patients with different facial types and clinical features that performed different treatment planning in orthognathic surgery by counterclockwise and clockwise rotations of the MMC, but the authors

disclosed to be more important the evaluation of the clinical features than clearly the obtainment of OP angulation during treatment planning.

In these case reports, two Class III patients with different clinical features and inclination of OP were presented, undergone different treatment planning, and submitted to alteration of OP by clockwise and counterclockwise rotations of the MMC for orthognathic surgery correction of DFD.

2. Case Reports

Two patients presented to the Oral and Maxillofacial Surgery Clinic of the University Hospital Pedro Ernesto (State University of Rio de Janeiro, Brazil) for treatment of dentofacial deformity, which complained of esthetic maxillary deficiency and functional masticatory restrictions. Patients underwent clinical examination (facial analysis and intraoral evaluation) associated with photographs and plaster models of dental arches. The patient signed an informed consent form for both treatment and use of images for publication.

2.1. Patient I. A healthy 25-year-old male was undergone to facial analysis which showed brachycephalic morphologic type and Class III malocclusion (Figures 1(a)–1(g)). The clinical features and cephalometric measures (McNamara Analysis) were presented in Table 1.

2.2. Patient II. A healthy 27-year-old female was undergone to facial analysis which showed dolichocephalic morphologic type and Class III malocclusion (Figures 2(a)–2(g)). The clinical features and cephalometric measures (McNamara Analysis) were presented in Table 1.

2.2.1. Treatment Planning. The treatment planning was aided by clinical examination (facial analysis and intraoral evaluation) associated with photographs, cone-beam computed tomography, and plaster models of dental arches.

TABLE 1: Comparison of clinical features and cephalometric measures between patients I and II.

(a)

Patient	Quantitative and qualitative data from facial analysis	
	Patient I Figures 1(a)–1(g)	Patient II Figures 2(a)–2(g)
Facial type (OP type)	Brachycephalic (low OP)	Dolichocephalic (high OP)
Upper incisor at rest	0 mm	7 mm
Dental and gingival display on the smile (mm*)	Vertical maxillary deficiency 7 mm e 0 mm	Vertical maxillary excess 13 mm e 3 mm
Maxillary dental midline to the midsagittal plane	Dental midline shifted to the left	Dental midline to the right
Paranasal fullness	Paranasal fullness little decreased	Paranasal fullness decreased
Upper lip support (Nasolabial angle)	Good upper lip support (normal)	Lack of upper lip support (obtuse)
Display among soft tissue of lips and chin	Chin forward of upper and lower lips	Lower lip forward upper lip and chin
Malocclusion Reverse overjet/overbite (mm*)	Class III −3 mm/0 mm	Class III −9 mm/0 mm

(b)

Skeletal sagittal relationship	Lateral cephalometric		
	Preoperative measurements		
	Patient I	Patient II	Range reference
SNA Angle	92.4°	75.5°	83.9° (±3.2°)
SNB Angle	94.3°	78.4°	81° (±3°)
ANB Angle	−2°	−2.9°	2° (±2°)
Point A to NPerp line	11.2 mm	−1.5 mm	1.1 mm (±2.7)
Pogonion to NPerp line	26.2 mm	4.2 mm	−0.3 mm (±3.8)
Mandible plane angle	18.4°	32.5°	21.3° (±3.9°)
Facial axis angle	10.8°	−1.9°	0.5 (±3.5°)
Maxilla incisor to point A	10.6 mm	3.4 mm	5.3 mm (±2)
Mandibular incisor to A-pogonion	8.7 mm	6.7 mm	2.3 mm (±2.1)

mm: millimeters; Nperp line: N perpendicular line.

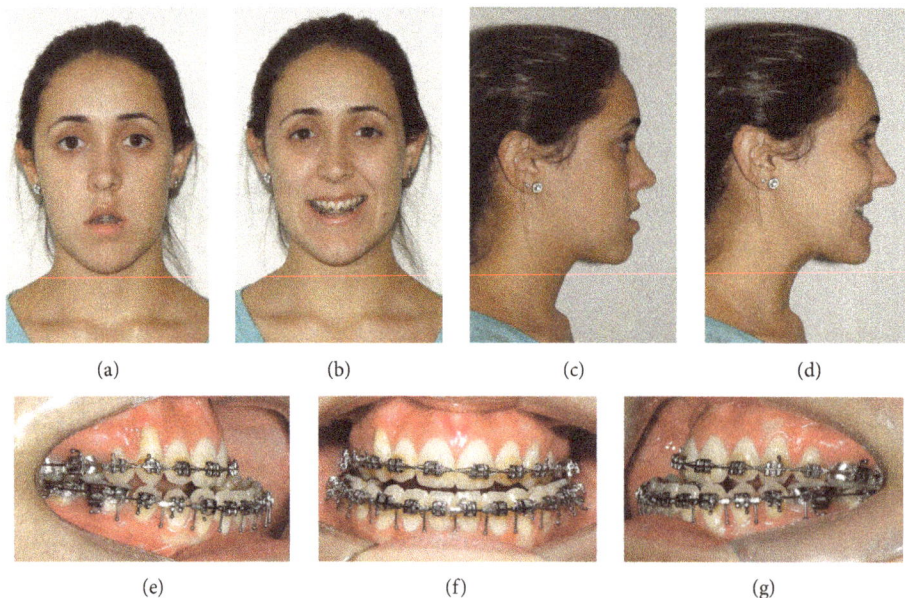

(a) (b) (c) (d)

(e) (f) (g)

FIGURE 2: (a–d) Preoperative evaluation at rest and smiling. (e–g) Intraoral images.

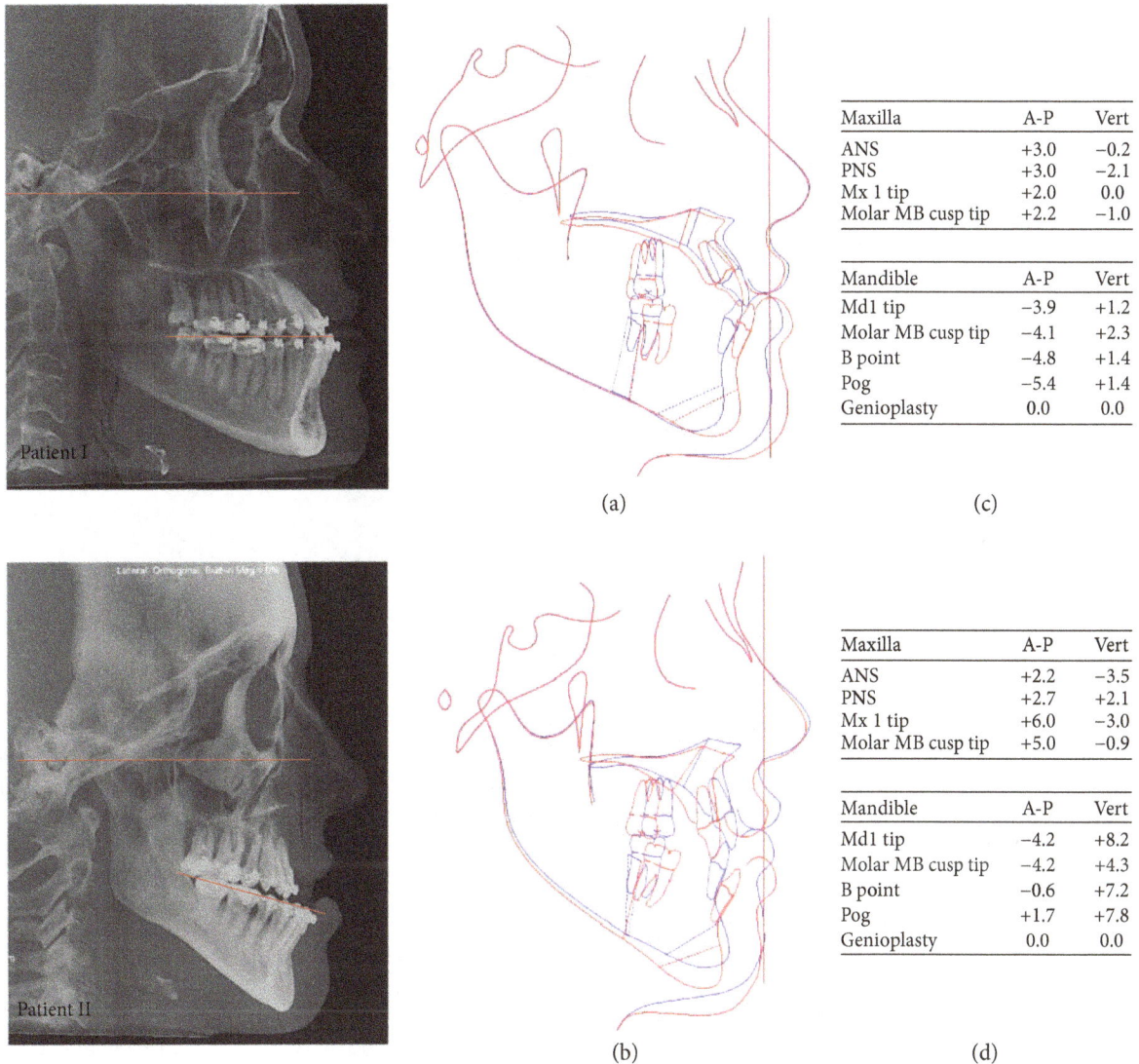

Maxilla	A-P	Vert
ANS	+3.0	−0.2
PNS	+3.0	−2.1
Mx 1 tip	+2.0	0.0
Molar MB cusp tip	+2.2	−1.0

Mandible	A-P	Vert
Md1 tip	−3.9	+1.2
Molar MB cusp tip	−4.1	+2.3
B point	−4.8	+1.4
Pog	−5.4	+1.4
Genioplasty	0.0	0.0

(a)   (c)

Maxilla	A-P	Vert
ANS	+2.2	−3.5
PNS	+2.7	+2.1
Mx 1 tip	+6.0	−3.0
Molar MB cusp tip	+5.0	−0.9

Mandible	A-P	Vert
Md1 tip	−4.2	+8.2
Molar MB cusp tip	−4.2	+4.3
B point	−0.6	+7.2
Pog	+1.7	+7.8
Genioplasty	0.0	0.0

(b)   (d)

FIGURE 3: Illustrations of the lateral radiographs and red lines showed a qualitative comparison of OP inclination. (a-b) Superimpositions of original and predictive tracings. (c-d) Surgical movements.

For planning, six facial features helped to plan for alteration of OP in orthognathic surgery: (I) facial type; (II) upper incisor display at rest regards to upper lip; (III) dental and gingival display on smile; (IV) fullness and soft tissue support in the lips and paranasal region; (V) chin projection regarding to lips; and (VI) lower lip projection.

The clinical facial characteristics of the patients were observed in a natural head position and properly registered (picture 1), correlating with the three-dimensional reconstructions of soft tissue and facial bone from the importation of DICOM (Digital Imaging and Communication in Medicine) from cone-beam computed tomography to Dolphin Imaging 11.7 Premium software (Dolphin Imaging and Management Solutions, Chatsworth, CA, USA). This software provided lateral radiographies and cephalometric measures that allowed bidimensional evaluation of the inclination of OP regards to Frankfort horizontal plane (Figure 3).

The plannings were based on the six clinical characteristics to obtain a harmony in facial appearance, considering patients' esthetic and functional complaints. Profile radiographs were performed for designing of original and predictive tracings (Figure 3) in a bidimensional evaluation. According to these factors, bimaxillary orthognathic surgeries were planned for both patients performed in an inverted sequence (mandible first). For patient I, it was planned alteration of OP in clockwise rotation of the MMC to decrease chin projection, to fill paranasal region, and to soften the mandibular contour. For patient II, it was planned alteration of OP of the MMC in counterclockwise rotation in order to improve chin posture in relation to the lower lip and to optimize the mandibular contour.

A conventional workflow was performed (wax bite registration under centric relation, facebow registration, and transfer of facebow registration to the semiadjustable articulator and model surgery). The surgical treatment plannings were simulated in model surgery, and the resulting postoperative model relationships were used to fabricate the intermediate and final splints. Theses splints were essential

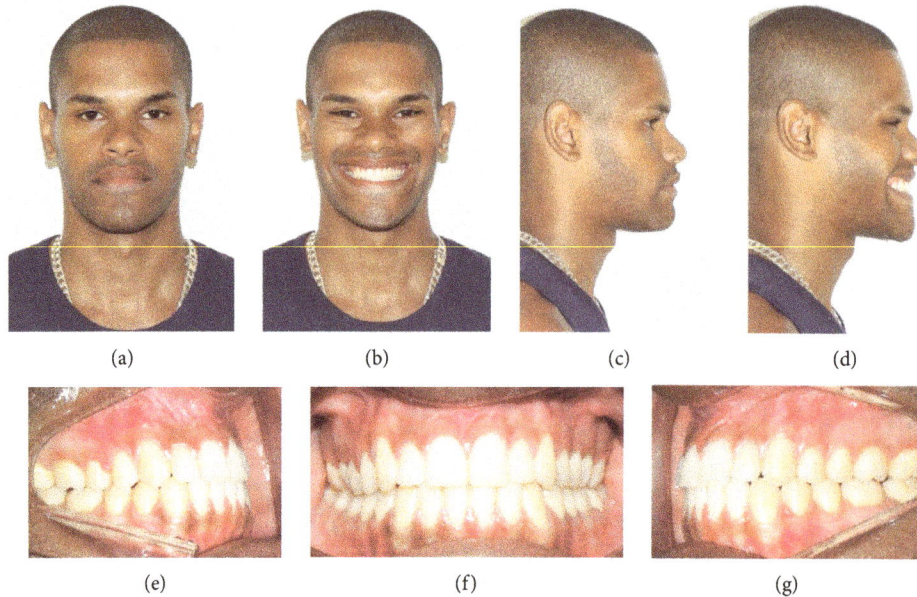

FIGURE 4: (a–d) Postoperative evaluation (2 years) at rest and smiling. (e–g) Intraoral images, postoperative occlusion after surgical and orthodontic treatment.

means to transfer the preoperative surgical treatment into accurate surgical procedure.

2.2.2. Surgical Procedure. In both patients, the surgical procedures were performed under general anesthesia. Initially, buccal access to the mandible was achieved through soft tissue incision on the external oblique line to the mesial aspect of the second molar laterally (a minimum of 5 mm of nonkeratinized mucosa maintained in the buccal region). Subperiosteal dissection of the buccal mucosa was then performed towards the internal oblique line in the retromolar region, aiming at partially exposing the medial region and lingula of the mandible. Using reciprocating saws (Stryker-CORE System), sagittal osteotomy of the bilateral mandible was performed and finished using chisels. The intermediate splint was then fixed to the orthodontic appliance for maxillomandibular splinting with steel wire. The mandible and maxilla were stabilized in intermediate occlusion, and the mandible was repositioned via rigid internal fixation with straight miniplates and monocortical (System 2.0—Neoface—Neoortho Orthopedic Products).

Surgical access to the maxilla was performed buccally and subperiosteal nonkeratinized mucosa detachment, extending from the floor of the nasal fossa to the pterygomaxillary region. Le Fort I osteotomy was performed using a reciprocating saw (Stryker-CORE System) and finished with chisels. After osteotomy in the pterygomaxillary regions and mobilization of the maxilla, the walls of the maxilla were leveled following the planning, using rougher forceps and rotatory burs. The final splint was inserted along with the orthodontic appliances and steel wire to stabilize the maxilla and the mandible in final occlusion. Finally, the maxilla was repositioned with rigid internal fixation using L-shaped miniplates in the zigomaticomaxillary regions and around the pyriform aperture (System

2.0—Neoface—Neoortho Orthopedic Products). Mentoplasty was performed for chin advancement to improve the contour of the mentolabial groove. The surgical procedures were considered according to the planning and without intercurrences.

2.2.3. Postoperative. The patient was evaluated weekly for the first 2 months and monthly thereafter until the sixth month. Postoperative orthodontic treatment was maintained through to completion.

Subjectively, the patients were satisfied with optimal esthetic and functional result. After 2 years of postoperative, the outcomes of the patients I and II showed, respectively, alterations of OP by clockwise (Figures 4(a)–4(g) and counterclockwise rotations of the MMC (Figures 5(a)–5(g)). The postoperative radiographies, lateral cephalometric tracings, and measures (McNamara Analysis) were presented at Figure 6 and Table 2, respectively.

3. Discussion

The bimaxillary orthognathic surgeries in both patients had been performed by alterations of OP, which proved to be a useful tool of planning to obtain favorable results. Thus, actual outcomes of Class III patients were based on planning and facial analysis of individual clinical features. The treatment planning of patients I and II was also based on the inclination of OP regarding to the Frankfort horizontal plane, but it was just qualitatively evaluated by comparing the posture of OP (Figure 3). Suchlike Parente et al. [14], similar planning to patients I and II were optimized by the clinical perception of the surgeons in detriment to the use of cephalometric tracings. Since 1993, Arnett and Bergman [15] had shown that performing orthognathic surgery planning only by cephalometric analysis could generate

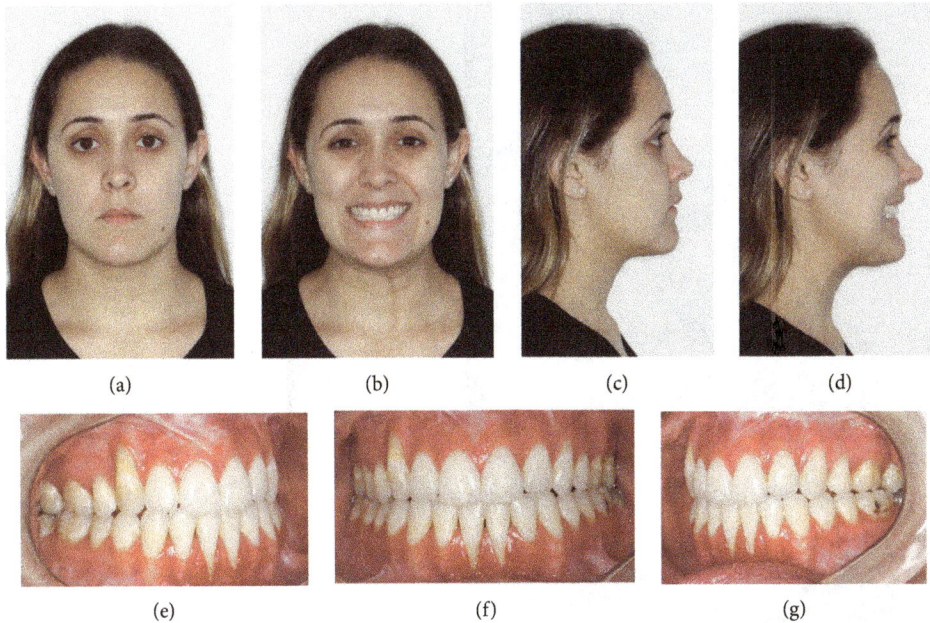

FIGURE 5: (a–d) Postoperative evaluation (2 years) at rest and smiling. (e–g) Intraoral images, postoperative occlusion after surgical and orthodontic treatment.

unfavorable esthetic results. Therefore, the planning cannot be based exclusively on cephalometric standards, as it could cause unfavorable esthetic results.

We also believe that lateral cephalometric analysis just quantifies dentoskeletal relationships in angular and linear measures (Tables 1 and 2). On the other hand, it cannot determine treatment planning in orthognathic surgery, because these measurements do not take into account the resting and dynamic relationships between hard and soft tissues, which are most critical aspects in treatment planning. Although the shortcoming of lateral cephalogram was determinant to not use as treatment goal, our case reports just were based on inclination of OP, there is matching with analysis of the facial morphologic form, soft tissue envelope, and the underlying facial bones integrated with dentition.

For Posnick et al. [16], facial esthetics can be achieved by changes in OP by counterclockwise or clockwise rotation of the MMC but emphasized that it is not a central point to quantify angular measurements of OP in the pre or post operatives, being more valid esthetic optimization by simply obtaining the most harmonic relations between skeletal structures and disposition of soft facial tissues. Marlière et al. [13] reinforced the idea that there was not an advantage to obtain the value of OP angulation, because OP angles may present wide variability in the population, there being more important to treatment planning based on surgeon's perceptions and clinical characteristics of each patient.

In this sense, six clinical characteristics observed in the patients were determinants for the planning of the surgical procedure. The facial type determined the way of OP alteration that was allowed by means of orthognathic surgery and counterclockwise rotation or clockwise rotation of the MMC. For patient I, clockwise rotation provided an increase in mandibular angle, and then, facial contour became more

harmonic and soften (Figure 4). When the OP change was set in counterclockwise rotation, as performed in patient II, there was a decrease in the mandibular angle and the facial contour was improved (Figure 5). The upper incisor display regards to upper lip margins were evaluated at rest and on smile that had managed the anterior vertical repositioning of the maxilla. For it, 3 mm was acceptable to display upper incisors, and on smile, gingival display regarding to bordering the cervical gingival contour of the upper incisors, through to 2 mm were considered harmonious [17]. The soft tissue support was evaluated in lips and paranasal region, due to the maxillary advancement to improve the upper lip support and to provide paranasal fullness, so both treatment planning was adequately sufficient to achieve appropriate soft tissue support. The chin projection regarding lower incisor inclination helped to regulate the amount of OP alteration; because we believe higher discrepancy between these structures, greater alteration of OP would be necessary. Therefore, patient I benefited from clockwise rotation because the chin rotated posteriorly, and patient II was favored from counterclockwise rotation for the chin rotated anteriorly. Lower lip projection was properly achieved for both patients after OP alterations, which got a better chin position regards to lower lip, without needing for genioplasty and more natural outcomes. The clinical features of orthognathic surgery were also described by Marlière et al. [13] and Parente et al. [14], who were successful in planning and achieved satisfactory esthetic and functional results.

After diagnosis, facial analysis, and planning, bimaxillary orthognathic surgeries were performed based on mandible first sequence, starting from sagittal osteotomy of the mandible bilaterally. According to Borba et al. [18], orthognathic surgery in the inverted sequence approach was described in the 1970s. However, to date, the decision regarding such

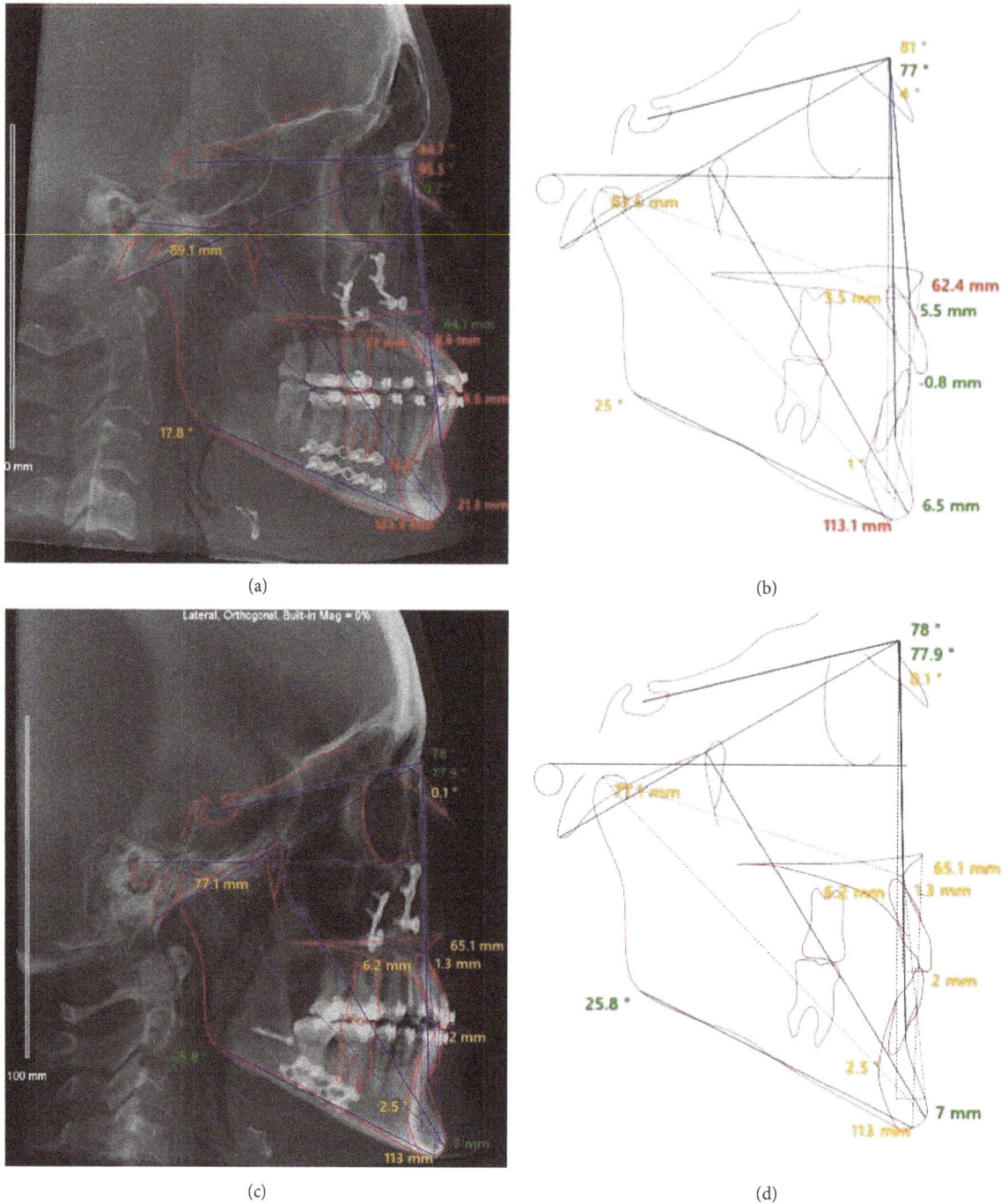

FIGURE 6: Illustrations of postoperative radiographs and lateral cephalometric. (a and b) Patient I. (c and d) Patient II.

mandible first is based on the experience and preference of the surgeon. In addition, the inverted surgical sequence would be beneficial in situations such as clockwise rotation of the MMC to avoid an anterior open bite intraoperatively (when intermaxillary fixation is impaired by a thick intermediate guide), inaccuracy of intercondylar registration, and uncertainty regarding condylar positioning [17]. Borba et al. [18] also highlighted that the inverted sequence might not be preferred in surgical movements with clockwise rotation of the MMC, because rotations using posterior maxillary

intrusion or anterior maxillary extrusion would require the mandible to be fixed in an "open bite" intermediate position with a thick intermediate splint in the incisor region, making the application of intermaxillary fixation difficult [19]. Another disadvantage, in cases undergoing the mandible first sequence in which an unfavorable split of the mandible occurs that is not correctable will have to postpone until a later date [20].

In terms of selection of surgical sequence, the inverted sequence of bimaxillary orthognathic surgery offered

TABLE 2: Comparison of postoperative cephalometric measures.

| | Lateral cephalometric | | |
| Skeletal sagittal relationship | Postoperative measurements | | |
	Patient I	Patient II	Range reference
SNA angle	94.7°	81°	83.9° (±3.2°)
SNB angle	95.5°	77°	81° (±3°)
ANB angle	−0.7°	4°	2° (±2°)
Point A to NPerp line	9.6 mm	5.5 mm	1.1 mm (±2.7)
Pogonion to NPerp line	21.3 mm	6.5 mm	−0.3 mm (±3.8)
Mandible plane angle	17.8°	25°	21.3° (±3.9°)
Facial axis angle	13.5°	1°	0.5 (±3.5°)
Maxilla incisor to point A	13 mm	3.5 mm	5.3 mm (±2)
Mandibular incisor to A-pogonion	6.6 mm	−0.8 mm	2.3 mm (±2.1)

mm: millimeters; Nperp line: N perpendicular line.

acceptable outcomes in patients I and II, regardless of whether clockwise rotation or counterclockwise rotation of the MMC. The traditional sequence of bimaxillary orthognathic surgery (maxilla first) was not preferred in surgical movements with clockwise rotation of the MMC, and we believe that the decision regarding which segment should be operated on first had relied on accurate preoperative planning based upon individual surgeon experience and preference.

A systematic review and meta-analysis published in 2016 compared postsurgical skeletal stability between counterclockwise and clockwise rotation of the MMC for correction of DFD. From screening and eligibility, three available studies were reviewed and showed that counterclockwise and clockwise rotations of the MMC are stable outcomes immediately after surgery and at longest follow-up, with no statistically significant difference between treatment planning, mainly, when there is no preexisting temporomandibular joint pathology [12]. Both Class III patients had similar skeletal stability because the postoperative outcomes have remained stable regarding facial esthetic and occlusal functionality in a follow-up over 2 years. Perhaps, they had treated by different planning based on alteration of OP from bimaxillary orthognathic surgery.

Finally, Class III patients had undergone same surgical treatment for correction of DFD, but different clinical features and inclination of OP helped to define treatment planning by clockwise rotation or counterclockwise rotation of the MMC. The clockwise and counterclockwise rotations of the MMC, also known as alteration of OP, should be considered to achieve soft tissue harmony among the subnasal, upper lip and lower lip support, and chin, because it influenced underlying facial skeleton integrated with the dental structures. These case reports showed that stable and harmonic outcomes between facial esthetics and occlusion are possible to achieve combining surgeon's clinical perception and qualitative evaluation of OP inclination, mainly, patients without facial asymmetry, because bidimensional images can represent the inclination bilaterally. Subjectively, outcomes after longest follow-up were associated with high patient satisfaction.

Acknowledgments

The authors thank Dr. Leonardo Koerich for his assistance in cephalometric analysis.

References

[1] F. Eslamipour, A. Borzabadi-Farahani, B. T. le, and M. Shahmoradi, "A retrospective analysis of dentofacial deformities and orthognathic surgeries," *Annals of Maxillofacial Surgery*, vol. 7, no. 1, pp. 73–77, 2017.

[2] M. R. Tucker and B. B. Farell, "Correction of dentofacial deformities," in *Contemporary Oral and Maxillofacial Surgery*, J. R. Hupp, M. R. Tucker, and E. Ellis, Eds., pp. 520–563, Elsevier Health Sciences, USA, 2016.

[3] J. C. Posnick, "Definition and prevalence of dentofacial deformities," in *Orthognathic Surgery, Principles and Practice*, J. C. Posnick, Ed., pp. 61–68, Elsevier Health Sciences, USA, 2013.

[4] E. M. Boeck, N. Lunardi, A. S. Pinto, K. E. D. C. Pizzol, and R. J. Boeck Neto, "Occurrence of skeletal malocclusions in Brazilian patients with dentofacial deformities," *Brazilian Dental Journal*, vol. 22, no. 4, pp. 340–345, 2011.

[5] A. Al–Deaiji, "Characteristics of dentofacial deformities in a Saudi population," *Saudi Dental Journal*, vol. 13, pp. 101–105, 2001.

[6] C. T. Lee, L. K. Cheung, B. S. Khambay, A. Y. Ayoub, and P. Benington, "Dentofacial deformities and orthognathic surgery in Hong Kong and Glasgow," *Annals of the Royal Australasian College of Dental Surgeons*, vol. 22, pp. 113–115, 2014.

[7] C. Harrington, J. R. Gallagher, and A. Borzabadi-Farahani, "A retrospective analysis of dentofacial deformities and orthognathic surgeries using the index of orthognathic functional treatment need (IOFTN)," *International Journal of Pediatric Otorhinolaryngology*, vol. 79, no. 7, pp. 1063–1066, 2015.

[8] L. Espeland, H. E. Hogevold, and A. Stenvik, "A 3-year patient-centred follow-up of 516 consecutively treated orthognathic surgery patients," *European Journal of Orthodontics*, vol. 30, no. 1, pp. 24–30, 2007.

[9] W. R. Proffit, T. H. Jackson, and T. A. Turvey, "Changes in the pattern of patients receiving surgical-orthodontic treatment," *American Journal of Orthodontics & Dentofacial Orthopedics*, vol. 143, no. 6, pp. 793–798, 2013.

[10] A. J. Ireland, S. J. Cunningham, A. Petrie et al., "An index of orthognathic functional treatment need (IOFTN)," *Journal of Orthodontics*, vol. 41, no. 2, pp. 77–83, 2014.

[11] A. Borzabadi-Farahani, F. Eslamipour, and M. Shahmoradi, "Functional needs of subjects with dentofacial deformities: a study using the index of orthognathic functional treatment need (IOFTN)," *Journal of Plastic, Reconstructive & Aesthetic Surgery*, vol. 69, no. 6, pp. 796–801, 2016.

[12] E. A. Al-Moraissi and L. M. Wolford, "Is counterclockwise rotation of the maxillomandibular complex stable compared with clockwise rotation in the correction of dentofacial deformities? A systematic review and meta-analysis," *Journal of Oral and Maxillofacial Surgery*, vol. 74, no. 10, pp. 2066.e1–2066.e12, 2016.

[13] D. A. A. Marlière, C. B. Lovisi, A. R. M. Schmitt, B. S. Sotto-Maior, and H. D. M. Chaves Netto, "Orthognathic surgery combined with partial lipectomy of the buccal fat pad: case report on optimization of esthetic outcome," *Journal of Pharmacy and Pharmacology*, vol. 5, no. 8, pp. 565–571, 2017.

[14] E. Parente, G. Lacerda, and M. G. Silvares, "Surgical manipulation of the occlusal plane in Class III deformities: 5 features to help planning," *Open Journal of Stomatology*, vol. 4, no. 5, article 45602, p. 5, 2014.

[15] G. W. Arnett and R. T. Bergman, "Facial keys to orthodontic diagnosis and treatment planning. Part I," *American Journal of Orthodontics and Dentofacial Orthopedics*, vol. 103, no. 4, pp. 299–312, 1993.

[16] J. C. Posnick, J. J. Fantuzzo, and J. D. Orchin, "Deliberate operative rotation of the maxillo-mandibular complex to alter the A point to B-point relationship for enhanced facial esthetics," *Journal of Oral and Maxillofacial Surgery*, vol. 64, no. 11, pp. 1687–1695, 2006.

[17] D. Sarver and R. S. Jacobson, "The aesthetic dentofacial analysis," *Clinics in Plastic Surgery*, vol. 34, no. 3, pp. 369–394, 2007.

[18] A. M. Borba, A. H. Borges, P. S. Cé, B. A. Venturi, M. G. Naclério-Homem, and M. Miloro, "Mandible-first sequence in bimaxillary orthognathic surgery: a systematic review," *International Journal of Oral and Maxillofacial Surgery*, vol. 45, no. 4, pp. 472–475, 2016.

[19] D. Perez and E. Ellis III, "Sequencing bimaxillary surgery: mandible first," *Journal of Oral and Maxillofacial Surgery*, vol. 69, no. 8, pp. 2217–2224, 2011.

[20] D. A. Cottrell and L. M. Wolford, "Altered orthognathic surgical sequencing and a modified approach to model surgery," *Journal of Oral and Maxillofacial Surgery*, vol. 52, no. 10, pp. 1010–1020, 1994.

14

Minimally Invasive Approach for Improving Anterior Dental Aesthetics: Case Report with 1-Year Follow-Up

H. Sevilay Bahadır ⓘ, Gökhan Karadağ ⓘ, and Yusuf Bayraktar ⓘ

Kırıkkale University Faculty of Dentistry, Department of Restorative Dentistry, Turkey

Correspondence should be addressed to Yusuf Bayraktar; yusufbayraktar@kku.edu.tr

Academic Editor: Andrea Scribante

Dental aesthetics have become highly important in recent years. Treating aesthetic demands with noninvasive or minimally invasive techniques can preserve the natural tissues. A 20-year-old female patient presented to the clinic with aesthetic concerns. After the clinical and radiographic examinations, hypomineralization was identified in the maxillary anterior teeth except the maxillary right canine. An external discoloration was also identified in the maxillary left canine tooth. Moreover, the right canine tooth was identified as a Turner's tooth according to the patient's anamnesis. The resin infiltration technique was applied to the maxillary anterior teeth except the maxillary right canine. The bleaching treatment was applied to the maxillary left canine tooth. Then, a laminate veneer restoration was applied to the upper right canine tooth with Turner's hypoplasia. Following the treatment, a satisfactory aesthetic restoration was achieved. After 1-year examination, no clinical failures were observed.

1. Introduction

Aesthetic dentistry has recently gained popularity with the aesthetic factors becoming highly important. More patients seek a visually pleasing smile, and the perception in the media about the concept of beauty has improved. Nowadays, patients' demands for invisible restorations performing with minimal invasive applications to dental tissues which provide a natural look have increased. Advanced restorative techniques along with biomimetic materials and the philosophy of preventive dentistry support the regaining of healthy, functional, and aesthetic smiles [1].

Tooth discolorations, hypocalcifications, and surface irregularities are important aesthetic concerns [2]. Tooth discolorations vary in etiology, appearance, localization, and tooth structure. They are classified as internal, external, and a combination of both. Vital bleaching treatment has been accepted for discoloration treatment [3].

Also, developmental defects of the enamel are important aesthetic concerns. Developmental defects of the enamel are basically classified under two main categories: enamel hypoplasia and enamel hypomineralization caused by an insult to the ameloblasts during amelogenesis. Hypomineralization (opacity) is a qualitative developmental defect of the enamel caused by incomplete enamel mineralization and maturation below the enamel surface that is intact at the time of eruption. The defect reveals a variable degree of alteration in the translucency of the enamel, which has initially a normal thickness and can be white, yellow, or brown. The border of the defect can be demarcated [4–6]. Hypoplasia is characterized as the decreased thickness of the enamel to varying degrees and pit and surface irregularities. Although the transparency and hardness of the enamel remain the same, the opacities may vary from small to large [2].

Turner's hypoplasia is a type of hypoplasia characterized by imperfections in a permanent tooth caused by trauma or periapical infections of deciduous teeth and commonly irritate patients aesthetically. The degree of hypoplasia can vary from light brown color to darker shades in the affected area. It may also affect the whole crown. This is often observed in maxillary incisors and maxillary and mandibular molar teeth [7].

"Dental fluorosis," a specific disturbance in tooth formation and an aesthetic condition, is defined as a chronic

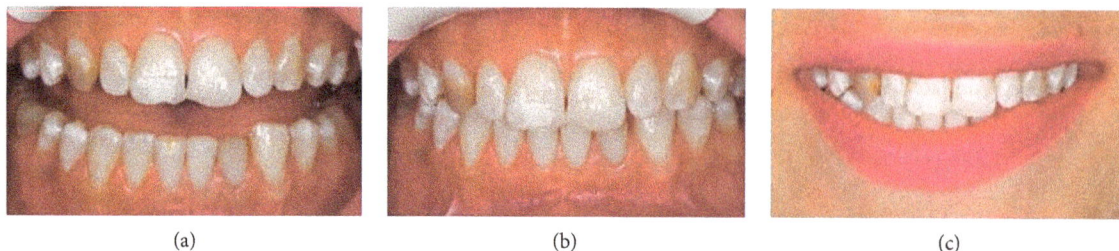

FIGURE 1: (a) Appearance of teeth in the half-open position. (b) Position of teeth in occlusion. (c) Lip position during a smile, smile line, and teeth visibility.

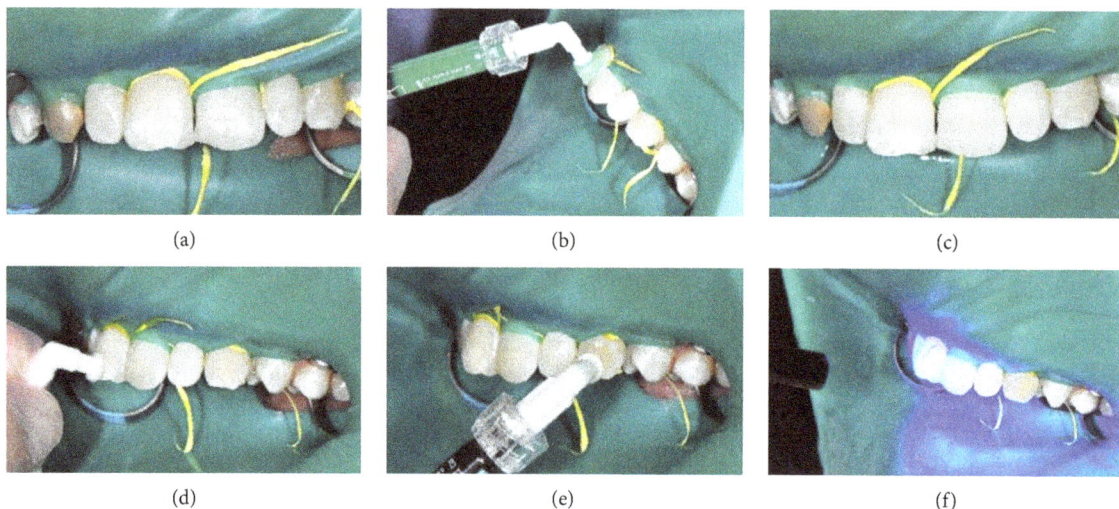

FIGURE 2: (a) Application of the acid gel. (b) Washing with a water spray. (c) Application of an ethanol drier. (d) Application of a low-viscosity resin infiltrate. (e) Polymerization. (f) Immediately after application.

fluoride-induced condition, in which enamel development is disrupted, and the enamel is hypomineralized. Clinically, enamel fluorosis is seen as white spots, brown stains, white opaque lines or striations, or a white parchment-like appearance of the tooth surface. Fluorosis is symmetrically distributed, but the severity varies among the different types of teeth. Teeth such as premolars have a higher prevalence of fluorosis and are more severely affected [8].

Many aesthetic treatments are used for these aesthetic imperfections. Problems such as Turner's hypoplasia, fluorosis, and external factors are usually treated with methods including bleaching, microabrasion technique, and laminate veneer restoration. The selection of the optimal treatment technique is related to the degree of discoloration [9].

This case report is aimed at reporting the treatment of a 20-year-old female patient with aesthetic concerns in the anterior teeth using a minimally invasive approach and evaluating the clinical performance after 1 year.

2. Case Report

A 20-year-old female patient was admitted to the Department of Restorative Dentistry, Faculty of Dental Medicine, Kırıkkale University, with aesthetic concerns. The anamnesis did not specify any systemic illnesses of the patient. After the clinical and radiographic examinations, hypomineralization

was identified in the maxillary anterior teeth except the right canine tooth. An external discoloration was also identified in the left canine tooth. Moreover, the right canine tooth was identified as a Turner's tooth according to the patient's anamnesis. (Figure 1).

A minimally invasive and aesthetically satisfactory treatment plan was made with the consent of the patient. The resin infiltration technique (Icon, DMG, Hamburg, Germany) was applied to the maxillary anterior teeth except the right canine. A rubber dam was implemented to protect the soft tissues and create a clean and dry working environment. The teeth were then cleaned with a cleaning pad, and the resin infiltration technique was applied step by step as follows. (1) A gel comprising 15% HCl, water, silica, and other additives was applied for 2 min with a special apparatus to ensure its homogenous application. Then, the acid gel was washed with a water spray for 30 s. (2) An ethanol drier was applied for 30 s to remove water in the lesion area and make the microporosity of the enamel surface more visible. (3) Finally, a low-viscosity resin infiltrate was applied for 3 min. Excess materials were removed with a cotton roll and a dental floss. Finally, a light curing accessory was used for polymerization and polishing for 40 s. (Figure 2).

Later on, the left canine tooth was identified to have a darker color and hence bleaching treatment was applied.

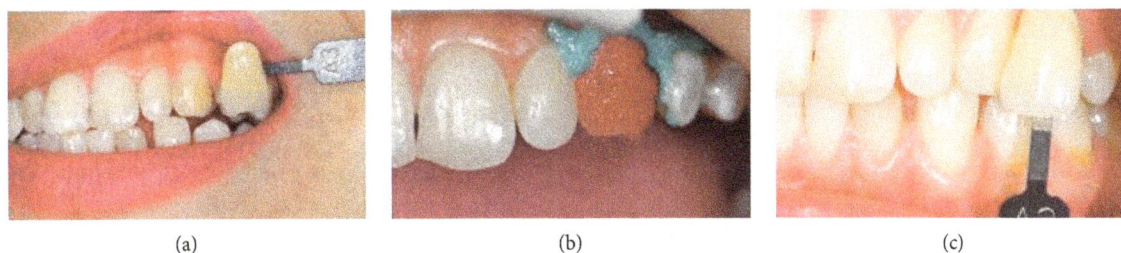

FIGURE 3: (a) Tooth was determined as A3 on the Vita scale. (b) Bleaching agent was applied. (c) Tooth was determined as A2 on the Vita scale.

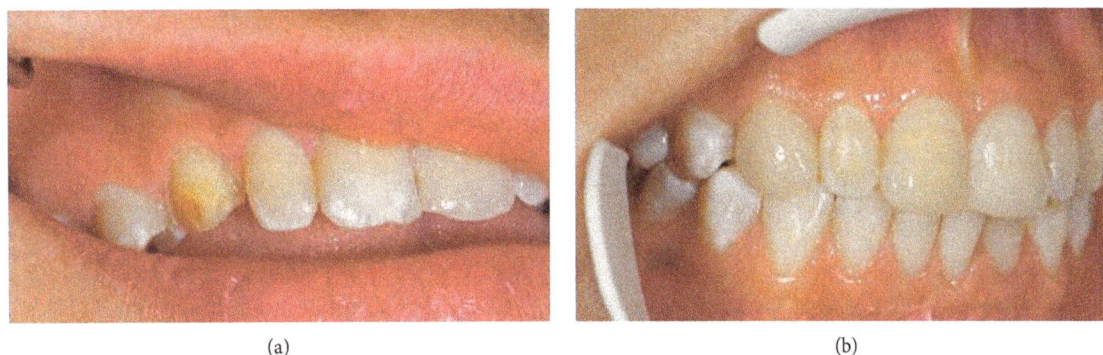

FIGURE 4: (a) Overlapped preparation. (b) Application of laminate veneer.

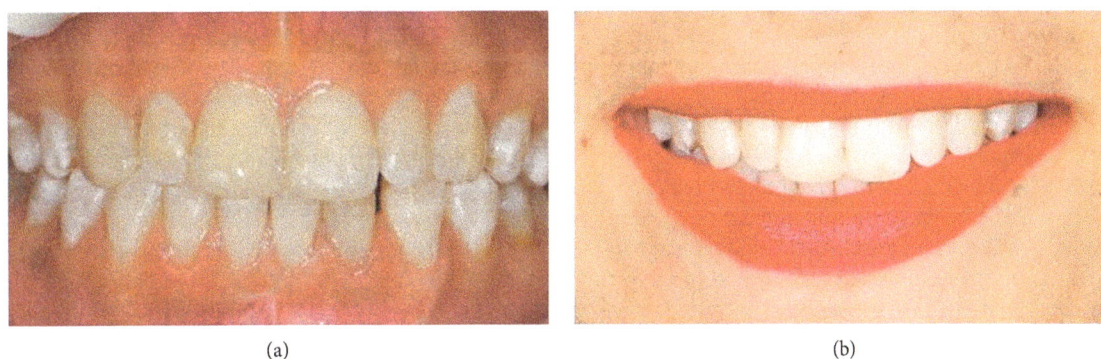

FIGURE 5: (a) Posttreatment. (b) One-year follow-up.

First, the color of the left canine tooth was determined as A3 on the Vita scale. Then, a gingival protective gel was applied to the contours of the gums following the manufacturer's protocol and polymerized with an LED light accessory. Two components of the whitening agent (Opalescence Boost PF, Ultradent, YT, USA) were mixed following the manufacturer's protocol and applied to the aforementioned area. The application took 40 min in one session, and the color of the tooth was determined as A2 on the Vita scale (Figure 3).

A laminate veneer restoration was planned for the upper right canine, which was a Turner's tooth according to the patient's anamnesis. The tooth was prepared (Komet Ceramic Veneer Kit, Komet Dental, Hamburg, Germany). The overlapped preparation was applied to exceed the incisal enamel contours by 2 mm. The gingival retraction was achieved using a combination of mechanical and chemical retraction methods. The prepared tooth and the opposite teeth were digitally measured with an intraoral scanner (TRIOS A/S, 3Shape Trios, Copenhagen, Denmark). The designed laminate veneer was produced with a CAM system (Coritec 550i, imes-icore, Eiterfeld, Germany) using lithium disilicate glass ceramic blocks (IPS e-max CAD, Ivoclar Vivadent, Schaan, Liechtenstein). The restorations were glazed in the laboratory and then cemented with adhesive cement (Panavia V5 Clear, Kuraray Noritake Dental, Tokyo, Japan) following the recommendations of the manufacturer (Figure 4).

Incisal irregularities on the maxillary central incisors were restored with a nanohybrid composite resin (Filtek Ultimate A2 Body, 3M ESPE, St. Paul, MN, USA). Following the treatment, a satisfactory aesthetic restoration was achieved. The examination of the restorations after 1 year did not reveal any clinical failures (Figure 5).

3. Discussion

Developmental defects of the enamel are caused by various etiological factors, such as amelogenesis imperfecta, overexposure to fluoride along the mineralization of the enamel, different disorders, or trauma. However, their origin is often unknown. Hypomineralization can occur independently or coexist with hypoplasia in one or more teeth depending on time, duration, susceptibility of the individual, and severity of the prenatal, perinatal, or postnatal insult [4, 6]. In this case report, the patient did not report any possible cause for the hypomineralization.

Reestablishing the visual dental aesthetics of a patient has been one of the chief purposes of modern dental medicine. Novel materials and treatment methods are being developed every day to reach this goal [10].

The resin infiltration technique is one of the methods for addressing aesthetic demands. Kielbassa et al. and Paris et al. first developed and applied this technique to cure proximal caries, which demonstrated the same grading level in histological caries extension [11, 12]. Later, this technique was used for white spot lesions and demonstrated to remove the white stains on the enamel [11, 13]. It was further implemented in cases of hypoplasia and fluorosis [2]. Defects such as white spot lesions, hypomineralization, and hypoplasia exhibit opacity because refractive indices of enamel crystals and the insides of the pores are different. The micropores of these lesions are filled with water or air. The resin infiltration technique infuses these micropores with a low-viscosity resin. Thus, the difference in the refractive indices between the micropores and the enamel is eliminated, and the lesion gains an enamel-like appearance [2, 14].

In this case report, the resin infiltration technique was applied to the maxillary anterior teeth except the right canine, all of which exhibited hypomineralization. The procedure yielded aesthetically satisfactory results, corroborating the findings of previous studies [2, 14–16]. Only the maxillary anterior six teeth were restored, as desired by the patient. The reason for the upper right central tooth not responding to the treatment as effectively might be that the thicker and more mineralized surface layers in lesions (pseudointact surface layer or sound enamel) and the pores of the lesion were contaminated with organic materials, such as proteins and carbohydrates, that hampered resin penetration [11, 12].

The resin infiltration technique has some limitations. These limitations are pseudointact surface layer of lesion, mineral content of lesion, amount of micropores of lesion, and structure of roughened surface of lesion. Furthermore, it has not been completely explained whether organic materials, such as biofilm remnants, carbohydrates, lipids, and proteins, attach to the inner enamel surfaces, thus possibly occluding the (underlying) pores in lesions and leading to an incomplete resin penetration of the porous structures. Additionally, deproteinization procedures using sodium hypochlorite should be implemented as procedural prerequisite with the infiltration technique because a cleaned surface would need to assure retention and bond strength to hamper biofilm formation and to impede further cariogenic

challenges to the infiltrated lesion and to increase ingress of the infiltrate's resinous matrix [17].

Additionally, bleaching treatment and laminate veneers are methods of addressing aesthetic demands. Bleaching treatment is a more conservative method compared with other methods used for treating discoloration. Office-type whitening treatment is one of the most popular methods. It involves the application of 25%–40% hydrogen peroxide or 16%–35% carbamide peroxide on the external surface of the teeth. The bleaching mechanism works on the principle that hydrogen peroxide penetrates the tooth and generates free radicals that oxidize the organic stains [18]. Several studies [19, 20] in the literature reported that the office-type whitening was successful.

Porcelain laminate veneers are nowadays commonly used for aesthetic purposes owing to their better aesthetic properties, higher resistance to abrasion and discoloration, and better biological harmony with the oral flora [21].

In this study, the porcelain laminate application was used for the upper right canine tooth with a CAD/CAM system. The CAD/CAM technology has improved significantly in clinical applications. It has been commonly used in the practical dental applications. Using this method, satisfactory aesthetic and functional results have been obtained in a short time, making the lives of both the patient and the dentist easier.

Composite resins or porcelain materials are generally preferred materials for aesthetic procedures. In this study, lithium disilicate glass ceramic material was used. Besides its satisfactory aesthetic quality, it also has high endurance against stretching, breaking, and chemicals. The rate of abrasion of the opposite teeth is lower, and the material has higher transparency compared with all other porcelain types [21, 22].

Nowadays, restorative treatment has achieved high aesthetic standards. It protects the dental structure maximally thanks to the development of adhesive systems, resin cement, and ceramics. The resin infiltration technique, bleaching treatment, and laminate veneer applications, among other minimally invasive treatments, have gained importance due to greater protection rates of the tooth and high aesthetic standards.

4. Conclusions

The resin infiltration technique, bleaching treatment, and laminate veneer treatment have been shown to be highly conservative methods that bring back a healthy and harmonious smile. The patient discussed in this case report was aesthetically and functionally satisfied with the treatment after 1-year follow-up.

Additional Points

Clinical Significance. Bleaching and resin infiltration techniques are noninvasive techniques for aesthetic dentistry. If these techniques are used in relevant cases, aesthetic results can be achieved.

Disclosure

This report was presented as oral presentation at the 21st International Congress of Esthetic Dentistry on 13–15 October 2017 in İstanbul (http://www.edad.org.tr/).

References

[1] G. N. Venâncio, G. Júnior, R. Rodrigues, and S. T. Dias, "Conservative esthetic solution with ceramic laminates: literature review," *RSBO*, vol. 11, no. 2, pp. 185–191, 2014.

[2] M. A. Muñoz, L. A. Arana-Gordillo, G. M. Gomes et al., "Alternative esthetic management of fluorosis and hypoplasia stains: blending effect obtained with resin infiltration techniques," *Journal of Esthetic and Restorative Dentistry*, vol. 25, no. 1, pp. 32–39, 2013.

[3] M. Q. Alqahtani, "Tooth-bleaching procedures and their controversial effects: a literature review," *The Saudi Dental Journal*, vol. 26, no. 2, pp. 33–46, 2014.

[4] B. Jälevik and J. G. Norén, "Enamel hypomineralization of permanent first molars: a morphological study and survey of possible aetiological factors," *International Journal of Paediatric Dentistry*, vol. 10, no. 4, pp. 278–289, 2000.

[5] E. Mahoney, F. S. M. Ismail, N. Kilpatrick, and M. Swain, "Mechanical properties across hypomineralized/hypoplastic enamel of first permanent molar teeth," *European Journal of Oral Sciences*, vol. 112, no. 6, pp. 497–502, 2004.

[6] N. Lygidakis, A. Chaliasou, and G. Siounas, "Evaluation of composite restorations in hypomineralised permanent molars: a four year clinical study," *European Journal of Paediatric Dentistry*, vol. 4, no. 3, pp. 143–148, 2003.

[7] G. Lavania and A. Lavania, "Endodontic and orthodontic interdisciplinary management of a patient with Turner's hypoplasia," *Journal of Interdisciplinary Dentistry*, vol. 5, no. 2, p. 75, 2015.

[8] A. K. Mascarenhas, "Risk factors for dental fluorosis: a review of the recent literature," *Pediatric Dentistry*, vol. 22, no. 4, pp. 269–277, 2000.

[9] E. S. Akpata, "Occurrence and management of dental fluorosis," *International Dental Journal*, vol. 51, no. 5, pp. 325–333, 2001.

[10] B. Korkut, F. Yanıkoğlu, and M. Günday, "Direct composite laminate veneers: three case reports," *Journal of Dental Research, Dental Clinics, Dental Prospects*, vol. 7, no. 2, pp. 105–111, 2013.

[11] A. M. Kielbassa, J. Muller, and C. R. Gernhardt, "Closing the gap between oral hygiene and minimally invasive dentistry: a review on the resin infiltration technique of incipient (proximal) enamel lesions," *Quintessence International*, vol. 40, no. 8, pp. 663–681, 2009.

[12] S. Paris, H. Meyer-Lueckel, and A. M. Kielbassa, "Resin infiltration of natural caries lesions," *Journal of Dental Research*, vol. 86, no. 7, pp. 662–666, 2007.

[13] S. Paris and H. Meyer-Lueckel, "Masking of labial enamel white spot lesions by resin infiltration–a clinical report," *Quintessence International*, vol. 40, no. 9, pp. 713–718, 2009.

[14] N. Gugnani, I. K. Pandit, V. Goyal, S. Gugnani, J. Sharma, and S. Dogra, "Esthetic improvement of white spot lesions and non-pitted fluorosis using resin infiltration technique: series of four clinical cases," *Journal of the Indian Society of Pedodontics and Preventive Dentistry*, vol. 32, no. 2, pp. 176–180, 2014.

[15] J.-H. Lee, D. G. Kim, C. J. Park, and L. R. Cho, "Minimally invasive treatment for esthetic enhancement of white spot lesion in adjacent tooth," *The Journal of Advanced Prosthodontics*, vol. 5, no. 3, pp. 359–363, 2013.

[16] H. Meyer-Lueckel and S. Paris, "Improved resin infiltration of natural caries lesions," *Journal of Dental Research*, vol. 87, no. 12, pp. 1112–1116, 2008.

[17] I. Ulrich, J. Mueller, M. Wolgin, W. Frank, and A. M. Kielbassa, "Tridimensional surface roughness analysis after resin infiltration of (deproteinized) natural subsurface carious lesions," *Clinical Oral Investigations*, vol. 19, no. 6, pp. 1473–1483, 2015.

[18] O. Polydorou, M. Wirsching, M. Wokewitz, and P. Hahn, "Three-month evaluation of vital tooth bleaching using light units—a randomized clinical study," *Operative Dentistry*, vol. 38, no. 1, pp. 21–32, 2013.

[19] S. Al Shethri, B. A. Matis, M. A. Cochran, R. Zekonis, and M. Stropes, "A clinical evaluation of two in-office bleaching products," *Operative Dentistry*, vol. 28, no. 5, pp. 488–495, 2003.

[20] T. Sari and A. Usumez, "Case report: office bleaching with Er: YAG laser," *Journal of the Laser and Health Academy*, vol. 1, pp. 4–6, 2013.

[21] J.-H. Jang, S.-H. Lee, J. Paek, and S.-Y. Kim, "Splinted porcelain laminate veneers with a natural tooth pontic: a provisional approach for conservative and esthetic treatment of a challenging case," *Operative Dentistry*, vol. 40, no. 6, pp. E257–E265, 2015.

[22] D. F. Alhekeir, R. A. Al-Sarhan, and A. F. Al Mashaan, "Porcelain laminate veneers: clinical survey for evaluation of failure," *The Saudi Dental Journal*, vol. 26, no. 2, pp. 63–67, 2014.

15

Maxillary Sinus Lift Using Autologous Periosteal Micrografts: A New Regenerative Approach and a Case Report of a 3-Year Follow-Up

Saturnino Marco Lupi ⓘ,[1] **Arianna Rodriguez y Baena,**[1] **Claudia Todaro,**[1]
Gabriele Ceccarelli ⓘ,[2] and **Ruggero Rodriguez y Baena** ⓘ[1]

[1]*Department of Clinical Surgical, Diagnostic and Pediatric Sciences, University of Pavia, Pavia, Italy*
[2]*Department of Public Health, Experimental Medicine and Forensic, Human Anatomy Unit, University of Pavia, Pavia, Italy*

Correspondence should be addressed to Ruggero Rodriguez y Baena; ruggero.rodriguez@unipv.it

Academic Editor: Gerardo Gómez-Moreno

This case report discusses about an innovative bone regeneration method that involves the use of autologous periosteal micrografts, which were used for a maxillary sinus floor lift in a 52-year-old female patient. This method allows for harvesting of a graft that is to be seeded on a PLGA scaffold and involves collection of a very little amount of palatal periosteal tissue in the same surgical site after elevation of a flap and disaggregation of it by using a Rigenera® filter. Histological samples collected at the time of implant installation demonstrate a good degree of bone regeneration. The clinical and radiographic outcomes at the 3-year follow-up visit showed an adequate stability of hard and soft tissues around the implants. This report demonstrates the possibility to obtain a sufficient quality and quantity of bone with a progenitor cell-based micrograft and in turn make the site appropriate for an implant-supported rehabilitation procedure, with stable results over a period of two years.

1. Introduction

Tooth loss causes alveolar bone resorption that often limits implant placement. In the superior maxilla, this process is associated with the pneumatization of the sinus [1–3].

Since the 60s, numerous surgical techniques have been proposed for the regeneration of maxillary bone defects. When the residual bone height is inadequate for implant placement, in case of favorable prosthetical spaces, a sinus lift is considered a safe procedure with predictable results [4–10]. Implant placement is contraindicated if the residual bone height is less than 5 mm [11].

Current treatment options for bone defects include autologous, homologous, xenologous, and allogenous grafts; artificial bone substitutes can be synthetic or bioceramic cements or a blend of two or more materials [12]. Although several studies have been conducted to identify the best graft material for sinus floor augmentation, a final consensus has not been reached [4]. Autologous bone grafts represent the gold

standard graft material because these exhibit osteoinductive, osteoconductive, and osteogenic properties. However, the use of this material remains limited owing to rapid resorption, collection of inadequate amounts of tissue if harvested intraorally, donor site morbidity, and high biologic cost [13]. Alternatively, the alloplastic bone substitutes and the xenologous bone show high availability, biocompatibility, and good mechanical support and also have adequate porosity that allows for penetration of blood capillaries, which is essential for the supply of oxygen, nutrients, and growth factors [14–19]. However, these bone substitutes are limited by the fact that they do not carry osteogenic cells and osteoinductive molecules, which are important for tissue regeneration [20–23].

In the last twenty years, researchers have shown renewed interest in developing new regeneration methods. Researchers are particularly focusing on mesenchymal stem cells because they represent a self-renewable reservoir of cells that can proliferate and differentiate at the same time.

CRANEX D

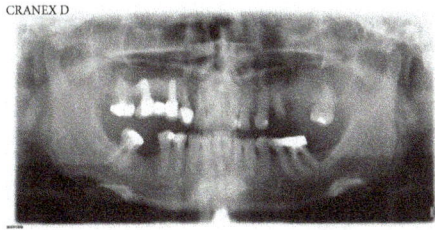

FIGURE 1: Preoperative panoramic radiograph of the patient.

Thus, if correctly transplanted, mesenchymal stem cells are able to regenerate a particular tissue [24–28].

Unfortunately, stem cell therapies require both highly developed technologies and methods, which are not yet allowed to be used in many countries (e.g., laboratory handling of stem cells to produce tissues). Moreover, a few researchers have reported that stem cell therapies could increase the risk for tumor growth [29–34].

Recently, a class I medical device (Rigeneracons®, Human Brain Wave S.R.L., Torino, Italy) has been introduced in clinical practice in order to disaggregate a portion of tissue and obtain 50 μm viable micrografts full of progenitor cells, while maintaining their regenerative and differentiation potentials. These micrografts can be obtained from a sample of autologous connective tissue few millimeters in length, which is harvested directly during the surgery, even from the same surgical site, and can be immediately used without any handling or cell culture [35].

The aim of this report is to present a clinical case in which autologous micrografts with a high percentage of progenitor cells were seeded on a PLGA hydroxyapatite- (HA-) enriched scaffold for a sinus floor lift augmentation procedure and to present the histological features shown by the sample collected at the implant site and the radiographic aspect obtained three years after the lift procedure.

2. Case Report

2.1. Materials and Methods. The procedure discussed in this case report was performed at the Department of Clinical Surgical, Diagnostic and Paediatric Sciences, University of Pavia, Italy, and the procedure was approved by the University Ethics Committee (recorded March 2014).

A 52-year-old woman, with a good health status (ASA score: 0), was enrolled for the study; written informed consent was obtained from the patient to have the case details and any accompanying images anonymously published. She was indicated for a prosthetic implant rehabilitation procedure in the second quadrant after a maxillary sinus lift procedure for atrophy of the maxillary bone at the bicuspid and molar level (1 mm residual bone crest height) in order to collect enough bone to install two endosseous implants (Figures 1 and 2).

The patient was prepared for the surgery with scaling and root planning two weeks prior to the sinus floor lift. The surgery was performed under antibiotic prophylaxis: amoxicillin plus clavulanic acid (Augmentin, GlaxoSmithKline S.p.A., Verona, Italy), 2 gr 1 hour before the surgery. For the

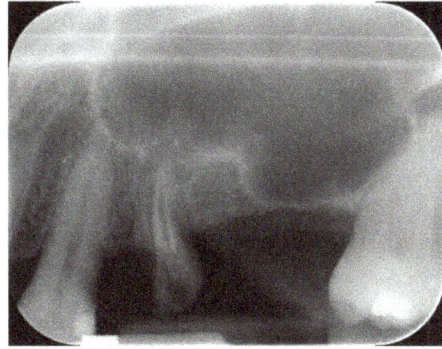

FIGURE 2: Intraoral radiograph (Rinn® collimator) of the surgery site.

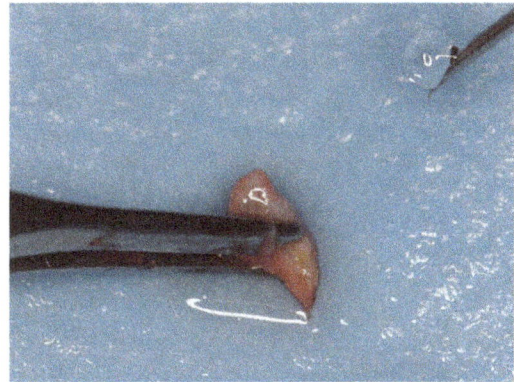

FIGURE 3: Connective tissue collected directly from the surgery site.

local anesthesia, articain 4% with 1/200000 epinephrine was used.

A full-thickness flap was lifted via mesial and distal relief incisions. From the palatal flap, a 3 mm periosteal sample was harvested and then washed with a sterile saline solution. Then, it was inserted in the Rigeneracons filter with 1 ml of sterile saline for the disaggregation process (Figures 3 and 4).

Tissue graft disaggregation was performed for 2 minutes at 70 rpm and 15 Ncm torque, and the cell suspension was withdrawn with a sterile syringe and added to the PLGA-HA scaffold (Alos®, Allmed srl, Lissone, MB, Italy) in order to be grafted into the new subantral cavity (Figure 5). In the meantime, the receiving site was prepared according to the standard protocol used for lateral sinus floor augmentation (Figure 6) [11, 14]. The wall osteotomy was performed with Piezosurgery® (Mectron S.p.A., Carasco, GE, Italy) using an OT5 insert. A resorbable membrane (Bio-Gide®, Geistlich Pharma AG, Wolhusen, Switzerland) was positioned in the newly formed subantral cavity to preserve the sinus membrane, and the space was then filled with the blend of PLGA and micrograft (Figures 6 and 7). The bone window was covered with collagen sponges (Gingistat®, Pierre Rolland Pharmaceutical, Merignac, Aquitaine, France) soaked in the cell suspension and a resorbable membrane (Bio-Gide, Geistlich Pharma, Wolhusen, Switzerland) (Figure 8). The flap was sutured with a 4-0 PTFE suture (Omnia S.p.A, Fidenza, PR, Italy).

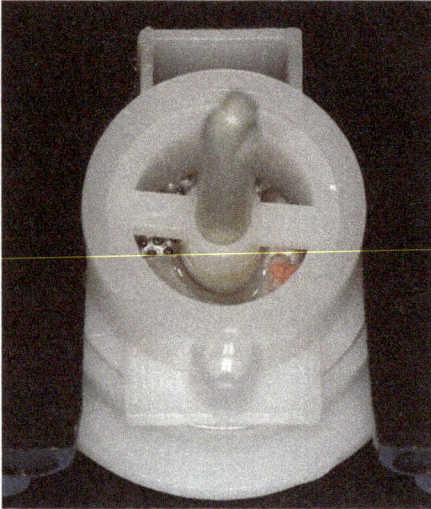

FIGURE 4: Tissue graft disaggregation with the Rigeneracons device, according to the manufacturer's instructions: 1 ml of sterile saline solution, performed for 120 seconds with implant contra-angle at 15 NCm and 70 rpm.

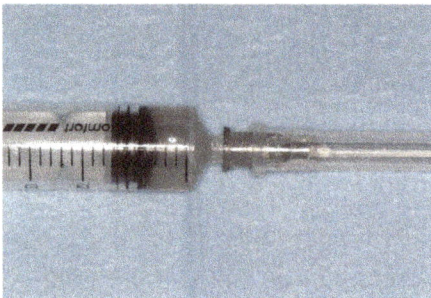

FIGURE 5: The syringe with progenitor cell-enriched suspension obtained via the periosteum disaggregation process.

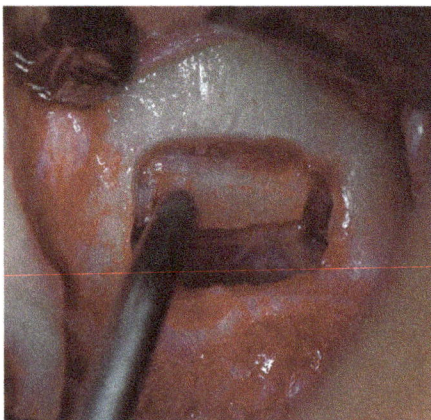

FIGURE 6: The window elevation.

During the postoperative period, the patient received antibiotic therapy (1 gr every 12 hours of amoxicillin + clavulanic acid for 7 days) and performed oral rinses with chlorhexidine 0.2% (Curasept®, Curaden Healthcare S.p.A.,

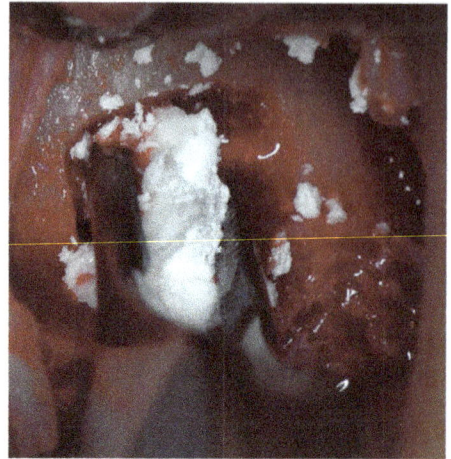

FIGURE 7: The biocomplex graft placement in the maxillary sinus, under the Schneider membrane.

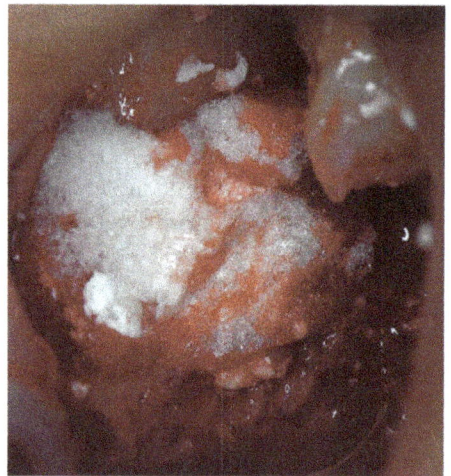

FIGURE 8: Covering the osteotomy access with collagen and resorbable membrane.

Saronno, VA, Italy), 3 times/day for 30 days, and she was administered nonsteroidal anti-inflammatory drugs (NSAIDs) if needed.

The healing was uneventful and the sutures were removed after 2 weeks.

At 4 months after the surgery, following a cone-beam CT examination demonstrating a good level of bone regeneration, a mucoperiosteal flap was elevated and two bone tissue carrots 3 mm in diameter were harvested from the implant sites using a trephine bur. Two 3.8 × 9 mm implants were installed (Camlog® Promote® Plus, Camlog Biotechnologies AG, Basel, Switzerland) according to the standard protocol [36]. The insertion torque was 25 N/cm. The mucosal flap covered the fixtures during the healing phase, and the sutures were removed after 10 days. No adverse events occurred (Figure 9).

The collected tissues were fixed in a 10% formalin solution and then prepared for microscopic observation in order to determine the ossification grade (Figure 10). Paraffin-embedded tissue sections were cut into 5 μm-thick slices,

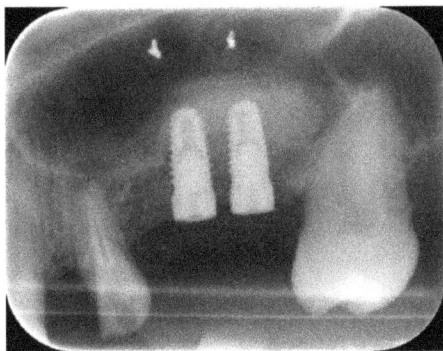

FIGURE 9: Radiograph taken postimplantation.

following which the paraffin slices were immersed in xylene and then in decreasing grades of ethanol (100% to 75%) and deionized water for deparaffinizing and rehydrating the sections. Subsequently, the slide sections were stained with hematoxylin for 1-2 minutes and rinsed in cold water to remove excess stain. The sections were then stained with eosin for 4-5 minutes and rinsed under running tap water. The tissue sections were then immersed in increasing grades of ethanol (from 50% to 100%), and finally after an immersion in xylene, they were coverslipped with a mounting medium. Histological analyses demonstrated that the combination of micrografts with the PLGA scaffold allowed the ossification process. In fact, at 40x magnification (Figure 10(b)), lamellar bone formation was observed, as seen by the presence of a typical Haversian system with the deposition of a calcified matrix.

8 weeks after the implant installation, the following standard prosthetic procedures were performed: implant impression, abutment and structure proof, and cemented prosthesis delivery.

After three years, during the follow-up visit [37], radiographs were taken, which demonstrated an excellent stability of the graft and of the regenerated bone and the success of the rehabilitation (Figure 11).

3. Discussion

Usually, a bone graft is the first therapeutic option in cases where the amount of bone is inadequate for implant installation. Autologous bone is considered the gold standard in sinus augmentation procedures but exposes to donor site morbidity. With the Rigenera protocol, the amount of tissue harvested is very little and the donor site is the surgical site itself, thus minimizing the risk of morbidity. In the presented clinical case, healing was uneventful and no sign of tissue harvesting resituated in the palatal flap. The authors did not observe any differences in postoperative soft tissue healing and patient morbidity with respect to the standard procedure due to soft tissue harvesting from the palatal flap. Synthetic materials exhibit a good capability to regenerate an adequate amount of bone, but they do not exhibit the osteoinductive and osteogenic properties needed for bone regeneration. Furthermore, some of these materials show a

lack of resorbability even after years from the time of production. This is the reason why the field of bone tissue engineering has focused on techniques such as the use of mesenchymal stem cells [38]. Although many reports suggest that stem cell-based tissue engineering is beneficial, general critiques of cell therapy approaches have included the lack of characterization of the cellular component of the graft [27]. Previous evaluation of micrografts produced by the Rigenera protocol indicated that these cells are positive to mesenchymal cell line markers and negative to hematopoietic and macrophage markers. In fact, cell characterization performed by FACS was positive for several mesenchymal cell markers, including CD90, CD105, and CD73, and negative for CD45 and CD14. Moreover, the Rigenera protocol demonstrated to be able to produce in a few minutes (about 2 min) a cell suspension containing millions of viable cells with a cutoff of $50 \mu m$, opportunely selected by filtration [35]. The behavior of these cells is not clearly known yet, and it could present some risks. However, many studies regarding this topic are being conducted and some researchers have also proposed to use patients' mesenchymal cell micrograft directly, so that the patient is the donor and the receiver at the same time.

A licit criticism related to the use of MSC in a therapeutic procedure is that the graft cell population is composed of nonclonal stromal cells containing stem cells, progenitor cells, and differentiated mesodermal cells, including fibroblasts, and that the advantages connected to their use are more related to their important role in modulating inflammation compared to any stem cell activity [39].

It was demonstrated that micrografts obtained by the Rigenera protocol are able to maintain the osteogenic and regenerative properties because of the content of the progenitor cells [35, 38]. In fact, histological analysis also suggested that the Rigenera protocol facilitates ossification process in the surgical site. In Figure 10, hematoxylin/eosin staining showed the formation of a new bone at 4 months after the maxillary sinus lift procedure, suggesting that the combination of the appropriate biomaterials and the micrografts accelerated the bone-healing process. In particular, the histological analysis showed the presence of bone lamellae, which are concentric rings of bone, surrounding a central channel, or the Haversian canal, containing nerves, blood vessels, and lymph (Figures 10(a) and 10(b)). These lamellae are produced by osteoblasts that secrete extracellular bone matrix with collagen fibers and inorganic phosphate.

The sinus lift surgery performed in this case was associated with a resorbable scaffold HA enriched with progenitor cell micrograft, which was harvested from the palatal periosteum. In particular, the small tissue sample was derived directly from the surgery flap, so the biologic cost was very low.

The scaffold is important to provide the stability and mechanical resistance required to maintain the viability of the cells. Different types of osteoconductive materials could be used as scaffolds. In this case, we chose the PLGA HA-enriched scaffold, which was completely resorbable, as PLGA without HA, but also offered more stability to the graft because of the presence of hydroxyapatite. The micrografts,

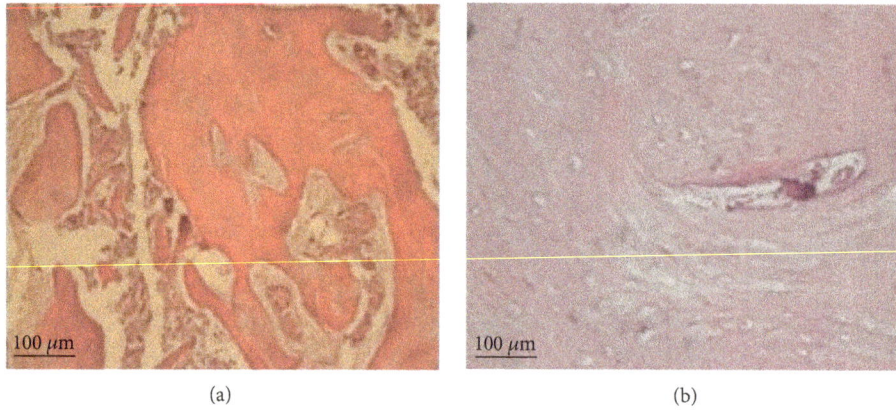

(a)   (b)

FIGURE 10: Hematoxylin/eosin staining of samples at 4 months (a, b) after grafting with the Rigenera system. (a) 10x magnification, (b) 40x magnification.

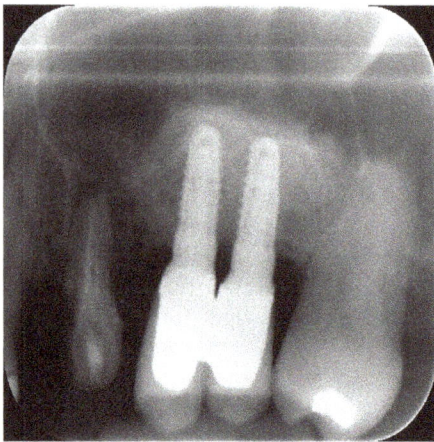

FIGURE 11: Intraoral radiograph taken after 3 years.

compared with the other bone grafts, are effective in the regeneration of bone required for implant surgery and are capable of supporting long-term prosthetical load [40, 41].

4. Conclusion

This case illustrates that the use of autologous micrografts, which are rich in progenitor cells, in the sinus floor lift procedure is effective in regenerating an adequate amount of bone tissue, with both excellent implant stability and minimum biological sacrifice.

Abbreviations

PLGA: Poly lactic-co-glycolic acid
NSAID: Nonsteroidal anti-inflammatory drugs
ASA: The American Society of Anesthesiologists.

References

[1] M. Peleg, Z. Mazor, and A. K. Garg, "Augmentation grafting of the maxillary sinus and simultaneous implant placement in patients with 3 to 5 mm of residual alveolar bone height,"

The International Journal of Oral & Maxillofacial Implants, vol. 14, no. 4, pp. 549–556, 1999.

[2] G. Tawil and M. Mawla, "Sinus floor elevation using a bovine bone mineral (Bio-Oss) with or without the concomitant use of a bilayered collagen barrier (Bio-Gide): a clinical report of immediate and delayed implant placement," *The International Journal of Oral & Maxillofacial Implants*, vol. 16, no. 5, pp. 713–721, 2001.

[3] M. J. Kim, U. W. Jung, C. S. Kim et al., "Maxillary sinus septa: prevalence, height, location, and morphology. A reformatted computed tomography scan analysis," *Journal of Periodontology*, vol. 77, no. 5, pp. 903–908, 2006.

[4] O. T. Jensen, L. B. Shulman, M. S. Block, and V. J. Iacono, "Report of the Sinus Consensus Conference of 1996," *The International Journal of Oral & Maxillofacial Implants*, vol. 13, pp. 11–45, 1998.

[5] S. S. Wallace and S. J. Froum, "Effect of maxillary sinus augmentation on the survival of endosseous dental implants. A systematic review," *Annals of Periodontology*, vol. 8, no. 1, pp. 328–343, 2003.

[6] M. Del Fabbro, T. Testori, L. Francetti, and R. Weinstein, "Systematic review of survival rates for implants placed in the grafted maxillary sinus," *The International Journal of Periodontics & Restorative Dentistry*, vol. 24, no. 6, pp. 565–577, 2004.

[7] M. Piattelli, G. A. Favero, A. Scarano, G. Orsini, and A. Piattelli, "Bone reactions to anorganic bovine bone (Bio-Oss) used in sinus augmentation procedures: a histologic long-term report of 20 cases in humans," *The International Journal of Oral & Maxillofacial Implants*, vol. 14, no. 6, pp. 835–840, 1999.

[8] P. Valentini, D. Abensur, B. Wenz, M. Peetz, and R. Schenk, "Sinus grafting with porous bone mineral (Bio-Oss) for implant placement: a 5-year study on 15 patients," *The International Journal of Periodontics & Restorative Dentistry*, vol. 20, no. 3, pp. 245–253, 2000.

[9] M. Yildirim, H. Spiekermann, S. Biesterfeld, and D. Edelhoff, "Maxillary sinus augmentation using xenogenic bone substitute material Bio-Oss® in combination with venous blood. A histologic and histomorphometric study in humans," *Clinical Oral Implants Research*, vol. 11, no. 3, pp. 217–229, 2000.

[10] M. Hallman, A. Cederlund, S. Lindskog, S. Lundgren, and L. Sennerby, "A clinical histologic study of bovine hydroxyapatite in combination with autogenous bone and fibrin glue for

maxillary sinus floor augmentation. Results after 6 to 8 months of healing," *Clinical Oral Implants Research*, vol. 12, no. 2, pp. 135–143, 2001.

[11] M. Chiapasco, M. Zaniboni, and L. Rimondini, "Dental implants placed in grafted maxillary sinuses: a retrospective analysis of clinical outcome according to the initial clinical situation and a proposal of defect classification," *Clinical Oral Implants Research*, vol. 19, no. 4, pp. 416–428, 2008.

[12] G. Ceccarelli, R. Presta, L. Benedetti, M. G. Cusella de Angelis, S. M. Lupi, and R. Rodriguez y Baena, "Emerging perspectives in scaffold for tissue engineering in oral surgery," *Stem Cells International*, vol. 2017, Article ID 4585401, 11 pages, 2017.

[13] C. J. Damien and J. R. Parsons, "Bone graft and bone graft substitutes: a review of current technology and applications," *Journal of Applied Biomaterials*, vol. 2, no. 3, pp. 187–208, 1991.

[14] S. Scaglione, P. Giannoni, P. Bianchini et al., "Order versus disorder: in vivo bone formation within osteoconductive scaffolds," *Scientific Reports*, vol. 2, no. 1, p. 274, 2012.

[15] D. Bollati, M. Morra, C. Cassinelli, S. M. Lupi, and R. Rodriguez y Baena, "In vitro cytokine expression and in vivo healing and inflammatory response to a collagen-coated synthetic bone filler," *BioMed Research International*, vol. 2016, Article ID 6427681, 10 pages, 2016.

[16] R. Rodriguez y Baena, S. M. Lupi, R. Pastorino, C. Maiorana, A. Lucchese, and S. Rizzo, "Radiographic evaluation of regenerated bone following poly(lactic-co-glycolic) acid/hydroxyapatite and deproteinized bovine bone graft in sinus lifting," *The Journal of Craniofacial Surgery*, vol. 24, no. 3, pp. 845–848, 2013.

[17] R. R. Betz, "Limitations of autograft and allograft: new synthetic solutions," *Orthopedics*, vol. 25, no. 5, pp. s561–s570, 2002.

[18] C. G. Finkemeier, "Bone-grafting and bone-graft substitutes," *The Journal of Bone & Joint Surgery*, vol. 84, no. 3, pp. 454–464, 2002.

[19] R. Rodriguez y Baena, R. Pastorino, E. Gherlone, L. Perillo, S. Saturnino, and A. Lucchese, "Histomorphometric evaluation of two different bone substitutes in sinus augmentation procedures: a randomized controlled trial in humans," *The International Journal of Oral & Maxillofacial Implants*, vol. 32, no. 1, pp. 188–194, 2017.

[20] Z. Zhang, "Bone regeneration by stem cell and tissue engineering in oral and maxillofacial region," *Frontiers in Medicine*, vol. 5, no. 4, pp. 401–413, 2011.

[21] S. P. Bruder and B. S. Fox, "Tissue engineering of bone. Cell based strategies," *Clinical Orthopaedics and Related Research*, vol. 367, pp. S68–S83, 1999.

[22] G. J. Meijer, J. D. de Bruijn, R. Koole, and C. A. van Blitterswijk, "Cell-based bone tissue engineering," *PLoS Medicine*, vol. 4, no. 2, article e9, 2007.

[23] R. Schmelzeisen, R. Schimming, and M. Sittinger, "Making bone: implant insertion into tissue-engineered bone for maxillary sinus floor augmentation—a preliminary report," *Journal of Cranio-Maxillo-Facial Surgery*, vol. 31, no. 1, pp. 34–39, 2003.

[24] D. Baksh, L. Song, and R. S. Tuan, "Adult mesenchymal stem cells: characterization, differentiation, and application in cell and gene therapy," *Journal of Cellular and Molecular Medicine*, vol. 8, no. 3, pp. 301–316, 2004.

[25] P. Bianco and P. G. Robey, "Stem cells in tissue engineering," *Nature*, vol. 414, no. 6859, pp. 118–121, 2001.

[26] M. F. Pittenger, A. M. Mackay, S. C. Beck et al., "Multilineage potential of adult human mesenchymal stem cells," *Science*, vol. 284, no. 5411, pp. 143–147, 1999.

[27] H. Egusa, W. Sonoyama, M. Nishimura, I. Atsuta, and K. Akiyama, "Stem cells in dentistry – part II: clinical applications," *Journal of Prosthodontic Research*, vol. 56, no. 4, pp. 229–248, 2012.

[28] G. Ceccarelli, R. Presta, S. Lupi et al., "Evaluation of poly(lactic-co-glycolic) acid alone or in combination with hydroxyapatite on human-periosteal cells bone differentiation and in sinus lift treatment," *Molecules*, vol. 22, no. 12, 2017.

[29] M. Battiwalla and P. Hematti, "Mesenchymal stem cells in hematopoietic stem cell transplantation," *Cytotherapy*, vol. 11, no. 5, pp. 503–515, 2009.

[30] G. Lucchini, M. Introna, E. Dander et al., "Platelet-lysate-expanded mesenchymal stromal cells as a salvage therapy for severe resistant graft-versus-host disease in a pediatric population," *Biology of Blood and Marrow Transplantation*, vol. 16, no. 9, pp. 1293–1301, 2010.

[31] A. Giordano, U. Galderisi, and I. R. Marino, "From the laboratory bench to the patient's bedside: an update on clinical trials with mesenchymal stem cells," *Journal of Cellular Physiology*, vol. 211, no. 1, pp. 27–35, 2007.

[32] R. Pal, N. K. Venkataramana, A. Bansal et al., "Ex vivo-expanded autologous bone marrow-derived mesenchymal stromal cells in human spinal cord injury/paraplegia: a pilot clinical study," *Cytotherapy*, vol. 11, no. 7, pp. 897–911, 2009.

[33] L. Sun, K. Akiyama, H. Zhang et al., "Mesenchymal stem cell transplantation reverses multiorgan dysfunction in systemic lupus erythematosus mice and humans," *Stem Cells*, vol. 27, no. 6, pp. 1421–1432, 2009.

[34] S. G. Hong, T. Winkler, C. Wu et al., "Path to the clinic: assessment of iPSC-based cell therapies in vivo in a nonhuman primate model," *Cell Reports*, vol. 7, no. 4, pp. 1298–1309, 2014.

[35] L. Trovato, M. Monti, C. del Fante et al., "A new medical device Rigeneracons allows to obtain viable micro-grafts from mechanical disaggregation of human tissues," *Journal of Cellular Physiology*, vol. 230, no. 10, pp. 2299–2303, 2015.

[36] S. Rizzo, P. Zampetti, R. Rodriguez Y Baena, D. Svanosio, and S. M. Lupi, "Retrospective analysis of 521 endosseous implants placed under antibiotic prophylaxis and review of literature," *Minerva Stomatologica*, vol. 59, no. 3, pp. 75–88, 2010.

[37] S. M. Lupi, M. Granati, A. Butera, V. Collesano, and R. Rodriguez Y Baena, "Air-abrasive debridement with glycine powder versus manual debridement and chlorhexidine administration for the maintenance of peri-implant health status: a six-month randomized clinical trial," *International Journal of Dental Hygiene*, vol. 15, no. 4, pp. 287–294, 2017.

[38] R. d'Aquino, L. Trovato, A. Graziano et al., "Periosteum-derived micro-grafts for tissue regeneration of human maxillary bone," *Journal of Translational Science*, vol. 2, no. 2, pp. 125–129, 2016.

[39] U. Galderisi and A. Giordano, "The gap between the physiological and therapeutic roles of mesenchymal stem cells," *Medicinal Research Reviews*, vol. 34, no. 5, pp. 1100–1126, 2014.

[40] D. Zaffe, R. Rodriguez y Baena, S. Rizzo et al., "Behavior of the bone-titanium interface after push-in testing: a morphological study," *Journal of Biomedical Materials Research*, vol. 64A, no. 2, pp. 365–371, 2003.

[41] R. Rodriguez y Baena, D. Zaffe, U. E. Pazzaglia, and S. Rizzo, "Morphology of peri-implant regenerated bone, in sheep's tibia, by means of guided tissue regeneration," *Minerva Stomatologica*, vol. 47, no. 12, pp. 673–687, 1998.

16

Single Sitting Surgical Treatment of Generalized Aggressive Periodontitis Using GTR Technique and Immediate Implant Placement with 10-Year Follow-Up

Fatme Mouchref Hamasni🄳, Fady El Hajj, and Rima Abdallah

Department of Periodontology, Faculty of Dental Medicine, Lebanese University, Hadath, Lebanon

Correspondence should be addressed to Fatme Mouchref Hamasni; fatmehamsni@gmail.com

Academic Editor: Sukumaran Anil

This case report exhibits a patient with generalized aggressive periodontitis who has been under maintenance for the past 12 years after being surgically treated in a single sitting and restored with dental implants. A 41-year-old systemically healthy male patient presented complaining of lower anterior teeth mobility and pain in the upper right quadrant. After clinical and radiographic examination, the upper right molars and lower anterior incisors were deemed unrestorable. Covered by doxycycline, the patient received a nonsurgical periodontal treatment. Three weeks later, teeth extraction, immediate implant placement, immediate nonloading provisional prosthesis, and a guided tissue regeneration were performed at indicated areas in a single sitting. The clinical decisions were based on patient compliance, the status of the existing periodontal tissues, and the prognosis of the remaining teeth. During the 12-year follow-up period, no residual pockets were observed and there was no exacerbation of the inflammatory condition. Marginal bone stability is present on all implants. For aggressive periodontal disease, a high risk of relapse as well as limited success and survival of dental implants should be considered. This case shows proper containment of the disease based on appropriate treatment planning and a strict maintenance program.

1. Introduction

In 1999, the term "aggressive periodontitis" (AgP) was introduced by the American Academy of Periodontology (AAP) to define a group of destructive periodontal diseases with a rapid progression. This definition was used to include previous terminologies of early-onset periodontitis, juvenile periodontitis, and rapidly progressive periodontitis, using "aggressive" nomenclature [1]. The emphasis was placed on the rapidity of progression, rather than on the age of onset (destruction is 2–5 times faster than in chronic periodontitis with an attachment loss of 4 to 5 micrometers per day) and perhaps also on the difficulty of maintaining it.

Lang et al. [2] classified the disease into localized and generalized forms. According to this report, the authors concluded that there are common features in both the localized and generalized forms of aggressive periodontitis. All symptoms can occur at any age in patients who follow regular dental care. A familial factor is present, and there is a possibility of self-arresting progression of attachment loss (AL) and bone loss.

Microbiological criteria were not mentioned as primary features separating chronic from aggressive periodontitis. However, for AgP, the secondary features that are generally, but not universally, present included elevated proportions of *Aggregatibacter actinomycetemcomitan* (AA) and, in some populations, *Porphyromonas gingivalis* (Pg), phagocyte abnormalities, and a hyper-responsive macrophage phenotype, including elevated levels of prostaglandin E2 and interleukin-1beta.

The following additional specific features were proposed for defining the localized and generalized forms. Localized aggressive periodontitis is usually circumpubertal onset,

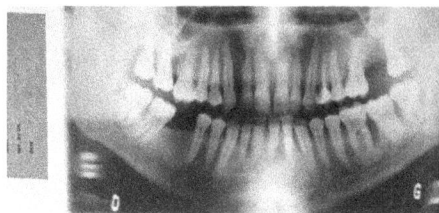

FIGURE 1: Preoperative panoramic X-ray showing generalized bone loss and missing teeth 27 and 46.

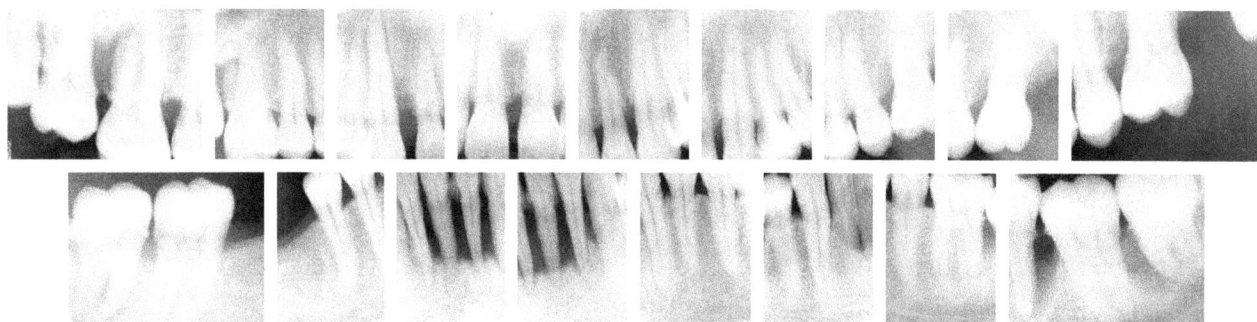

FIGURE 2: Full mouth periapical X-rays showing severe bone loss at lower anterior sextant and vertical bone loss at 13 and 37.

localized to first molar and incisor presentation with interproximal attachment loss on at least two permanent teeth (one of which is a first molar) and involving no more than two teeth other than first molars and incisors. Generalized aggressive periodontitis usually affects adult persons between 20 and 30 years of age, but patients may be older. There is generalized interproximal attachment loss affecting at least three permanent teeth other than first molars and incisors. The disease has a pronounced episodic nature of the destruction of attachment and alveolar bone with a history of relapse.

Although success in implant dentistry depends on marginal bone stability and health, patient systemic factors and susceptibility to periodontal diseases play a role in achieving long-term stability.

Many studies have shown the negative effect of previously treated and untreated periodontal disease on marginal bone stability around implants, including higher frequency of mucositis and peri-implantitis and lower success and survival rates of implants placed in patients with history of chronic or aggressive periodontitis [3–12].

Swierkot et al. [13] reported in a prospective study with a follow-up period of 5–16 years that GAgP patients had five times greater risk of implant failure, three times greater risk of mucositis, and 14 times greater risk of peri-implantitis.

This case report exhibits a 41-year-old systemically healthy male patient with GAgP who has been maintained for the past 12 years after being treated periodontally in a single sitting and restored with dental implants. He has been compliant for 10 years with supportive and maintenance therapy since the conclusion of his treatment in 2007.

2. Case Presentation

2.1. Patient History and Chief Complaint. An engineer living abroad sought a second opinion at our office in 2005.

The patient's oral surgeon had previously recommended extraction and immediate implantation of all compromised teeth including any tooth with a vertical defect. He sought an alternative treatment option after being shocked that at only 41 years of age, the only treatment will be losing 16 of his teeth. The patient's chief complaint was that he is not able to bite on his front teeth and that his esthetics are compromised due too increased crown length.

2.2. Initial Assessment. Diagnostics included radiographic examination (Figures 1 and 2) and a thorough clinical examination. Probing was done at the affected sites, and it was noted that there was probing depth of more than 10 mm at 11 sites and between 6 and 9 mm at 6 sites. He was missing teeth number 27 and 46.

A conventional supra gingival scaling and subgingival root planing was performed under the coverage of antibiotics having a significant action against AA (doxycycline (Doxylag)® 100 mg 2 tabs first day and 1 tab daily for 21 days) [14, 15] and a chlorohexidine mouth wash (0.1% chlorohexidine and 0.5% chlorobutanol) for a period of 14 days to assess the periodontal tissue response and to stabilize the condition. This initial assessment led to the establishment of the prognosis for the remaining teeth and identification of those that could not be treated. The patient returned for definitive treatment after 3 weeks.

2.3. Surgical Treatment. Upon the patients' return, teeth 18, 17, and 16 all had class III furcation involvement with grade 3 mobility; they were extracted under full thickness flap allowing visibility of a 3-wall defect of 10 mm at the mesial of tooth number 13 which was then treated with guided tissue regeneration technique using bovine xenograft bone substitute Bioss® and resorbable collagen membrane Resolute®.

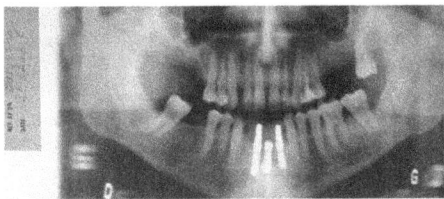

FIGURE 3: Panoramic X-ray after 3 months of first visit showing bone formation at the site of extracted molars and bone stability around Straumann mandibular implants.

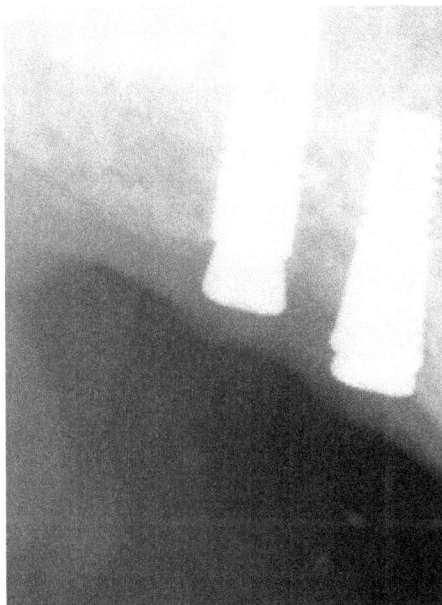

FIGURE 4: Astra* implants (4.5 × 11, 4.0 × 11) replacing teeth 16 and 17.

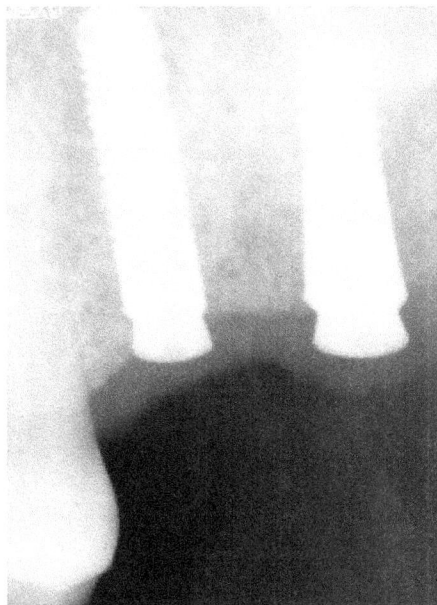

FIGURE 5: Astra* implants (4.0 × 13, 5 × 11) replacing teeth 26 and 27.

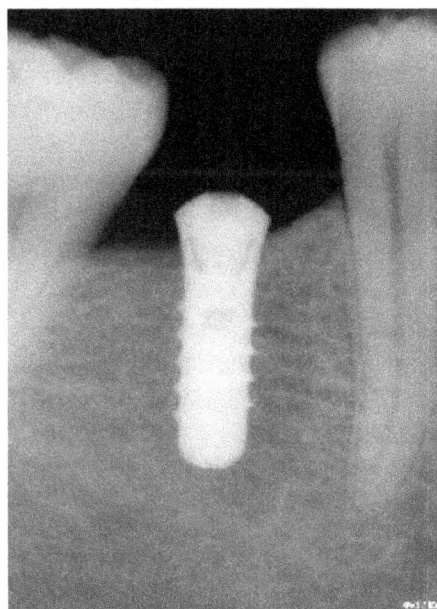

FIGURE 6: Straumann (4.1 × 10) replacing tooth 46.

At the same visit, extraction of tooth number 26 was performed as it presented with a 9 and 10 mm bone loss at the mesial and distal sites, respectively, with a class III furcation involvement.

At the lower right quadrant, tooth number 48 was extracted, and scaling and root planing was performed at the distal of tooth number 47 which presented with a wide shallow bony defect.

At the lower left quadrant, extraction of tooth number 38 was done, and the full thickness flap showed a narrow and deep bone defect until the apex of tooth number 46 distally maintaining the mesial bone peak at tooth number 47 which presented as well with a wide moderate bone defect distally. Scaling and root planing was done, due to the contained geometry of the defect on the 46; the bone substitute Bioss was used as a filling materiel, without the need for a membrane.

Teeth 32, 31, 42, and 41 were extracted and immediately replaced with 3 narrow neck SLA Straumann dental implants (3.3 × 12 mm at site 41 and 31 and 3.3 × 10 mm at site 32). The choice of cantilevering was based on the presence of a wide intrabony defect surrounding tooth number 42; immediate nonloading temporization was provided on implants number 41 and 32 to maintain the esthetic appearance.

No provisional prosthesis was delivered for molar areas, and an association of amoxicillin 500 mg and metronidazole 250 mg was prescribed 3 times a day for 8 days [16].

Almost 5 months later, the clinical exam showed a perfect soft tissue integrity, and the radiographic evaluation revealed total bone formation at the site of extracted molars and bone stability around Straumann mandibular implants (Figure 3). Four osseospeed Astra* implants were used in the maxilla replacing the first and second molars: (4.5 × 11 mm, 4.0 × 11 mm) implants were inserted on the right side, and (4.0 × 13 mm, 5.0 × 11 mm) implants on the left side (Figures 4 and 5). One Straumann SLA tissue level

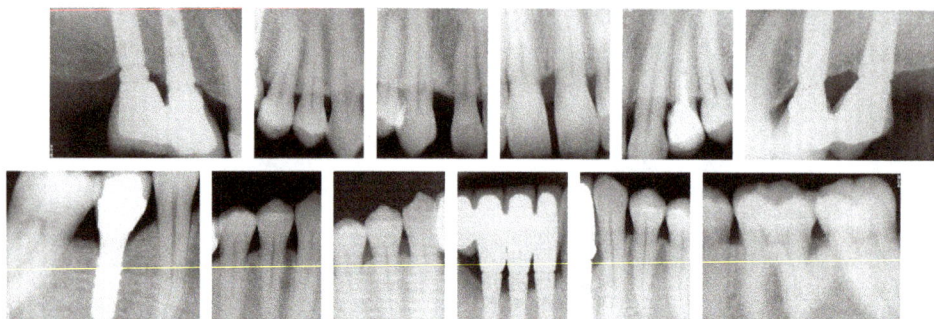

FIGURE 7: Radiographic evaluation 10 years after prosthesis insertion.

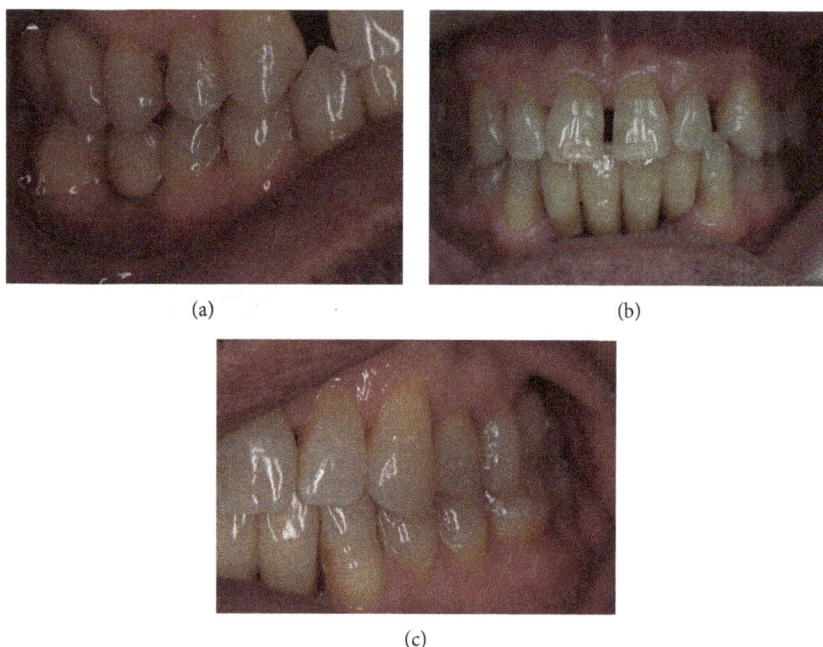

(a)

(b)

(c)

FIGURE 8: Clinical photos 12 years after periodontal surgery and 10 years after final implant prothesis.

implant (4.1 ×10 mm) was inserted to replace tooth 46 (Figure 6).

The patient could not return until 16 months after the implant surgery, and for the realization of final fixed prosthesis, all prosthesis were delivered within 10 days and the case was documented radiographically and clinically and follow-up maintenance program was scheduled after this visit.

2.4. Maintenance and Supportive Therapy. The patient is placed on a strict maintenance schedule; prophylaxis is performed every 3 to 6 months and periapical follow-up radiographs are done every year to follow-up on the surgical sites. During the 12 year follow-up period, no residual pockets were observed, and there was no exacerbation of the inflammatory condition. Marginal bone stability is present on all implants. Since the case was done, there was no need for the adjunct use of antibacterial mouth rinses or systemic antibiotic use (Figures 7 and 8).

3. Discussion

The high risk of relapse as well as limited success and survival rate of dental implants is considered as a severe complication related to aggressive periodontal disease, and this case showed a perfect bone stability, after guided tissue regeneration and around implants, over 10 years after treatment without any sign of inflammation, and the stability of such results is maybe related to the strict supportive therapy program or the choice of doing full mouth surgery in one day which may assure the complete eradication of bacteria and prevent the contamination of treated areas when surgeries are usually done at variable intervals. To the best of our knowledge, this is the first case report treating surgically a case of generalized aggressive periodontitis with GTR and immediate implantation in one single day. The successful treatment is maybe related to the choice of the treatment; however, additional clinical studies with more patients are necessary in order to support this choice.

References

[1] G. C. Armitage, "Development of a classification system for periodontal diseases and conditions," *Annals of Periodontology*, vol. 4, no. 1, pp. 1–6, 1999.

[2] N. Lang, P. M. Bartold, M. Cullinan et al., "Consensus report–aggressive periodontitis," *Annals of Periodontology*, vol. 4, no. 1, p. 53, 1999.

[3] A. Mombelli, M. Marxer, T. Gaberthuel, U. Grunder, and N. P. Lang, "The microbiota of osseointegrated implants in patients with a history of periodontal disease," *Journal of Clinical Periodontology*, vol. 22, pp. 124–130, 1995.

[4] M. Quirynen, M. De Soete, and D. van Steenberghe, "Infectious risks for oral implants: a review of the literature," *Clinical Oral Implants Research*, vol. 2, no. 13, pp. 1–19, 2002.

[5] M. Quirynen, M. Abarca, N. Van Assche, M. Nevins, and D. Van Steenberghe, "Impact of supportive periodontal therapy and implant surface roughness on implant outcome in patients with a history of periodontitis," *Journal of Clinical Periodontology*, vol. 34, no. 9, pp. 805–815, 2007.

[6] I. K. Karoussis, S. Muller, G. E. Salvi, L. J. Heitz-Mayfield, U. Bragger, and N. P. Lang, "Association between periodontal and peri-implant conditions: a 10-year prospective study," *Clinical Oral Implants Research*, vol. 15, no. 1, pp. 1–7, 2004.

[7] I. K. Karoussis, S. Kotsovilis, and I. Fourmousis, "A comprehensive and critical review of dental implant prognosis in periodontally compromised partially edentulous patients," *Clinical Oral Implants Research*, vol. 18, no. 6, pp. 669–679, 2007.

[8] J. M. Albandar and E. M. Tinoco, "Global epidemiology of periodontal diseases in children and young persons," *Periodontology 2000*, vol. 29, no. 1, pp. 153–176, 2002.

[9] J. M. Albandar, "Aggressive periodontitis: case definition and diagnostic criteria," *Periodontology 2000*, vol. 65, no. 1, pp. 13–26, 2014.

[10] S. Schou, P. Holmstrup, H. V. Worthington, and M. Esposito, "Outcome of implant therapy in patients with previous tooth loss due to periodontitis," *Clinical Oral Implants Research*, vol. 17, no. 2, pp. 104–123, 2006.

[11] S. Matarasso, G. Rasperini, S. V. Iotio, G. E. Salvi, N. P. Lang, and M. Aglietta, "A 10-year retrospective analysis of radiographic bone-level changes of implants supporting single-unit crowns in periodontally compromised vs. periodontally healthy patients," *Clinical Oral Implants Research*, vol. 21, pp. 898–903, 2010.

[12] S. Rinke, S. Ohl, D. Ziebolz, K. Lange, and P. Eickholz, "Prevalence of periimplant disease in partially edentulous patients: a practice-based cross-sectional study," *Clinical Oral Implants Research*, vol. 22, no. 8, pp. 826–833, 2011.

[13] K. Swierkot, P. Lottholz, L. Flores-de-Jacoby, and R. Mengel, "Mucosistis, peri-implantitis, implant success, and survival of Implants in patients with treated generalized aggressive periodontitis: 3- to 16-year results of a prospective long-term cohort study," *Journal of Periodontology*, vol. 83, no. 10, pp. 1213–1225, 2012.

[14] J. Slots and T. E. Rams, "Antibiotics and periodontal therapy: Advantages and disadvantages," *Journal of Clinical Periodontology*, vol. 17, p. 479, 1990.

[15] A. Prakasam, S. S. Elavarasu, and R. K. Natarajan, "Antibiotics in the management of aggressive periodontitis," *Journal of Pharmacy and Bioallied Sciences*, vol. 4, no. 2, pp. S252–S255, 2012.

[16] A. J. van Winkelhoff, C. J. Tijhof, and J. D. Graaff, "Microbiological and clinical results of metronidazole plus amoxicillin therapy in actinobacillus actinomycetemcomitans–associated periodontitis," *Journal of Periodontology*, vol. 63, no. 1, pp. 52–57, 1992.

17

Endodontic Management of a Severely Dilacerated Mandibular Third Molar: Case Report and Clinical Considerations

Suraj Arora,[1] Gurdeep Singh Gill ⓘ,[2] Priyanka Setia,[2] Anshad Mohamed Abdulla ⓘ,[3] Ganapathy Sivadas ⓘ,[4] and Vaishnavi Vedam ⓘ[5]

[1]Department of Restorative Dentistry, College of Dentistry, King Khalid University, Abha, Asir Province, Saudi Arabia
[2]Department of Conservative Dentistry & Endodontics, JCD Dental College, Sirsa, Haryana, India
[3]Department of Pediatric Dentistry and Orthodontic Sciences, College of Dentistry, King Khalid University, Abha, Asir Province, Saudi Arabia
[4]Department of Pedodontics and Preventive Dentistry, Faculty of Dentistry, Asian Institute of Medicine, Science and Technology (AIMST) University, Kedah, Malaysia
[5]Department of Oral Pathology, Faculty of Dentistry, Asian Institute of Medicine, Science and Technology (AIMST) University, Kedah, Malaysia

Correspondence should be addressed to Anshad Mohamed Abdulla; anshad2004@gmail.com

Academic Editor: Jiiang H. Jeng

This article aims at providing an insight to the clinical modifications required for the endodontic management of severely dilacerated mandibular third molar. A 35-year-old patient was referred for the root canal treatment of the mandibular left third molar. An intraoral periapical radiograph revealed a severe curvature in both the canals. A wide trapezoidal access was prepared following the use of intermediate-sized files for apical preparation. Owing to increased flexibility, Hero Shaper NITI files were used for the biomechanical preparation and single cone obturation was carried out. Third molars owing to their most posterior location-limited access coupled with a severe curvature pose utmost clinical challenges require meticulous skill, advanced technology, and patience to achieve success.

1. Introduction

Endodontic treatments of third molars are considered an ordeal owing to their most posterior location, unpredictable internal anatomy, bizarre occlusal anatomy, and aberrant eruption patterns [1]. Though the extraction of third molars is often the treatment of choice, few clinical situations might demand the retention of these teeth. Third molars might serve as abutments for removable partial denture of fixed prosthesis, where second molars are lost. Moreover, the principle of endodontics is directed at the preservation of each and every functional component of the dental arch [2]. The anatomical variations confronted in third molars range from curved roots, bayonet roots, fused canals, C-shaped canals, etc. The prevalence of curved canals has been found to be relatively higher in mandibular third molars, ranging from 3.3 to 30.92%, compared to maxillary molars that range from 1.33 to 8.46%. Curved root canals pose great difficulty in cleaning, shaping, and obturation of the root canal system with an exponential rise in difficulty with an increase in curvature. Predictability of treatment is ensured from a blend of profound knowledge and meticulous skill of the practitioner. The following article presents a case report of the endodontic treatment of a mandibular third molar with severely curved canals and highlights the various disciplines and modifications employed for its management.

2. Case Report

A 35-year-old male patient reported to the dental clinic with a history of sharp pain in the left lower back region for the last two days. Clinical examination revealed a deep carious lesion in the left mandibular third molar and a missing left mandibular second molar, extracted two years back. The oral findings were confirmed with an intraoral periapical (IOPA) radiograph depicting a deep carious lesion approaching the pulp in the left mandibular third molar. The IOPA radiograph further revealed curved mesial and distal canals, a sickle-shaped curvature extending from the middle half of the root till apex (Figure 1). Pulp vitality tests (cold and electric pulp test) confirmed the diagnosis of symptomatic irreversible pulpitis. The patient had an intention to restore the missing mandibular second molar; hence, an endodontic treatment was planned for mandibular first and third molar in view of providing a fixed partial denture.

After adequate local anaesthesia and isolation with a rubber dam, the access cavity was prepared using Endo Access kit (Dentsply) in the mandibular left third molar. After gaining an adequate access, initial scouting of all the root canals was done with K-file no. 10, and the patency of root canals was established. Gates Glidden (GG) drills were placed sequentially in a step-back fashion (i.e., nos. 1, 2, and 3) to allow easy placement of instruments and to gain a straight line access to the apex. The working length was confirmed using an apex locator (Root ZX J. Morita) and SS K-file no. 15 through an IOPA radiograph (Figure 2). Succeeding, path finder files (Dentsply) of intermediate sizes, i.e., no. 13, no. 16, and no. 19, were used in order to closely follow the curvature and maintain the apical spatial orientation. Each filing sequence was accompanied with 17% EDTA (Glyde, Dentsply) followed by copious irrigation with saline and 3.2% NaOCl. The rotary Hero Shaper files were subsequently used in the fashion as instructed by the manufacturer (20-0.6, 20-0.4). Following the biomechanical preparation, the canals were irrigated, flushed with EDTA 17%, and dried prior to obturation. Single cone 4% taper gutta percha cones (Dentsply) were used to obturate all the canals (Figure 3). The post obturation restoration was done with a composite to maintain a good coronal seal (Figure 4). Similarly, endodontic treatment was executed for 36. A three-unit bridge was given to the patient finally.

3. Discussion

As a general consensus, endodontic treatment of third molars is avoided and these teeth are doomed for extraction. But for certain clinical situations, the retention of third molars is preferable as where second molars are already missing or need extraction owing to a large carious lesion or third molars are indicated options for transplantations or orthodontic translations. In the aforementioned case, the third molar could serve as an excellent abutment of the fixed prosthesis for restoring the missing second molar. Moreover, the mouth opening and gag reflex of the patient were favourable. Therefore, an endodontic treatment was planned for the concerned third molar.

The posterior-most location of the third molar makes it a clinical dilemma, compromises access of vision and instrumentation, and often presents with bizarre occlusal anatomy and internal patterns. The incidence of curved canals, fused roots, and C-shaped canals is generously

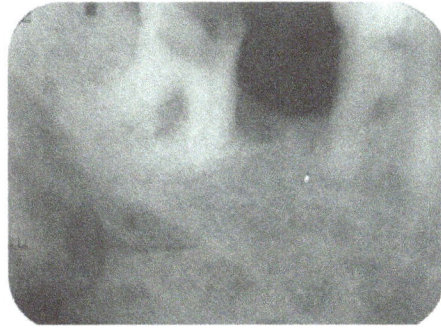

FIGURE 1: Diagnostic radiograph showing severely curved canals.

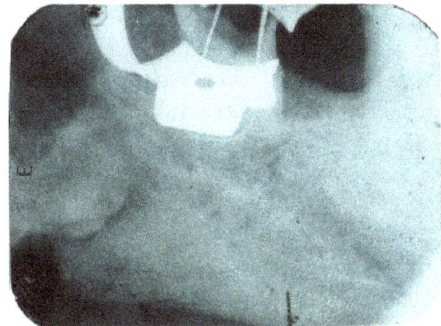

FIGURE 2: Working length radiograph.

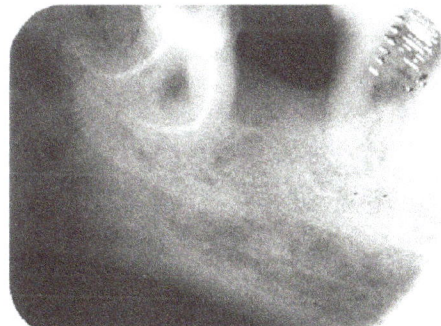

FIGURE 3: Post obturation radiograph.

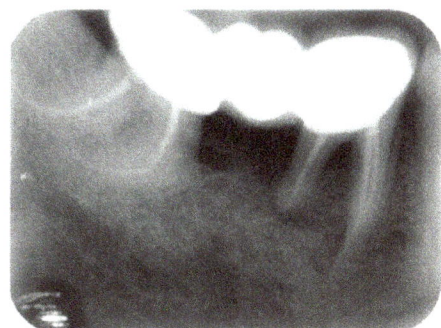

FIGURE 4: Radiograph showing final restoration.

reported in the literature. Gulabivala et al. [3] found 10.9% of single-rooted mandibular third molars having C-shaped variants. Hamasha et al. [4] reported the prevalence of dilacerations to be 3.8% and it was the highest in lower third molars, 19.2%. Similarly, the prevalence of curved canals has been found to be relatively higher in mandibular third molars, ranging from 3.3 to 30.92%, compared to maxillary molars that range from 1.33 to 8.46%. A tooth is considered dilacerated when there is a mesial or distal tilt of the root and the angle is equal or exceeds 90 in relation to the tooth or root axis. Another school of thought considers a dilaceration when its apical deviation is equal or exceeds 200 in relation to the normal tooth axis [5].

Root canal curvatures may be apical, gradual, sickle-shaped, severe-moderate-straight curve, bayonet/S-shaped curve, and dilacerated curve [6]. Curved root canals present as a challenge in cleaning, shaping, and obturation of the root canal system [7]. These curves must always be valued and maintained strictly. The clinical strategy alters with the degree of dilacerations. Various attempts have been made for measuring the extent of curvatures. The most accepted one is given by Schneider. This method involves drawing a line parallel to the long axis of the canal in the coronal third of the root canal and another line drawn from the apical foramina to intersect the first line on a hard copy of the diagnostic radiographic printout. Schneider's angle is formed from the intersection of these lines. Accordingly, the degree of root canal curvature is categorized as straight: $5°$ or less moderate: $10–20°$ and severe: $25–70°$. Gunday et al. [8] introduced the term "canal access angle" (CAA), another parameter, which provides more information about the coronal geometry of canal curvature. Abiding by Schneider's method, the aforementioned third molar exhibited severe dilacerations (Figure 5) and demanded a cautious preparation at each step. While preparing the curved canals, the following principles were closely followed:

(1) To maintain the apical foramen in its original spatial location

(2) To gain a straight line access to the site of curvature

(3) To respect the anatomical danger zone in curved canals: the inner wall of the middle third and outer aspect of the apical third

(4) To use an instrument that closely adapts to the original shape of the canal, respecting its anatomy [9]

The access cavity was prepared using an Endo Access kit (Dentsply). A slight wide tapered access cavity was prepared to allow easy access of instruments. No 10 k file was used as the scouting files as smaller files exhibit sufficient flexibility and control over movement to prepare a glide path. Subsequently, the orifice widening and coronal flaring were achieved using Gates Glidden drill in crown down fashion up to nos. 3, 2, and 1. Guttman [10] suggested preflaring the coronal 1/3 of the canal (at the expense of the tooth structure) to reduce the angle of curvature. Working length was established using file no. 15 and apex locator (Root ZX, Dentsply). This was followed by the usage of intermediate size files, namely, Pathfinder file nos. 13, 17, and 19 (Dentsply). The standardized instruments increase in size

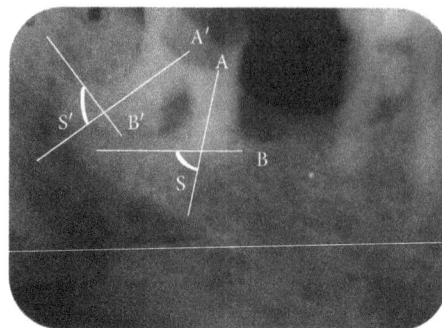

FIGURE 5: Measurement of Schneider's angle using radiograph. Both S and S' are more than $70°$ (severely curved canals).

by fixed, absolute increments (0.05 mm in diameter, 1.0 mm from the tip end), but increases in size are not constant. For example, there is a 50% increase in size from no. 10 to no. 15 and a 33% increase in size from no. 15 to no. 20, which is tremendous [11]. Such a mismatch of sizes of successive files tends to place excessive force on each file and may lead to the straightening of curvature, "direct perforation," "ledges" or "false canals," creation of a "teardrop foramen," stripping, and blockage of canals. Thus, it becomes imperative to use files of intermediate sizes, precurved files, and anticurvature filing technique.

The final results of the instrumentation of curved root canals may be influenced considerably by the flexibility and diameter of the endodontic instruments. The Hero Shaper nickel-titanium rotary files provide excellent flexibility and centric ability. The canals were prepared using Hero Shaper files up to 20 apical size with a minimal taper of 4%. Copious irrigation was carried out with the repeated use of 3.2% NaOCl and 17% EDTA. NaOCl helps in loosening and flushing out the organic fibrous content, and EDTA manages to dissolve the inorganic matter within the canal [12]. Profuse irrigation was employed to ensure the maintenance of working length and avoid undue debris clogging within the canal. After the final rinse of EDTA and saline, the canals were dried with paper points and obturation was carried out using 4% taper gutta percha cones and a zinc oxide eugenol sealer.

To ensure optimum sealing, the access cavity was sealed with composite restoration. In the subsequent visits, crown preparations were performed and a fixed three-unit prosthesis was delivered to the patient.

4. Conclusion

Severely curved canals cannot be an indication for the extraction of a restoratively important third molar. Following the basic principles and taking advantage of new innovations (usage of intermediate precurved sequential filing and flexible rotary systems) in the field of endodontics, even most severely curved canals can be negotiated and treated successfully as in the present case.

References

[1] H. M. A. Ahmed, "Management of third molar teeth from an endodontic perspective," *European Journal of General Dentistry*, vol. 1, no. 3, p. 148, 2012.

[2] J. Cosić, N. Galić, M. Vodanović et al., "An in vitro morphological investigation of the endodontic spaces of third molars," *Collegium Antropologicum*, vol. 37, no. 2, pp. 437–442, 2013.

[3] K. Gulabivala, A. Opasanon, Y. L. Ng, and A. Alavi, "Root and canal morphology of Thai mandibular molars," *International Endodontic Journal*, vol. 35, no. 1, pp. 56–62, 2002.

[4] A. A. Hamasha, T. Al-Khateeb, and A. Darwazeh, "Prevalence of dilaceration in Jordanian adults," *International Endodontic Journal*, vol. 35, no. 11, pp. 910–912, 2002.

[5] S. W. Schneider, "A comparison of canal preparations in straight and curved root canals," *Oral Surgery, Oral Medicine, and Oral Pathology*, vol. 32, no. 2, pp. 271–275, 1971.

[6] N. Jain and S. Tushar, "Curved canals: ancestral files revisited," *Indian Journal of Dental Research*, vol. 19, no. 3, pp. 267–271, 2008.

[7] F. J. Vertucci, "Root canal morphology and its relationship to endodontic procedures," *Endodontic Topics*, vol. 10, no. 1, pp. 3–29, 2005.

[8] M. Gunday, H. Sazak, and Y. Garip, "A comparative study of three different root canal curvature measurement techniques and measuring the canal access angle in curved canals," *Journal of Endodontia*, vol. 31, no. 11, pp. 796–798, 2005.

[9] H. Jafarzadeh and P. Abbott, "Dilaceration: review of an endodontic challenge," *Journal of Endodontics*, vol. 33, no. 9, pp. 1025–1030, 2007.

[10] J. L. Guttman, *Problem Solving in Endodontics*, Mosby - Year book Inc, Missouri, 3rd edition, 1997.

[11] C. U. Donald and H. Schilder, "Cleaning and shaping the apical third of a root canal system," *General Dentistry*, vol. 3, pp. 267–270, 2001.

[12] E. S. J. Pereira, I. F. C. Peixoto, R. K. L. Nakagawa, V. T. L. Buono, and M. G. A. Bahia, "Cleaning the apical third of curved canals after different irrigation protocols," *Brazilian Dental Journal*, vol. 23, no. 4, pp. 351–356, 2012.

18

Approach and Treatment of Giant Luminal Unicystic Ameloblastoma

George Borja de Freitas (D),[1] **Evelyne Pedroza de Andrade,**[1] **Riedel Frota Sá Nogueira Neves,**[2]
Stefanny Torres dos Santos,[2] **Daniella Cristina da Costa Araújo,**[2]
and **Victor Ângelo Montalli** (D)[1]

[1]Department of Oral Pathology, São Leopoldo Mandic Institute and Research Center, Campinas, SP, Brazil
[2]Department Maxillofacial Surgery, Hospital Getúlio Vargas, Recife, PE, Brazil

Correspondence should be addressed to George Borja de Freitas; george_borja@hotmail.com
and Victor Ângelo Montalli; victormontalli@gmail.com

Academic Editor: Gerardo Gómez-Moreno

Unicystic ameloblastoma is an odontogenic tumor that affects mainly young patients and usually involves the posterior region of the mandible. In this article, we report on the case a 12-year-old girl presenting with an 8-month history of facial swelling in her lower right quadrant. Radiographic examination revealed a unilocular radiolucent lesion extending from the body of the mandible through to the angle and ascending ramus. An incisional biopsy was performed, and a diagnosis of luminal unicystic ameloblastoma was made based on clinicopathological features. The lesion was treated in two stages, namely, an initial conservative approach via decompression and subsequent excision. The patient has been followed up for 6 months without clinical and radiographic evidence of recurrence. In conclusion, conservative timely intervention combined with a conservative surgical approach has proven efficacious in the treatment of ameloblastoma in this young patient.

1. Introduction

Unicystic ameloblastoma is a cystic lesion that shows clinical and radiographic features that resemble those of odontogenic cysts, though histological features are crucial to ascertain the presence of ameloblastic epithelium and its variants [1].

This lesion mainly affects the posterior regions of the mandible in young patients. Its radiographic features include a single unilocular and radiolucent lesion generally associated with the crown of an unerupted third molar [1].

Such lesions tend to grow slowly, though locally invasive, which may cause bone deformities and painless swelling [2, 3]. They may be classified into three histological variants: luminal, intraluminal, and mural. Treatment planning and prognosis are based on the histological subtype [1, 3].

Several treatment approaches have been reported, such as enucleation, marsupialization, and resection of the affected area; however, conservative measures tend to be preferred in young patients [4].

2. Case Report

A 12-year-old Brazilian female, with no systemic comorbidities, attended the oral and maxillofacial surgery service with a chief complaint of a painless growing facial swelling for 8 months (Figure 1). On extraoral examination, a unilateral expansive lesion was detected on the lower right aspect of her face. On intraoral examination, the swelling could be seen affecting the body and the angle of the mandible on the right side associated with her lower right third molar. Panoramic radiographic examination revealed a unilocular radiolucent lesion extending from the body of the mandible through to the angle and right ascending

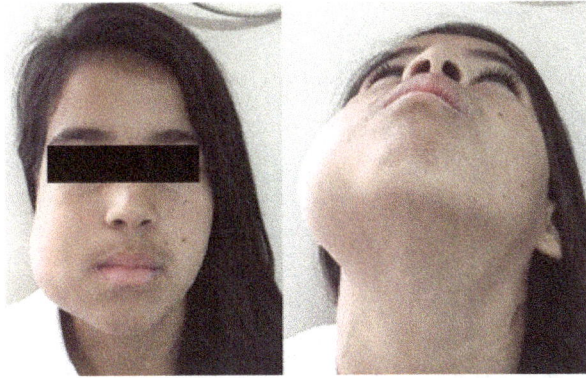

Figure 1: A 12-year-old Brazilian female with a chief complaint of a painless growing facial swelling for 8 months.

ramus, causing displacement of the second molar towards the base of the mandible and the third molar towards the ascending ramus (Figure 2). A CT scan revealed that the lesion caused expansion of the buccal and lingual aspects of the cortical bone with areas of fenestration. Needle aspiration was performed to evaluate the contents of the swelling, mainly to exclude the possibility of a vascular lesion. An incisional biopsy was then performed, and the specimen was sent for histological evaluation (Figure 3). The access window left from the biopsy was used to accommodate a flexible tube for decompression and subsequent volume reduction of the lesion in an attempt to minimize the need for mutilating surgery in such a young patient. In view of the clinical and radiographic characteristics, two differential diagnoses were raised, namely, unicystic ameloblastoma or dentigerous cyst (Figure 3). The histological diagnosis confirmed the suspicion of a unicystic ameloblastoma. A decision was made to continue with the assisted decompression approach using daily irrigations of sterile saline solution intercalated with 0.12% chlorhexidine digluconate to remove debris and decontaminate the site, which was followed up both clinically and radiographically. After 5 months of decompression, a significant reduction of the lesion was observed radiographically, with evidence of bone neoformation in the periphery of the lesion. In view of the favorable progression, complete enucleation of the lesion combined with peripheral osteotomy and cryotherapy was performed under general anesthesia to reduce the risk of recurrence. The excised specimen was sent for histopathological evaluation, which reiterated the previous diagnosis of unicystic ameloblastoma. The patient has been followed up for 6 months, with no clinical or radiographic evidence of recurrence (Figure 4). A supernumerary tooth in the right maxilla was also observed in the panoramic radiograph. This tooth was not removed since cone beam computed tomography was not available for a better surgical planning due to financial reasons. However, the patient remains in close follow-up.

The histological sections showed the presence of a fibrous capsule lined by nonkeratinized stratified pavement epithelium exhibiting spongiosis, reverse polarization of the basal layer, and areas that resembled the stellate reticulum. The fibrous capsule consisted of dense connective tissue, presenting moderate to severe lymphoplasmacytic inflammatory infiltrate and hemorrhagic areas (Figure 5).

3. Discussion

Unicystic ameloblastoma usually presents as slow growing, persistent, and locally invasive lesions, which may lead to bone deformation [1]. These expansive lesions exhibit well-defined radiolucent areas, which are surrounded by sclerotic borders, mainly in the posterior region of the mandible [5]. In this report, a unilocular radiolucent lesion was clearly outlined extending from the body of the mandible, through to the angle and ascending ramus, causing displacement of the teeth 47 and 48, which corroborates the descriptions for this type of lesions in the literature.

Most such cases are diagnosed in the second decade of life [1, 2, 5]. Painful lesions are associated with older patients and do not seem to correlate directly with tumor growth [5]. Thus, as in this report, a young patient (12 years old), asymptomatic, exhibiting root resorption corroborated previous published reports describing a mean age of 13 years at diagnosis, predominantly affecting the mandible [1].

Unicystic ameloblastomas may present three histological variants, where the luminal subtype of the tumor is confined to the luminal surface of the cyst and the cystic wall is totally or partially lined by ameloblastic epithelium; the intraluminal variant presents ameloblastoma nodules protruding into the lumen of the cyst and finally, in the third variant, known as mural, the cystic wall is infiltrated by ameloblastoma [5, 6]. The histological characteristics described on the excised specimen of the present case are compatible with the luminal subtype.

Despite there being a consensus that ameloblastomas should be treated radically to prevent recurrence, one is often faced with a dilemma whenever the treatment plan involves children, since the mandibular lesions at this age are usually benign, and, therefore, conservative surgery should be the treatment of choice, especially in a context of bone growth and unerupted teeth [1, 7–9].

Still regarding management, it is worth mentioning enucleation, marsupialization followed by enucleation, enucleation and chemical cauterization (Carnoy's solution), cryotherapy, decompression followed by enucleation, and peripheral osteotomy. Indeed, rare are the cases for which block resection has been the treatment of choice [1]. Such findings are pertinent with the approach selected for the case presented herein, where decompression was performed using a flexible device installed on the occasion of the incisional biopsy, followed by enucleation and peripheral osteotomy, in order to minimize the risk of recurrence. The patient has been followed up for six months without evidence of relapse.

4. Conclusion

Conservative timely intervention and conservative surgery combined with local adjuvants such as liquid nitrogen

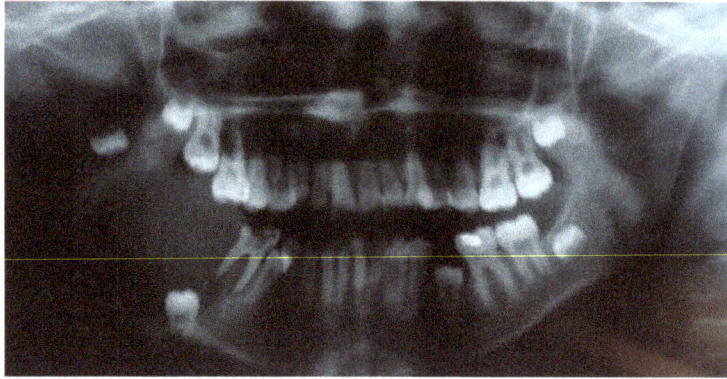

FIGURE 2: Panoramic radiographic examination revealed a unilocular radiolucent lesion extending from the body of the mandible through to the angle and right ascending ramus.

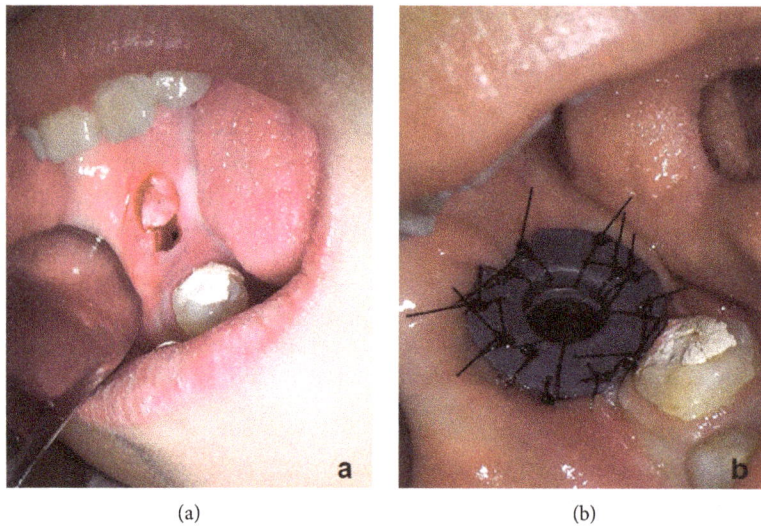

(a)

(b)

FIGURE 3: Incisional biopsy (a). Flexible tube for decompression (b).

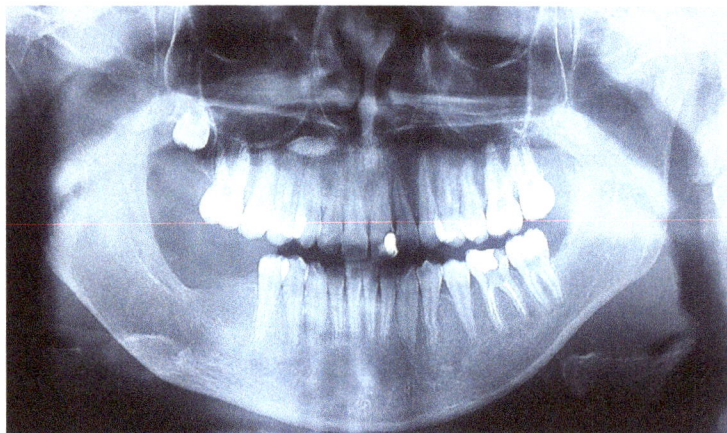

FIGURE 4: The patient has been followed up for 6 months, with no clinical or radiographic evidence of recurrence.

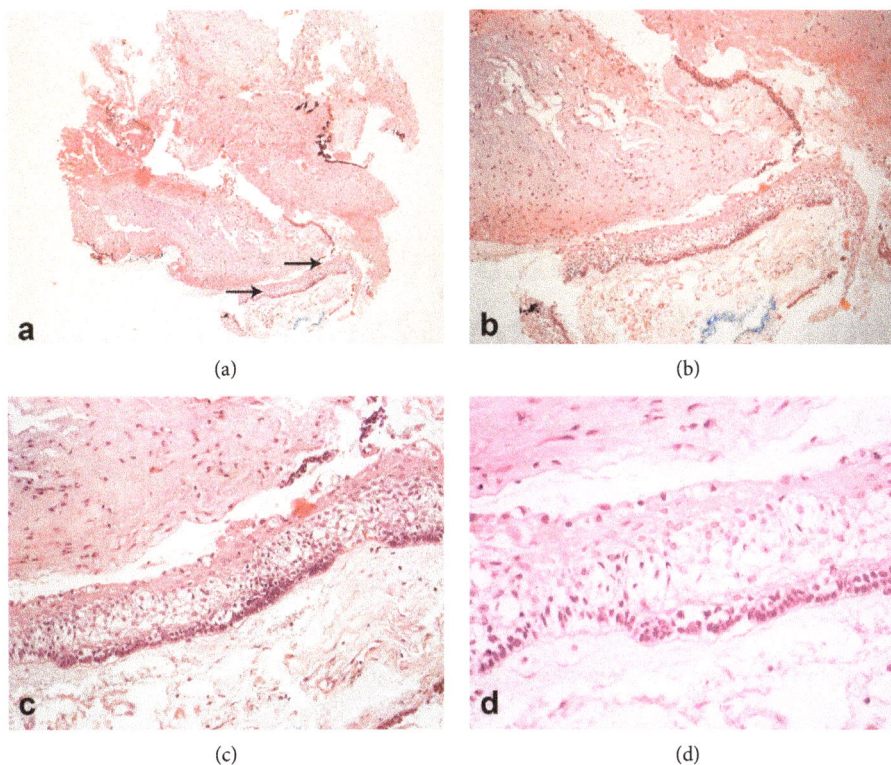

FIGURE 5: Photomicrograph showing ameloblastic epithelium. Hematoxylin and eosin. Original magnification 40x (a). Original magnification 100x (b). Original magnification 200x (c). Original Magnification 400x (d).

cryotherapy, peripheral osteotomy, and exodontia should be the first treatment option for ameloblastoma in young patients. Such an approach has often been associated with positive outcomes, including from the esthetic, psychological, and functional viewpoints, when compared to major resections.

References

[1] M. Meshram, L. Sagarka, J. Dhuvad, S. Anchlia, S. Vyas, and H. Shah, "Conservative management of unicystic ameloblastoma in young patients: a prospective single-center trial and review of literature," *Journal of Maxillofacial and Oral Surgery*, vol. 16, no. 3, pp. 333–341, 2017.

[2] K. Jain, G. Sharma, P. Kardam, and M. Mehendiratta, "Unicystic ameloblastoma of mandible with an unusual diverse histopathology: a rare case report," *Journal of Clinical and Diagnostic Research*, vol. 11, no. 4, pp. ZD04–ZD05, 2017.

[3] S. L. Pereira de Castro Lopes, I. L. Flores, T. de Oliveira Gamba et al., "Aggressive unicystic ameloblastoma affecting the posterior mandible: late diagnosis during orthodontic treatment," *Journal of the Korean Association of Oral and Maxillofacial Surgeons*, vol. 43, no. 2, pp. 115–119, 2017.

[4] S. Kalaiselvan, A. V. Dharmesh Kumar Raja, B. Saravanan, A. S. Vigneswari, and R. Srinivasan, ""Evaluation of safety margin" in

ameloblastoma of the mandible by surgical, radiological, and histopathological methods: an evidence-based study," *Journal of Pharmacy & Bioallied Sciences*, vol. 8, Supplement 1, pp. S122–S125, 2016.

[5] A. I. Filizzola, T. Bartholomeu-dos-Santos, and F. R. Pires, "Ameloblastomas: clinicopathological features from 70 cases diagnosed in a single oral pathology service in an 8-year period," *Medicina Oral, Patología Oral y Cirugía Bucal*, vol. 19, no. 6, pp. e556–e561, 2014.

[6] S. Ghattamaneni, S. Nallamala, and V. R. Guttikonda, "Unicystic ameloblastoma in conjunction with peripheral ameloblastoma: a unique case report presenting with diverse histological patterns," *Journal of Oral and Maxillofacial Pathology*, vol. 21, no. 2, pp. 267–272, 2017.

[7] E. Okoturo, O. V. Ogunbanjo, and G. T. Arotiba, "Spontaneous regeneration of the mandible: an institutional audit of regenerated bone and osteocompetent periosteum," *Journal of Oral and Maxillofacial Surgery*, vol. 74, no. 8, pp. 1660–1667, 2016.

[8] N. G. Garcia, D. T. Oliveira, and M. T. V. Rodrigues, "Unicystic ameloblastoma with mural proliferation managed by conservative treatment," *Case Reports in Pathology*, vol. 2016, Article ID 3089540, 4 pages, 2016.

[9] Z. Agani, V. Hamiti-Krasniqi, J. Recica, M. P. Loxha, F. Kurshumliu, and A. Rexhepi, "Maxillary unicystic ameloblastoma: a case report," *BMC Research Notes*, vol. 9, no. 1, p. 469, 2016.

19

Combination of Medical and Surgical Treatments for Masseter Hypertrophy

M. Ayhan ⓘ, Sabri Cemil İşler, and C. Kasapoglu

Faculty of Dentistry, Department of Oral and Maxillofacial Surgery, Istanbul University, Istanbul, Turkey

Correspondence should be addressed to M. Ayhan; drmustafaayhan@gmail.com

Academic Editor: Maria Beatriz Duarte Gavião

Masseter hypertrophy (MH) is one of the uncommon conditions that swelling can be seen in the angular mandibular region of the face. The etiology of MH includes several factors, and various treatment methods are mentioned in the literature. Botulinum toxin type A application is most commonly used for the treatment because of its less invasive feature. As a surgical method, some treatment alternatives that aim to reduce muscle mass or reshape the bone tissue in the angular region are considered. In this case report, a 21-year-old male patient with unilateral masseter hypertrophy on the right side is presented. After the patient was diagnosed with MH, botulinum toxin treatment in two sessions at one-month intervals was done. Since the reduction in muscle volume was not in satisfactory dimensions after the botulinum toxin application, the masseter was reduced on the right side through an intraoral approach. At the same time, bone enlargements on each side of the angulus mandibula were reshaped and smoothened through an extraoral retro mandibular approach. Clinical and radiographic evaluation of the patient revealed more aesthetic and symmetrical appearance in the regular controls.

1. Introduction

Masseter hypertrophy (MH) is an uncommon condition that can cause aesthetic and functional problems. Aesthetic problems consist of prominent masseter muscle in the face, rectangular face shape, and wide mandibular angle. Patients may suffer psychological issues due to an unattractive look [1]. Differential diagnosis requires clinical history and physical examination and may even include complementary imagination resources such as magnetic resonance (MR) and computed tomography (CT) scans to exclude other disorders. Differential diagnosis must consist of muscle tumors, salivary gland disorders, and intrinsic masseter myopathy. In some cases, patients may report signs and symptoms of well-localized pain [1, 2]. However, it is asymptomatic, and patients' chief complaint is about aesthetics. Moreover, masseteric musculature is inserted in the mandibular angle anatomically and can cause overdevelopment of these angles because of its traction forces [2]. The etiology of MH has been attributed to many factors such as tensions and clenching caused by emotional stress, chronic bruxism, masseteric hyperfunction, and parafunction. It is essential to make the differential diagnosis of head and neck mass, particularly unilateral mass located in the cheek. The possible underlying pathologic factors should be assessed carefully with detailed patient history and imaging techniques before deciding on treatment [3]. Treatment of MH is controversial. Varying degrees of success have been reported for some of the treatment options for MH which range from simple pharmacotherapy to more invasive surgery. Reduction of the masseter muscle, osteotomy, botulinum toxin, and splint therapy are options for managing this problem [2, 3]. Injection of botulinum toxin type A into the masseter muscle is considered as a less invasive modality and has been reported to be successfully used for cosmetic sculpting of the lower face [4]. Botulinum toxin type A (botulinum toxin) is a potent neurotoxin which is produced by the anaerobic organism *Clostridium botulinum* and when injected into a muscle causes interference with the neurotransmitter mechanism, producing selective paralysis and subsequent atrophy of the muscle [3–5]. Results showed the efficiency of botulinum in MH, but many times in MH concomitant with bone enlargement in the angulus; therefore, the best aesthetic results may be gained with manipulation of the bony structure. The

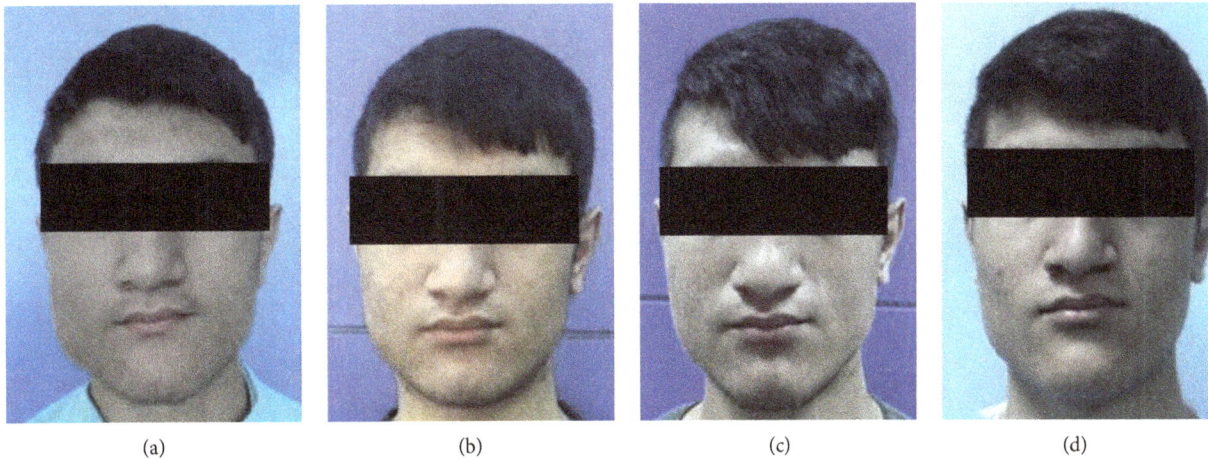

FIGURE 1: (a) Initial profile image; (b) profile image after one month of the first botulinum toxin application; (c) profile image after one month of the second botulinum toxin application; (d) profile image after six months of the surgery.

traditional method of treatment for MH is the partial surgical excision of the masseter muscle and osteotomy of the mandibular angle region and reshaping the curvature of the bone under general anaesthesia [5]. The use of an intraoral approach was first suggested by Wood. He recommended the removal of bone enlargement of the mandibular angle without any masseter muscle manipulation. Tabrizi et al. advocated an intraoral approach including masseter muscle reduction and partially monocortical and bicortical osteotomy in the mandibular angle in the treatment of MH [3–6].

2. Case Presentation

A 22-year-old male patient applied to our clinic for painless asymmetric swelling on the right side of the face for five years (Figure 1(a)). The history of the patient revealed that there are no parafunctional habits, functional and mouth opening limitation, bruxism, and trauma. And also, the masseteric region was nontender and normal in tone, and the temporomandibular joints and mandibular angulus region were not painful on palpation. The patient said that the only complaint was aesthetic and he wanted to have a more attractive facial appearance. Computed tomography, MR imagination, and panoramic radiographs were taken to make a differential diagnosis of MH. In MR examination, significant enlargement of the right masseter muscle compared to the left side was naturally detectable. There was also no pathological formation in the muscle. In CT and panoramic radiographs, reactive bone formation and significant asymmetry compared to the left side were observed in the mandibular angular region on the right side (Figure 2(a)). The patient was diagnosed with masseter hypertrophy. It was decided to apply botulinum toxin as the first step of the treatment.

2.1. Botulinum Toxin Application. Botulinum toxin type A (Botox; Allergan Inc., Irvine, CA) was supplied as a freeze-dried powder of 100 units and was reconstituted with 2 ml of sterile saline solution, giving a concentration of 100 units.

Percutaneous intramuscular injection of botulinum toxin type A was performed to the hypertrophic muscle using 2 ml syringe with 25G needle. 75 units of botulinum toxin type A was injected equally into five points at the centre of the lower third of the masseter muscle (Figure 1(b)). Determining the number of injection points is based on our clinical experience and previous satisfactory results as injections are more homogenously located in the masseter muscle. A month later, an additional 60 units of botulinum toxin were applied to the muscle at the second visit. A decrease in the size of the masseter muscle was seen after one month of the application (Figure 1(c)). Within the six months' follow-up period, severe masseter muscle atrophy occurred, but although clinically significant atrophy has occurred, the patient was not entirely satisfied with his appearance. Thus the decision to perform surgery has made with permission of the patient and his family in order to reduce the volume of the right masseter muscle and soften the couture of the patients face.

2.2. Surgery. The patient underwent surgery involving bilateral resection of mandibular angles and unilateral resection of the masseter muscle through intraoral and extraoral submandibular approaches. Under general anaesthesia, on the right side of the patient, an intraoral incision was made supraperiostally, slightly lateral to the external oblique line, and extended mandibular first molar region. The anterior portion of the masseter muscle was exposed, and the inner belly of the muscle was removed by the method described by Beckers [7]. The intraoral incision was closed with absorbable sutures. Next, by using the extraoral submandibular approach on both sides, after the skin incision was made 1.5 cm below the mandibular border, the platysma muscle and the superficial layer of the deep cervical fascia were sectioned, and with taking care of the marginal mandibular branch of the facial nerve, facial vein, and facial artery, the pterygomasseteric connection was reached. The pterygomasseteric connection was cut from the bottom of the mandible to the angular region. A bone cut

(a)

(b)

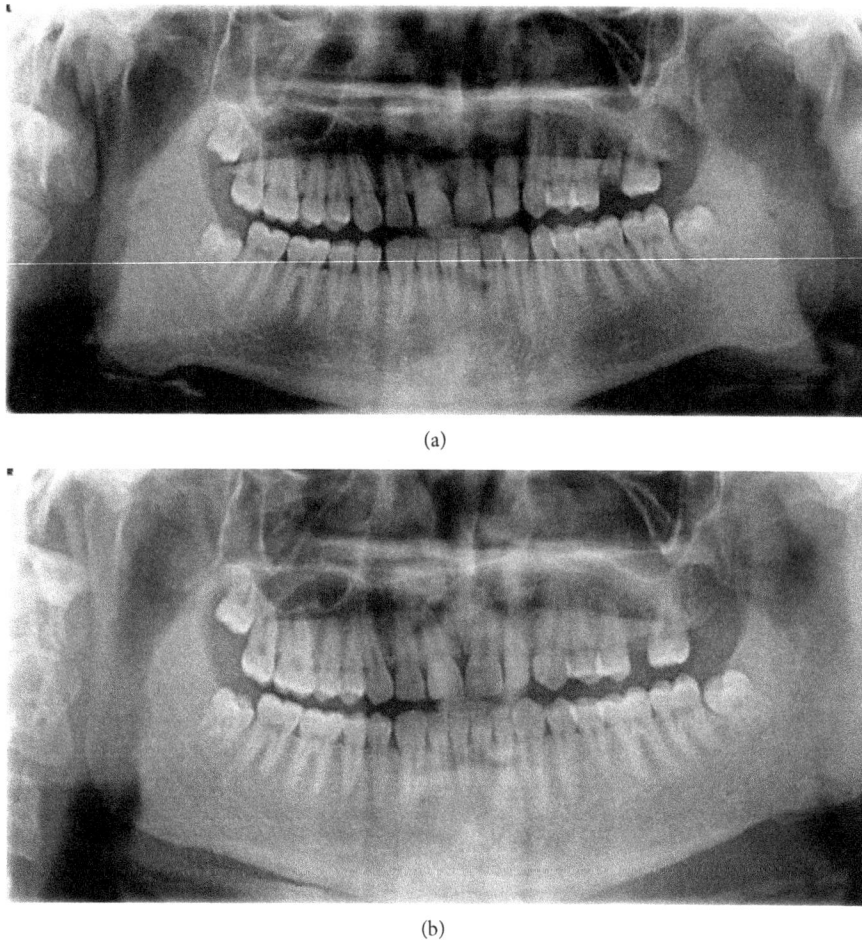

FIGURE 2: (a) Initial panoramic view; (b) panaromic view after six months of the surgery.

was made on the lateral surface of the ramus via a piezo-electric surgery device on a curve shape line connecting a point about one-third height of the posterior border of the ramus and the anterior portion of the antegonial notch. Complete separation and removal of the segment from mandible were accomplished using a periosteum retractor (Figures 3(a) and 3(b)). The pterygomasseteric connection was closed with single absorbable suture, while the platysma was covered with absorbable continuous suture. Particular attention was shown to ensure that the underlying vascular structures and the mandibular nerve were not damaged during closure and the skin was closed. No drain was used in the surgery zone, and primary closure was performed. A pressure bandage and ice pack were applied for 72 hours. Antibiotic and analgesic therapy was prescribed. From MR views which were taken one year following the surgery, the decreased volume of the right masseter muscle can be seen apparently (Figures 4(a) and 4(b)). The patient was followed for one year without any problems (Figure 1(d)).

3. Discussion

There are many factors in the etiology of masseter hyper-trophy, such as tensions and clenching caused by emotional stress and parafunctional habits. It is observed that none of the etiologic factors in the literature are present in our patient such as dental attrition, and therefore, we can refer to this condition as idiopathic masseter hypertrophy. Especially in the diagnosis of the clinical situation in unilateral hy-pertrophy, the differential diagnosis of head and neck soft tissue pathologies should be made [5, 7]. Before deciding on the treatment plan, MR and CT, thanks to their high imaging capacity, should be used to exclude possible pathologies such as muscle tumors, salivary gland disorders, parotid tumors, parotid inflammatory diseases, and intrinsic masseter my-opathy. MR images of the patient in our case showed that the masseter muscle and surrounding soft tissues had a regular structure, but the right masseter muscle was significantly larger than the left side. Also, in panoramic radiographs of the patient, reactive bone formation and significant asym-metry compared to the left side were observed in response to the abnormal activity of the masseter muscle in the man-dibular angular region on the right side. After the patient was diagnosed with MH, two options for treatment became prominent. One of them is the injection of botulinum toxin type A, and the other one is the respective surgery of the masseter muscle and angulus of the mandible. The use of botulinum toxin in the treatment of masseter hypertrophy is

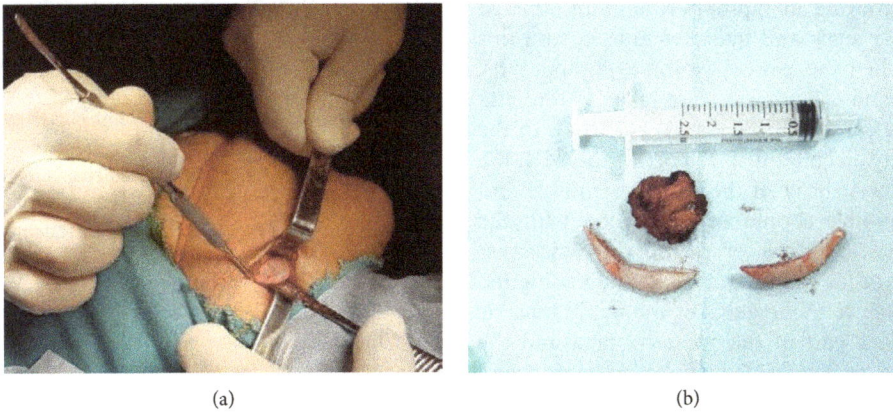

(a)   (b)

FIGURE 3: (a) Intraoperative view of the resected fragments of the right and left angulus of the mandible and 2/3 inner belly of the right masseter muscle; (b) extraoral submandibular approach.

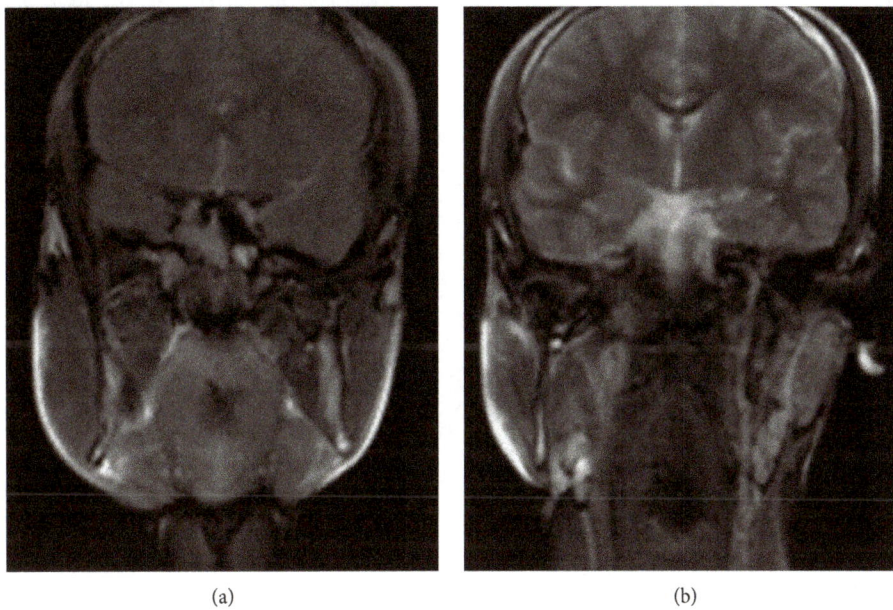

(a)   (b)

FIGURE 4: Pre-op (a) and post-op (b) MR views. Decreased volume of the right masseter muscle can be seen obviously.

a frequently preferred treatment option since 1994. The minimally invasive nature of this procedure and the fact that the risk ratio is meager are the most important reasons why botulinum toxin is used for many years with success for cosmetic purposes [4, 8]. In the literature, botulinum toxin has been shown to cause muscle atrophy by blocking neurotransmission at the neurotransmitter junction. But, as the botulinum toxin activity declines over time, atrophic muscle tends to return to its former size, as neural conduction in the neurotransmitter junction will return to normal, so the injection should be repeated approximately every 4–8 months; however, there are various techniques and protocols for extending this lasting duration in the literature [8], which constitutes the biggest disadvantage of botulinum toxin treatment [4, 7]. On the other hand, surgical treatment, although providing more permanent results than botulinum toxin, has various complication risks such as hematoma formation, facial nerve paralysis, infection,

mouth opening limitation, and appearance of scar [9]. After discussing the possible advantages and risks of both treatment options with the patient, botulinum toxin application was agreed as the first treatment option. 75 units of botulinum toxin was given at the first visit. One month later, at the second visit, 60 units of botulinum toxin were applied to the muscle. After six months, it was observed that the muscles had diminished to the initial position, but the symmetrical condition was still found to be unsatisfactory by the patient, and the surgical option was on the table. Some authors claim the partial removal of the masseter muscle is enough to correct MH. According to Beckers, the insertion of hypertrophic masseter muscle causes an abnormal growing mandibular angle. Other authors confirmed that, in order to reach satisfactory results, a mandibular angle resection should be performed [5, 7–10]. In our case, a more permanent and lighter facial contouring could be achieved compared to botulinum toxin treatment since the surgical procedure entails removing an appropriate amount of tissue from the mandibular angle and masseter muscle, and this can be observed when the patient's profile photographs, panoramic graphs, and MR images were taken before and after the surgery are compared (Figures 1, 2, and 4). In the literature, it is widely accepted that, to correct the MH, the resection of the inferior belly of the masseter muscle and angulus of the mandible should be performed with the intraoral approach [9–11]. However, despite the easy access to the inferior belly of the masseter muscle when using the intraoral approach, since the angulus of the mandibular is located in the thickest part of the operative area and the strong tension of the masseter muscle makes retraction very difficult, the surgeon's vision is limited in a sagittal direction [12, 13]. In our case, taking this limited access to the mandibular angular region when using the intraoral approach into account and since under these circumstances making the bone cut in the desired amount would be extremely difficult, the extraoral submandibular approach was chosen during the bone resection. The primary disadvantage of the extraoral approach is the risk of a scar on the face. The skin incision should be thrown parallel to the Langers lines and should be kept as short as possible to minimize this risk [13]. We have experienced no complication and scar with removal of the enlarged mandibular angle when using the combination of extraoral and intraoral approaches.

4. Conclusion

There is not yet a standard protocol in the literature about the treatment of masseter hypertrophy. When treatment is planned, the patient's expectations and physical findings should be evaluated thoroughly. In cases where masseter hypertrophy causes appositional changes in the bone, the success rate with botulinum toxin treatment alone is low, and the surgical option should be considered. Further experimental and clinical studies are necessary to estimate the success of surgical treatment in the short and long term.

References

[1] R. Roncevic, "Masseter muscle hypertrophy—aetiology and therapy," *Journal of Maxillofacial Surgery*, vol. 14, pp. 344–346, 1986.

[2] R. R. Addante, "Masseter muscle hypertrophy: report of case and literature review," *Journal of Oral and Maxillofacial Surgery*, vol. 52, no. 11, pp. 1199–1202, 1994.

[3] G. D. Wood, "Masseteric hypertrophy and its surgical correction," *British Dental Journal*, vol. 152, no. 12, pp. 416–417, 1982.

[4] A. G. Smyth, "Botulinum toxin treatment of bilateral masseteric hypertrophy," *British Journal of Oral and Maxillofacial Surgery*, vol. 32, no. 1, pp. 29–33, 1994.

[5] G. D. S. Trento, L. S. Benato, N. L. B. Rebellato, and L. E. Klüppel, "Surgical resolution of bilateral hypertrophy of masseter muscle through intraoral approach," *Journal of Craniofacial Surgery*, vol. 28, no. 4, pp. 400–402, 2017.

[6] R. Tabrizi, B. T. Ozkan, and S. Zare, "Correction of lower facial wideness due to masseter hypertrophy," *Journal of Craniofacial Surgery*, vol. 21, no. 4, pp. 1069–1097, 2010.

[7] H. L. Beckers, "Masseteric muscle hypertrophy and its intraoral surgical correction," *Journal of Maxillofacial Surgery*, vol. 5, pp. 28–35, 1977.

[8] R. Rauso, M. Santagata, G. Colella, N. Nesi, G. Gherardini, and G. Tartaro, "Can occlusal devices prolong the effect of botulinum toxin type A in the contouring of the lower face?," *European Journal of Plastic Surgery*, vol. 33, no. 1, pp. 35–40, 2010.

[9] B. Bas, B. Ozan, M. Muglali, and N. Celebi, "Treatment of masseteric hypertrophy with botulinum toxin: a report of two cases," *Medicina Oral Patología Oral y Cirugia Bucal*, vol. 1, no. 15, pp. 649–652, 2010.

[10] R. J. de Holanda Vasconcellos, D. M. de Oliveira, B. C. do Egito Vasconcelos, and R. V. Nogueira, "Modified intraoral approach to removal of mandibular angle for correction of masseteric hypertrophy: a technical note," *Journal of Oral and Maxillofacial Surgery*, vol. 63, no. 7, pp. 1057–1060, 2005.

[11] M. Nishida and T. Iizuka, "Intraoral removal of the enlarged mandibular angle associated with masseteric hypertrophy," *Journal of Oral and Maxillofacial Surgery*, vol. 53, no. 12, p. 1479, 1995.

[12] A. R. Andreishchev, R. Nicot, and J. Ferri, "Mandibular angle resection and masticatory muscle hypertrophy—a technical note and morphological optimization," *Revue de Stomatologie, de Chirurgie Maxillo-faciale et de Chirurgie Orale*, vol. 115, no. 5, p. 301, 2014.

[13] D. Z. Rispoli, P. M. Camargo, J. L. Pires et al., "Benign masseter muscle hypertrophy," *Revista Brasileira de Otorrinolaringologia*, vol. 74, no. 5, pp. 790–793, 2008.

20

Bilateral Maxillary Dentigerous Cysts in a Nonsyndromic Child

Rakshit Vijay Khandeparker ⓘ,[1] **Purva Vijay Khandeparker,**[1] **Anirudha Virginkar,**[2] **and Kiran Savant**[3]

[1]Department of Oral and Maxillofacial Surgery, Goa Dental College and Hospital, Bambolim, Goa, India
[2]ICU Horizon Hospital, Margao, Goa, India
[3]Rejoice Aesthetic Centre, Bangalore, Karnataka, India

Correspondence should be addressed to Rakshit Vijay Khandeparker; rockdotcom1386@gmail.com

Academic Editor: Daniel Torrés-Lagares

Dentigerous cysts represent the second most common odontogenic cysts of the jaws after radicular cysts and are usually associated with the crowns of unerupted permanent teeth and rarely deciduous teeth. They are usually solitary in their presentation. Multiple and bilateral dentigerous cysts are an extremely rare presentation in the absence of developmental syndromes or systemic diseases or the use of prescribed certain medications. We hereby present a case of a bilateral dentigerous cyst of the maxilla in a 10-year-old child involving the crowns of unerupted permanent second premolar on the right side and the unerupted permanent canine on the left side. An effort has also been made to review the existing literature on this entity and to stress the importance of radiographic and histopathological examinations in diagnosing such an entity.

1. Introduction

Dentigerous cyst (DC) is an epithelial-lined developmental cavity that encloses the crown of an unerupted tooth at the cementoenamel junction. It accounts for nearly 24% of all the true cysts in the jaws, thus being only the second most common to radicular cysts in the frequency of occurrence [1, 2]. The usual presentation is that of a solitary lesion; however, in the presence of developmental syndromes or systemic diseases or the concurrent use of certain drugs, bilateral or multiple lesions are seen to occur [3–6]. Having said that, the occurrence of the bilateral DC in the absence of any of these factors is an extremely rare occurrence. We hereby present a rare case of a bilateral DC of the maxilla in a nonsyndromic 10-year-old child. The authors believe that this is one of the only four cases to have presented in the maxilla bilaterally and therefore needs a special mention. In fact, the review of existing English literature and extensive search on PubMed database from 1943 to 2017 brought to light a total of 30 cases of the bilateral DC, 3 of which have been reported in the maxilla so far, while 24 have been reported in the mandible and the remaining 3 in both the maxilla and the mandible [2, 6]. These statistics only point towards the true rarity of the condition.

2. Case Presentation

A 10-year-old child reported to our unit with the chief complaint of swelling in relation to the right middle third of the face since one month. On extraoral examination, except for the facial symmetry on the right side and deviation of the nasal dorsum to the left side, no other relevant clinical findings were present (Figures 1(a)–1(c)). Intraoral examination revealed a mixed dentition with vestibular obliteration present from the maxillary right lateral incisor extending posteriorly towards the right maxillary permanent molar (Figure 2). The mucosa over the swelling appeared normal, and there was no evidence of discharge from the swelling. A panoramic radiograph was advised that revealed a well-defined unilocular radiolucent lesion with sclerotic

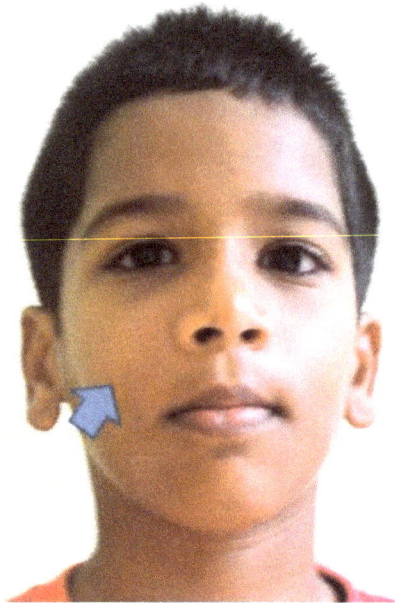

(a)

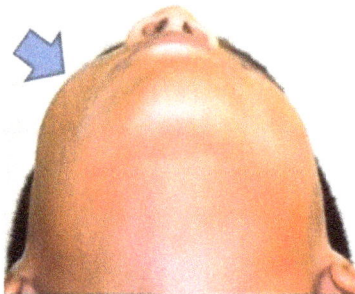

(b)

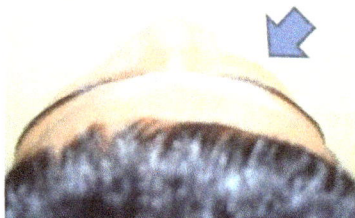

(c)

FIGURE 1: (a–c) Extraoral photographs with arrows depicting the facial swelling. (a) Frontal view. (b) Basal view. (c) Bird's eye view.

margins measuring roughly 4 cm × 3 cm in greatest dimensions and arising from the cementoenamel junction of the unerupted right maxillary permanent second premolar and extending to involve the entire maxillary sinus with displacement of the unerupted right maxillary permanent canine towards the medial aspect of the orbital floor. There was radicular resorption seen in relation to the right maxillary deciduous canine and right maxillary deciduous second molar as well as in the right maxillary permanent first premolar. What was interesting to note was the presence of

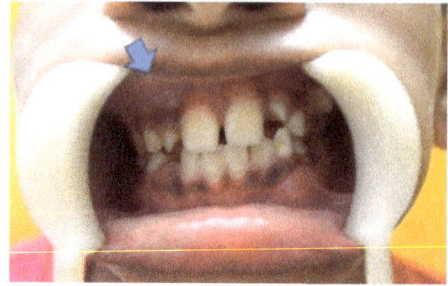

FIGURE 2: Intraoral photograph showing vestibular obliteration in relation to the right maxillary vestibule as depicted by an arrow.

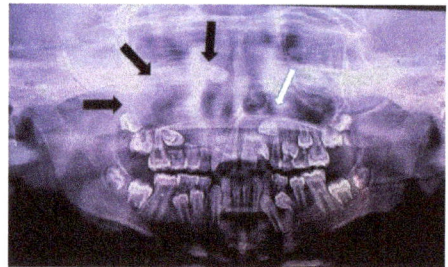

FIGURE 3: Panoramic radiograph showing bilateral unilocular radiolucencies depicted by black arrows on the right side and by a white arrow on the left side.

an occult well-defined unilocular radiolucent lesion with sclerotic margins in relation to the unerupted left maxillary permanent canine measuring roughly 1.5 × 1.5 cm in greatest dimensions (Figure 3). The extensive involvement of the right maxillary bone prompted us to perform advanced imaging in the form of cone beam computed tomography (CBCT) with three-dimensional reconstruction. The presence of bilateral maxillary lesions and the origin, size, bony destruction, expansion of the cortical plates, and involvement of the adjacent teeth were all confirmed using the axial, sagittal, and coronal views of CBCT (Figures 4(a)–4(e) and 5(a)–5(e)). The right maxillary lesion was extensive involving the entire maxillary bone with encroachment into the right nasal cavity and up to the right orbital floor (Figures 4(a)–4(e)). The aspiration of the bilateral lesions was attempted for the purpose of protein estimation which revealed a straw-coloured fluid with shiny cholesterol crystals with protein estimation values of 7.34 g/dl and 6.95 g/dl from the right and left lesions, respectively (Figure 6). A thorough systemic examination and laboratory testing ruled out the presence of any associated syndromes or systemic disease. We decided to carry out incisional biopsies of the bilateral lesions under general anesthesia to get a clearer picture of the pathology. Both specimens submitted for histopathological examination revealed a thin fibrous cystic wall lined by the 2-3 cell layer thick nonkeratinised stratified squamous epithelium. Rete pegs were absent, and the connective tissue showed mild inflammatory cell infiltrates. The subepithelial layers showed parallel bundles of collagen fibres at the periphery. These findings were consistent with the DC (Figures 7(a) and 7(b)). Under general anesthesia, enucleation of the bilateral cystic lesions

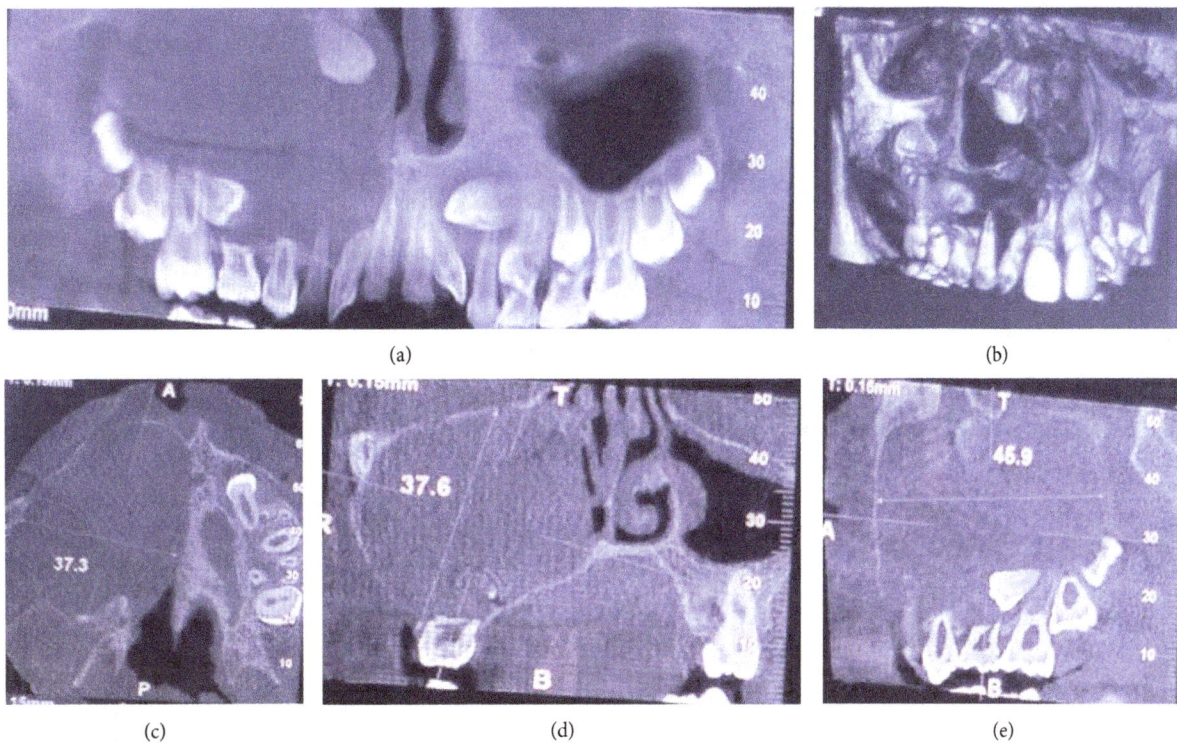

FIGURE 4: CBCT views with 3D reconstructed view showing more precisely the right maxillary radiolucency in relation to the crown of the unerupted permanent second premolar.

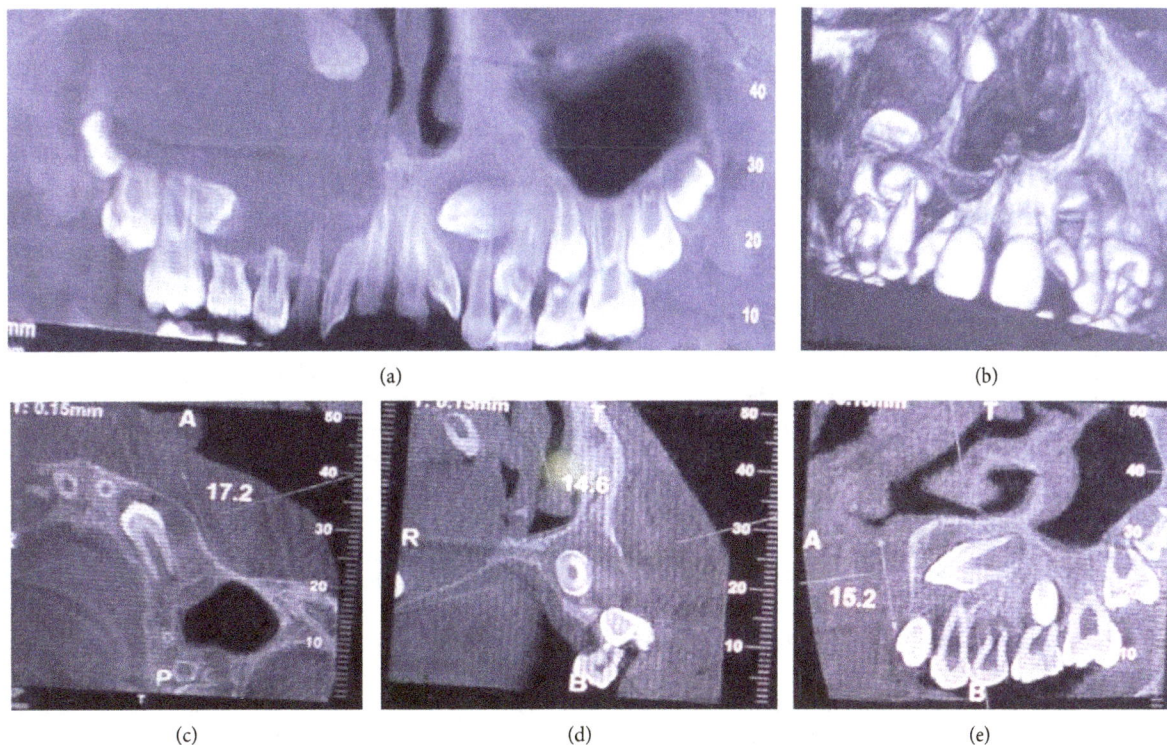

FIGURE 5: CBCT views with 3D reconstructed view showing the left maxillary radiolucency more precisely in relation to the unerupted permanent maxillary canine.

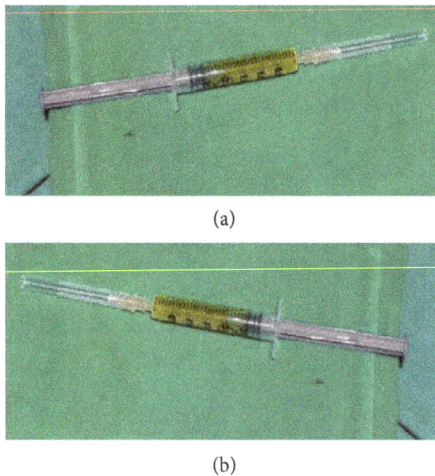

(a)

(b)

Figure 6: Aspiration of the cystic lesions revealing a straw-coloured fluid. (a) Aspirate from the right maxillary lesion. (b) Aspirate from the left maxillary lesion.

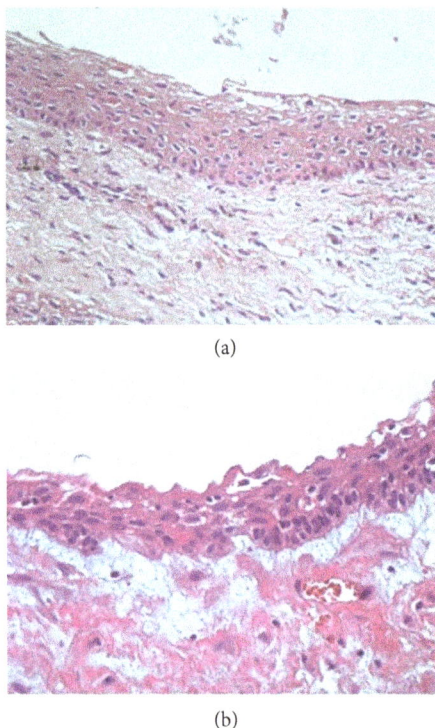

(a)

(b)

Figure 7: Histopathological examination of the bilateral maxillary lesions showing features of dentigerous cysts. (a) Histopathological picture of the right maxillary lesion. (b) Histopathological picture of the left maxillary lesion.

was carried out together with extraction of the involved teeth, and closure was affected using 4-0 Vicryl sutures in a watertight manner (Figures 8(a)–8(c)). The specimens were submitted for histopathological examination that confirmed the diagnosis of the bilateral DC (Figures 9(a) and 9(b)). No dysplastic or metaplastic changes were noted when the entire specimen was examined histopathologically. Unfortunately, the patient was lost to follow-up almost immediately

following the discharge, and therefore, no postoperative photographs or radiographs could be presented in this case to understand the treatment outcome. Nevertheless, considering the fact that bilateral DCs are rarely reported in the literature, this case deserves to be reported despite this minor pitfall.

3. Discussion

DCs represent benign odontogenic cysts associated with crowns of either unerupted or impacted permanent teeth or supernumerary teeth or odontomas but rarely deciduous teeth [3, 7]. They mostly present in the second or third decades of life and are rarely seen during childhood [3]. Seventy-five percent of the cases are seen to occur in the mandible. The substantial majority of DCs involve mandibular third molars followed by the maxillary permanent canine followed by mandibular premolars, maxillary third molars, and rarely maxillary premolars. In our case, the cysts were seen encircling the crowns of the unerupted right maxillary permanent second premolar and the permanent left canine. Studies have shown that the incidence of the DC involving the maxillary premolar was 2.7% as compared to 45.7% involving the mandibular third molar [2]. Mourshed stated that 1.44% of the impacted teeth undergo DC transformation, so DCs involving premolars are rare [8]. Daley et al. reported an incidence rate of 0.1–0.6%, whereas Shear found the incidence to be 1.5% [1, 2, 9].

The exact histogenesis of this entity is not clearly understood. It is seen to develop by accumulation of the fluid between the reduced enamel epithelium and enamel or within the enamel organ. The venous outflow is seen to get obstructed due to the pressure exerted by the empty tooth on an impacted tooth follicle, leading to rapid transudation of serum across capillary walls. This leads to the increase in hydrostatic pressure of the pooling fluid with resultant separation of the follicle from the crown with or without the reduced enamel epithelium. The development of the DC is also seen to be influenced by an intrafollicular spread of periapical infection from the deciduous tooth [4, 10].

DCs usually occur solitarily in most instances, and bilateral occurrence is an extremely rare finding. Bilateral and multiple DCs have been reported to occur in association with the number of syndromes or systemic diseases including basal-cell nevus syndrome, Gardner's syndrome, Maroteaux–Lamy syndrome (mucopolysaccharidosis type IV), cleidocranial dysplasia, and Klippel–Feil syndrome [3–6]. Sometimes, this entity is induced by prescribed medications like the combined use of cyclosporine A and calcium channel blockers [2, 4]. Pleomorphism in chromosome 1qh+ has also been reported with this condition [2, 4]. In our case, syndromic association or history of systemic medication was clearly ruled out through the absence of abnormal physical findings or laboratory results and through the absence of the use of any systemic medications.

A comprehensive search of PubMed and English literature could locate a total of 30 cases of nonsyndromic bilateral DC, 24 of which occurred in the mandible, 3 in the maxilla, and 3 in both the maxilla and the mandible [2, 6]. The age range for reported cases was seen to vary from

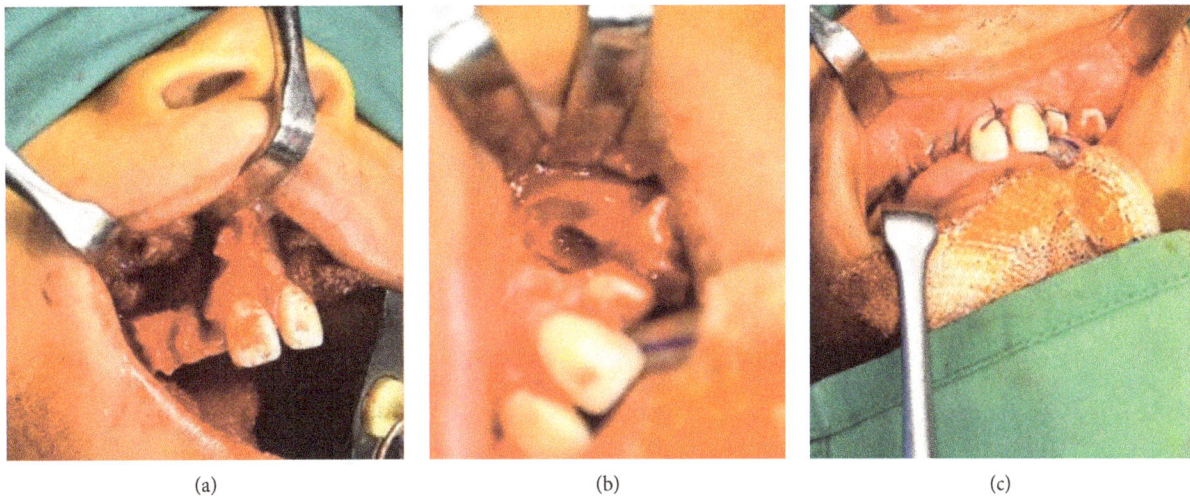

FIGURE 8: Intraoperative photographs of the patient. (a) Enucleation of the right maxillary lesion. (b) Enucleation of the left maxillary lesion. (c) Closure.

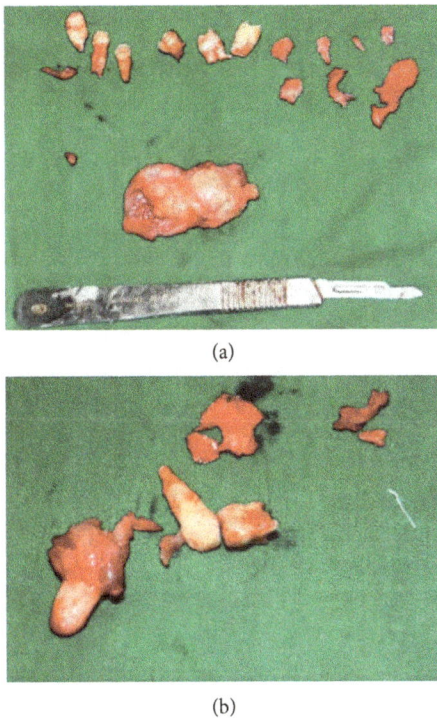

FIGURE 9: Specimens following enucleation submitted for histopathological examination. (a) The enucleated right specimen together with extraction of involved teeth. (b) The enucleated left specimen together with extraction of involved teeth.

5 to 57 years, and the mandibular teeth were most frequently involved in the majority of the cases [2, 6]. The most common site was the mandibular third molar (11 cases), followed by the mandibular first molar (10 cases), maxillary third molar (2 cases), maxillary cuspid (2 cases), mandibular first premolar (2 cases), mandibular second premolar (1 case), mandibular central incisor (1 case), and maxillary central incisor (1 case) [6, 11, 12]. In our case, the age of the presentation was 10 years, and the cysts were seen to involve

the right maxillary permanent second premolar and the left permanent canine. Only 3 cases of bilateral maxillary involvement have been reported so far in the literature. To the best of our knowledge, this is only the fourth case of the simultaneous presentation of the DC bilaterally in the maxilla. This finding points towards the true rarity of the condition, and it is therefore conceivable that bilateral DCs are either underreported or underrecognised as sometimes they are known to regress spontaneously.

DCs are usually painless unless secondarily infected and may cause facial swelling only when they have reached grotesque proportions. Therefore, early detection can be challenging. Delayed eruption of teeth is also seen [3, 5, 7]. It is imperative to perform radiographic examination in cases of unerupted teeth. In fact, DCs are frequently discovered when the radiographs are taken to investigate a missing tooth, malalignment, or the failure of tooth eruption [3, 5]. A panoramic radiograph is an excellent option for this examination. The advantage of this imaging modality is that occult lesions in either of the jaws can be clearly delineated as was the case in our patient. The classical radiographic picture is that of a unilocular radiolucent lesion of various sizes with well-defined sclerotic borders associated with the crown of an unerupted tooth. This modality also helps in differentiating a normal follicular space from that of a DC. While normal follicular space is 3-4 mm, a follicular space more than 5 mm points towards the possibility of the DC [4, 5]. Displacement of adjacent teeth and resorption of teeth roots can also be observed radiographically [4, 13]. In our case, resorption was seen in the roots of the right maxillary deciduous canine and the right maxillary deciduous second molar as well as in the right maxillary permanent first premolar with displacement of the impacted right maxillary canine towards the medial aspect of the right orbital floor. Other lesions may share the same radiological features as DCs such as periapical cysts, odontogenic keratocysts, or unicystic ameloblastomas. Although involvement of the tooth, cortical expansion, and radicular resorption are characteristics more related to DCs, other lesions were not excluded until the results of pathological analysis were known. Odontogenic keratocysts do not expand the bone to the same degree as DCs and are less likely to produce teeth resorption. Clinically and radiographically, unicystic ameloblastomas and DCs cannot be differentiated, and therefore, in such cases, the histopathological analysis serves as the only means of differentiating the two lesions. In cases of extensive bony involvement and the presence of complex cystic lesions such as our case, advanced imaging in the form of CBCT or computed tomography becomes necessary. In the maxilla, DCs may be destructive, may be occupying the maxillary sinus and nasal cavities, and may encroach on the orbit as observed in our case. Advanced imaging helps in ruling out solid or fibro-osseous lesions, displays bony details, and gives the exact information about the size, origin, content, expansion of cortical plates, and relationship of lesions to adjacent anatomical structures [3, 14, 15].

Although radiographic examination provides valuable information, histopathological examination is paramount for definite diagnosis and for ruling out the possibility of other pathologies included in the differential diagnosis. The cystic lining has an inherent ability for metastatic change largely due to areas of orthokeratinisation, ciliated cells, or mucin-secreting cells present in the cystic lining. As a result of this, some DCs may progress to odontogenic keratocysts, ameloblastomas, mucoepidermoid carcinomas, or squamous cell carcinomas which are more aggressive lesions [4]. In the present case, both the cystic linings were devoid of any metaplastic or dysplastic changes.

As far as treatment is concerned, most DCs are treated with enucleation and removal of associated teeth as was advocated by us. Large DCs have also been treated by marsupialization when enucleation might otherwise result in neurosensory dysfunction or predispose to increased chances of pathological fracture. Some authors have suggested that surgery is not the only treatment modality for DC [16, 17]. Two rare cases of bilateral DCs treated with the conservative approach have been reported, both of which progressed to spontaneous resolution preventing unnecessary surgical procedures. Although, the mechanism involved in such a spontaneous resolution is still unknown. The prognosis is usually excellent, and recurrence has been nonexistent with this entity. Unfortunately, we could not comment on the prognosis as the patient was lost to follow-up immediately following discharge from the hospital.

In conclusion, the bilateral DC not associated with any syndrome or systemic disease is an extremely rare finding and therefore necessitates a special mention. Thorough clinical examination aided with systemic examination is paramount to rule out any associated syndromes or systemic diseases. Early diagnosis using both conventional and advanced imaging modalities is important to reduce morbidity and avoid more aggressive surgical procedures.

References

[1] T. D. Daley, G. P. Wysocki, and G. A. Pringle, "Relative incidence of odontogenic tumors and oral and jaw cysts in a Canadian population," *Oral Surgery, Oral Medicine, Oral Pathology*, vol. 77, no. 3, pp. 276–280, 1994.

[2] A. Dhupar, S. Yadav, V. Dhupar, H. C. Mittal, S. Malik, and P. Rana, "Bi-maxillary dentigerous cyst in a non-syndromic child: review of literature with a case presentation," *Journal of Stomatology, Oral and Maxillofacial Surgery*, vol. 118, no. 1, pp. 45–48, 2017.

[3] E. Ustuner, S. Fitoz, C. Atasoy, I. Erden, and S. Akyar, "Bilateral maxillary dentigerous cysts: a case report," *Oral Surgery, Oral Medicine, Oral Pathology, Oral Radiology, and Endodontology*, vol. 95, no. 5, pp. 632–635, 2003.

[4] P. Devi, V. B. Thimmarasa, V. Mehrotra, and A. Agarwal, "Multiple dentigerous cyst: a case report and review," *Journal of Maxillofacial and Oral Surgery*, vol. 14, no. 1, pp. 47–51, 2015.

[5] K. S. Ko, D. G. Dover, and R. C. Jordan, "Bilateral dentigerous cysts: report of an unusual case and review of the literature," *Journal of Canadian Dental Association*, vol. 65, no. 1, pp. 49–51, 1999.

[6] J. Y. Jeon, C. J. Park, S. H. Cho, and K. G. Hwang, "Bilateral dentigerous cysts that involve all four dental quadrants: a case report and literature review," *Journal of the Korean Association of Oral and Maxillofacial Surgeons*, vol. 42, no. 2, pp. 123–126, 2016.

[7] C. S. Miller and L. R. Bean, "Pericoronal radiolucencies with and without radiopacities," *Dental Clinics of North America*, vol. 38, no. 1, pp. 51–61, 1994.

[8] F. Mourshed, "A roentgenographic study of dentigerous cysts. Incidence in a population sample," *Oral Surgery, Oral Medicine, Oral Pathology*, vol. 18, no. 1, pp. 47–53, 1964.

[9] M. Shear and P. M. Speight, *Cysts of the Oral and Maxillofacial Regions*, Blackwell Publishing, Hoboken, New Jersey, USA, 4th edition, 2007.

[10] V. B. Ziccardi, T. I. Eggleston, and R. E. Schneider, "Using fenestration technique to treat a large dentigerous cyst," *Journal of the American Dental Association*, vol. 128, no. 2, pp. 201–205, 1997.

[11] S. Shirazian and F. Agha-Hosseini, "Non-syndromic bilateral dentigerous cysts associated with permanent second premolars," *Clinics and Practice*, vol. 1, no. 3, p. e64, 2011.

[12] S. E. Cury, M. D. Cury, S. E. Cury et al., "Bilateral dentigerous cyst in a nonsyndromic patient: case report and literature review," *Journal of Dentistry for Children*, vol. 76, no. 1, pp. 92–96, 2009.

[13] U. Ertas and M. Selim, "Interesting eruption of four teeth associated with a large dentigerous cyst in mandible by only marsupialisation," *Journal of Oral and Maxillofacial Surgery*, vol. 61, no. 6, pp. 728–730, 2003.

[14] M. H. Han, K. H. Chang, C. H. Lee, D. G. Na, K. M. Yeon, and M. C. Han, "Cystic expansile masses of the maxilla: differential diagnosis with CT and MR," *American Journal of Neuroradiology*, vol. 16, no. 2, pp. 333–338, 1995.

[15] D. Q. Freitas, L. M. Tempest, E. Sicoli, and F. C. Lopes-Neto, "Bilateral dentigerous cyst: review of the literature and report of an unusual case," *Dentomaxillofacial Radiology*, vol. 35, no. 6, pp. 464–468, 2006.

[16] Y. S. Chew and B. Aghabeigi, "Spontaneous regression of bilateral dentigerous cysts: a case report," *Dental Update*, vol. 35, no. 1, pp. 63–65, 2008.

[17] N. Shah, H. Thuau, and I. Beale, "Spontaneous regression of bilateral dentigerous cysts associated with impacted mandibular third molars," *British Dental Journal*, vol. 192, no. 2, pp. 75–76, 2002.

21

Maturogenesis of an Immature Dens Evaginatus Nonvital Premolar with an Apically Placed Bioceramic Material (EndoSequence Root Repair Material®): An Unexpected Finding

S. Nagarajan M. P. Sockalingam ⓘⒹ, Mohd Safwani Affan Alli Awang Talip, and Ahmad Shuhud Irfani Zakaria

Centre for Family Oral Health, Faculty of Dentistry, The National University of Malaysia (UKM), Kuala Lumpur, Malaysia

Correspondence should be addressed to S. Nagarajan M. P. Sockalingam; drnaga67@gmail.com

Academic Editor: Jose López-López

Dens evaginatus is a dental developmental anomaly that arises due to the folding of the inner dental epithelium that leads to the formation of an additional cusp or tubercle on the occlusal surface of the affected tooth. This accessory tissue projection may carry with it a narrow and constricted pulp horn extension. Occasionally, the tubercle easily fractures, thus leading to microexposure of the pulp horn and eventual pulp necrosis. Often, the pulp necrosis occurs at a time the root development of the affected tooth is incomplete. Apexification with calcium hydroxide and mineral trioxide aggregates has been the mainstay of treatment options before root canal obturation in immature nonvital permanent teeth. Lately, regenerative endodontics (maturogenesis) is becoming one of the preferred treatment modalities to manage such teeth. The current case highlights the possibility of a bioceramic material (EndoSequence Root Repair Material, BC RRM-Fast Set Putty™, Brasseler, USA) which supposed to provide apical root closure (apexification) and could also induce continuation of root growth (maturogenesis).

1. Introduction

Dens evaginatus (DE) is a rare dental anomaly that is common in 1–4% people of Asian descent and mainly observed in the premolars. The mandibular premolars are five times most likely to have this developmental anomaly than the maxillary premolars [1]. The outward projection of the tooth may appear as tubercle on the occlusal surface and consists of a dentine core with outer enamel coverage. There are four anatomical variations to the DE tubercle types, namely, smooth, grooved, terraced and ridged, as classified by Lau in 1955 [2]. Oehlers et al. in 1967 reported that 70% of tubercles have pulp tissue extensions into them [3].

One of the major clinical issues related to DE is the possible traumatic occlusion of the adjacent erupted tooth in contact. The traumatic forces may cause either attrition or fracture of the tubercle, thus resulting in inevitable pulp exposure [2]. Pulp exposure often leads to signs and symptoms of pulpitis, pulp necrosis, and apical periodontitis. In

some of the reported DE cases, apical periodontitis had progressed into facial cellulitis and osteomyelitis [4].

The current case describes the management of a nonvital immature mandibular right second premolar tooth with DE that developed pulp necrosis and symptomatic apical periodontitis. Although apexification was performed successfully with a newly available bioceramic root repair material (Endo-Sequence®, BC RRM-Fast Set Putty, Brasseler, USA), the use of this material also resulted in the unexpected continued root growth (maturogenesis).

2. Case Report

A healthy 11-year-old girl was presented to the National University of Malaysia (UKM) Paediatric Dental Clinic with a referral for further management of pulp necrosis of an immature lower right second premolar (tooth 45), secondary to the fractured tubercle of dens evaginatus. Two weeks earlier, she had treatment at a general dental clinic for pain

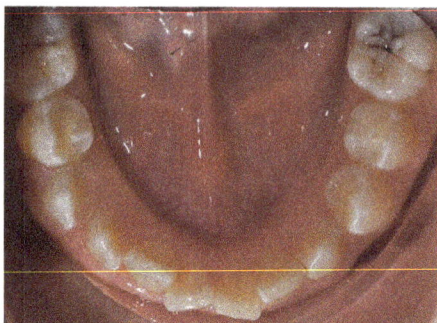

FIGURE 1: Clinical photograph of tooth 45 with an occlusal restoration of the access cavity and fractured dens evaginatus tubercle of tooth 35.

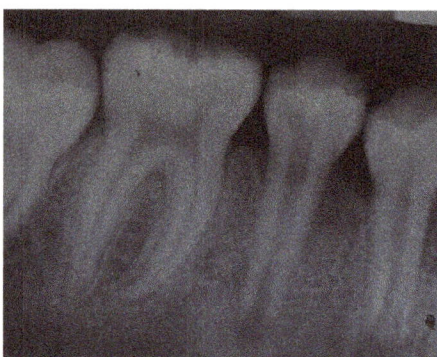

FIGURE 3: Periapical radiograph of tooth 45 after apexification with EndoSequence Root Repair Material.

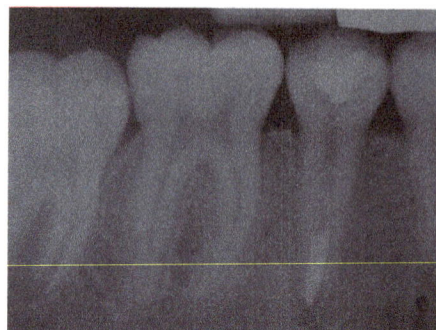

FIGURE 2: Periapical radiograph of tooth 45 showing immature root apex.

related to tooth 45. Tooth 45 had spontaneous and lingering pain following cold and thermal stimuli. The tooth was diagnosed to have symptomatic irreversible pulpitis, and root canal therapy was initiated. The canal was accessed, and pulp extirpation performed before the placement of intracanal nonsetting calcium hydroxide by the general dental practitioner (GDP).

At the time of current assessment, her tooth-related symptoms had completely resolved. General oral examination showed the presence of generalised mild gingivitis with a basic periodontal examination (BPE) score of 1 in all sextants. The patient's oral hygiene was fair with a plaque score of 30%. The patient is still in her mixed dentition with the presence of the primary maxillary canines. Her upper dental arch was well aligned, and mild crowding of anterior teeth was noted in the lower arch. Tooth 45 has an occlusal glass ionomer dressing of the access cavity made for the pulp extirpation earlier by the GDP (Figure 1). Cold and electric pulp sensibility testings showed positive responses to all fully erupted premolars indicative of tooth vitality expect for tooth 45. Tooth 45 also has slight tenderness to percussion. Periapical radiograph of tooth 45 showed an immature root with convergent open apex and small periapical radiolucency. The pulp space of tooth 45 is of an even width from the coronal to the apical portion (Figure 2). Based on the

assessments, tooth 45 was diagnosed with pulp necrosis secondary to fractured dens evaginatus and symptomatic apical periodontitis.

On the day of initial assessment, tooth 45 was isolated with rubber dam after infiltration of local anaesthetic solution (2% lidocaine with 1 : 80000 adrenaline). Pulp chamber was reentered through the previously prepared access cavity. The root canal was exposed and irrigated with saline. After that, the canal was dried with paper points and the tooth working length was estimated with a K-file No. 60. A working length, 2 mm short of the apical opening, was determined (17 mm). The canal was gently prepared with the K-file No. 60 and then irrigated with a copious volume of 1.5% sodium hypochlorite (NaOCl). After drying the wet canal with paper points, nonsetting calcium hydroxide was placed into the canal and the access cavity was double sealed with Cavit™ 3M, USA, and glass ionomer cement (GIC) (Riva Self Cure™ SDI, Australia).

Two weeks later, the tooth was reassessed for any signs and symptoms of infection. The tooth was no longer tender to percussion, and there was no indication of infection-related signs and symptoms. After isolation with a rubber dam, the root canal of tooth 45 was reaccessed and irrigated with a copious volume 1.5% NaOCl to remove the nonsetting calcium hydroxide. Then, the canal was irrigated with sterile water and dried with paper points. Subsequently, the canal was irrigated with 17% EDTA (Pulpdent™, Watertown, Massachusetts) for a minute and dried with paper points. Finally, under the guidance of a dental operating microscope (Carl Zeiss Surgical GmbH, S100), the apical region was filled using the EndoSequence (BC RRM-Fast Set Putty, Brasseler, USA) material up to 4 mm thickness to create an apical seal (Figure 3). The orifice of the root canal was double sealed with a cotton pellet, temporary filling material (Cavit 3M, USA), and GIC (Riva Self Cure SDI, Australia).

Once again, the root canal was reaccessed two weeks later, irrigated with 1.5% NaOCl, and dried with paper points. Next, the dried canal was obturated with thermoplasticised gutta-percha using the Obtura III Max System (Obtura Spartan® Endodontics) (Figure 4). After that, the access cavity was double sealed with GIC (Riva Self Cure SDI, Australia) and nanohybrid composite (AURA™ SDI, Australia), respectively.

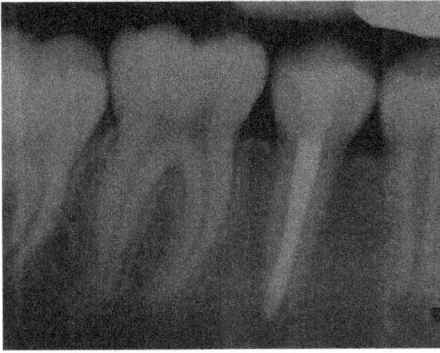

FIGURE 4: Periapical radiograph of tooth 45 after root canal obturation with thermoplasticised gutta-percha.

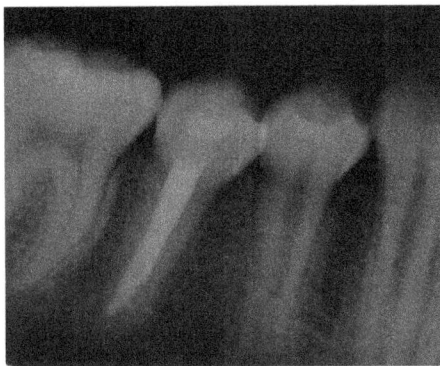

FIGURE 5: Periapical radiograph of tooth 45, 6-month postapexification showing complete root maturogenesis.

Following the obturation, tooth 45 was reviewed at three-month and six-month intervals. During both reviews, tooth 45 was asymptomatic. However, at the six-month review, a periapical radiograph of tooth 45 showed an unexpected finding. The apical root of tooth 45 continued to grow beyond the apexification level with a normal periodontal ligament space and lamina dura. No evidence of periapical radiolucency was noted (Figure 5). However, regular annual monitoring of tooth 45 is essential to ensure that the coronal seal is intact and no apical complication further arises.

3. Discussion

Numerous treatment modalities are available to treat teeth with dens evaginatus (DE) [2, 4, 5]. However, the treatment selection depends mainly on the stage of root development and symptomatic status of the affected tooth. Levitan and Himel in 2006 proposed a possible treatment protocol to manage teeth with DE based on whether the treatment is for teeth with healthy or diseased pulp. Dens evaginatus tooth with healthy pulp is treated either by reducing the occlusal contact of the opposing tooth or by strengthening its tubercle with a flowable composite resin regardless of whether the tooth has a mature or immature root. If the tooth has an inflamed pulp, partial pulpotomy with MTA is suggested for an immature tooth and conventional root canal treatment for the mature tooth. If the DE tooth has a necrotic pulp, apexification is proposed for an immature tooth and conventional root canal treatment for a mature tooth [2].

Necrotic teeth with immature roots provide significant challenges to clinicians especially with their wide open apices which do not allow successful canal obturation and thin dentine walls which are prone to fracture and compromised crown-root ratio [6]. Over the years, apexification with calcium hydroxide has been the mainstay of treatment for the immature teeth. Apexification allows apical barrier formation that enables condensation of root filling materials against it. However, the usage of calcium hydroxide for apexification had declined currently due to its shortcomings such as prolonged treatment time to achieve apical barrier, and it has hygroscopic and proteolytic properties that induce the desiccation of dentinal proteins [7–10]. In the last decade, mineral trioxide aggregates (MTA) have been used widely in the apexification of nonvital immature teeth. Although MTA has reduced the treatment time and had shown higher success rate than calcium hydroxide [11], nevertheless, it too has some setbacks such as tooth discolouration and weakening of the dentine wall due to the similarity in its effect to calcium hydroxide [10, 12, 13]. Of late, many other materials such calcium-enriched cement, bioaggregate, Biodentine, and EndoSequence Root Repair Material have been marketed for various endodontic procedures [14]. These materials showed some promising results, but the long-term evidence of their success is still scanty.

The regenerative endodontic technique (RET) is another treatment option that has received wide coverage in the literature regarding the management of nonvital permanent teeth in recent times. Although this technique is initially known as the vascularisation [15], other names for this technique are revitalisation, repopulation, regeneration, or even maturogenesis [6]. However, Wigler et al. in 2013 argued that this technique not only promotes blood vessel formation but also leads to continued root development; therefore, maturogenesis is a better term to use to describe the root growth [16]. This technique allows repopulation of the root canal with pluripotent cells from the apical papilla of the immature tooth and initiation of root development [15]. Maturogenesis is said to promote continued root development with increased dentine thickness, thus improving the long-term prognosis of the affected teeth [6]. This treatment technique has caused a paradigm shift in our management thoughts regarding nonvital immature teeth. Nevertheless, it is still premature to conclude that this method is successful in all cases.

In the described case, we performed an apexification procedure on necrotic immature tooth 45 after discussing the various treatment options with the child's parents. In this procedure, the EndoSequence Root Repair Material (ERRM) was used to create an apical barrier. This material is a premixed bioceramic material which is composed of calcium silicates, zirconium oxide, tantalum oxide, calcium phosphate monobasic, and filler agents [17]. The material has a putty-like consistency that allows easy placement through a syringe. It has high tissue compatibility, antibacterial action (pH > 12), and excellent sealing properties [18–21]. Besides these advantageous properties, the material also has both the osteoconductive and osteoinductive potentials. Hydration of the material leads to the release of calcium and hydroxide ions into the surroundings. Over time, with the presence of phosphate ions in the surroundings, osteoconduction occurs with hydroxyapatite crystal-like structures being deposited over the placed ERRM material, and this results in the apical barrier formation.

Though the intended treatment for this patient is to create an apical barrier for root canal obturation, an unexpected finding was observed during the follow-up stages after the root canal obturation. We found that the root continued to grow and achieved its matured development. A normal lamina dura with an even periodontal space was noted around the apex of the tooth. One of the reasons for this occurrence is probably due to the osteoinductive property of the ERRM. The osteoinductivity of ERRM could have attracted the pluripotent cells from the surroundings to form preosteoblasts. The presence of preosteoblasts leads to the secretion of the bone matrix that later calcified into bone [17]. Based on a literature search, this appears to be the first case that reports maturogenesis of the root of a necrotic nonvital immature permanent tooth using ERRM as an apexification material.

4. Conclusion

The current case showed that ERRM is not only successful in creating an apical barrier in a nonvital immature permanent tooth for root canal obturation but also able to promote continued root growth. However, the potential of ERRM in fostering continued root growth on nonvital immature permanent teeth needs further clinical and research evidence.

References

[1] E. A. Echeverri, M. M. Wang, C. Chavaria, and D. L. Taylor, "Multiple dens evaginatus: diagnosis, management, and complications: case report," *Pediatric Dentistry*, vol. 16, no. 4, pp. 314–317, 1994.

[2] M. E. Levitan and V. T. Himel, "Dens evaginatus: literature review, pathophysiology, and comprehensive treatment regimen," *Journal of Endodontics*, vol. 32, no. 1, pp. 1–9, 2006.

[3] F. A. Oehlers, K. W. Lee, and E. C. Lee, "Dens evaginatus (evaginated odontome). Its structure and responses to external stimuli," *The Dental Practitioner and Dental Record*, vol. 17, no. 7, pp. 239–244, 1967.

[4] Y. Ju, "Dens evaginatus–a difficult diagnostic problem?," *Journal of Clinical Pediatric Dentistry*, vol. 15, no. 4, pp. 247–248, 1991.

[5] F. J. Hill and W. J. Bellis, "Dens evaginatus and its management," *British Dental Journal*, vol. 156, no. 11, pp. 400–402, 1984.

[6] M. Duggal, H. J. Tong, M. Al-Ansary, W. Twati, P. F. Day, and H. Nazzal, "Interventions for the endodontic management of non-vital traumatised immature permanent anterior teeth in children and adolescents: a systematic review of the evidence and guidelines of the European Academy of Paediatric Dentistry," *European Archives of Paediatric Dentistry*, vol. 18, no. 3, pp. 139–151, 2017.

[7] J. O. Andreasen, B. Farik, and E. C. Munksgaard, "Long-term calcium hydroxide as a root canal dressing may increase risk of root fracture," *Dental Traumatology*, vol. 18, no. 3, pp. 134–137, 2002.

[8] G. E. Doyon, T. Dumsha, and J. A. von Fraunhofer, "Fracture resistance of human root dentin exposed to intracanal calcium hydroxide," *Journal of Endodontics*, vol. 31, no. 12, pp. 895–897, 2005.

[9] B. Rosenberg, P. E. Murray, and K. Namerow, "The effect of calcium hydroxide root filling on dentin fracture strength," *Dental Traumatology*, vol. 23, no. 1, pp. 26–29, 2007.

[10] W. A. Twati, D. J. Wood, T. W. Liskiewicz, N. S. Willmott, and M. S. Duggal, "An evaluation of the effect of non-setting calcium hydroxide on human dentine: a pilot study," *European Archives of Paediatric Dentistry*, vol. 10, no. 2, pp. 104–109, 2009.

[11] D. P. Pradhan, H. S. Chawla, K. Gauba, and A. Goyal, "Comparative evaluation of endodontic management of teeth with unformed apices with mineral trioxide aggregate and calcium hydroxide," *Journal of Dentistry for Children*, vol. 73, no. 2, pp. 79–85, 2006.

[12] D. Felman and P. Parashos, "Coronal tooth discoloration and white mineral trioxide aggregate," *Journal of Endodontics*, vol. 39, no. 4, pp. 484–487, 2013.

[13] G. Krastl, N. Allgayer, P. Lenherr, A. Filippi, P. Taneja, and R. Weiger, "Tooth discoloration induced by endodontic materials: a literature review," *Dental Traumatology*, vol. 29, no. 1, pp. 2–7, 2013.

[14] S. Utneja, R. R. Nawal, S. Talwar, and M. Verma, "Current perspectives of bio-ceramic technology in endodontics: calcium enriched mixture cement - review of its composition, properties and applications," *Restorative Dentistry & Endodontics*, vol. 40, no. 1, pp. 1–13, 2015.

[15] F. Banchs and M. Trope, "Revascularization of immature permanent teeth with apical periodontitis: new treatment protocol?," *Journal of Endodontics*, vol. 30, no. 4, pp. 196–200, 2004.

[16] R. Wigler, A. Y. Kaufman, S. Lin, N. Steinbock, H. Hazan-Molina, and C. D. Torneck, "Revascularization: a treatment for permanent teeth with necrotic pulp and incomplete root development," *Journal of Endodontics*, vol. 39, no. 3, pp. 319–326, 2013.

[17] N. Shokouhinejad, M. H. Nekoofar, H. Razmi et al., "Bioactivity of EndoSequence Root Repair Material and bioaggregate," *International Endodontic Journal*, vol. 45, no. 12, pp. 1127–1134, 2012.

[18] A. Z. AlAnezi, J. Jiang, K. E. Safavi, L. S. W. Spangberg, and Q. Zhu, "Cytotoxicity evaluation of endosequence root repair material," *Oral Surgery, Oral Medicine, Oral Pathology, Oral Radiology, and Endodontology*, vol. 109, no. 3, pp. e122–e125, 2010.

[19] J. Ma, Y. Shen, S. Stojicic, and M. Haapasalo, "Biocompatibility of two novel root repair materials," *Journal of Endodontics*, vol. 37, no. 6, pp. 793–798, 2011.

[20] K. F. Lovato and C. M. Sedgley, "Antibacterial activity of endosequence root repair material and proroot MTA against clinical isolates of Enterococcus faecalis," *Journal of Endodontics*, vol. 37, no. 11, pp. 1542–1546, 2011.

22

Conservative Treatment of Dentigerous Cyst by Marsupialization in a Young Female Patient

Layal Ghandour,[1] **Hisham F. Bahmad**ⓘ**,**[2] **and Samar Bou-Assi**ⓘ[1,3]

[1]Department of Orthodontics and Dentofacial Orthopedics, Faculty of Dentistry, Lebanese University, Hadath, Lebanon
[2]Department of Anatomy, Cell Biology, and Physiological Sciences, Faculty of Medicine, American University of Beirut, Beirut, Lebanon
[3]Division of Orthodontics and Dentofacial Orthopedics, Department of Otolaryngology-Head and Neck Surgery, Faculty of Medicine, American University of Beirut Medical Center, Beirut, Lebanon

Correspondence should be addressed to Samar Bou-Assi; assisamar@hotmail.com

Academic Editor: Daniel Torrés-Lagares

Dentigerous cysts (DCs) are the most prevalent developmental odontogenic cysts that occur in middle-aged individuals. They frequently originate from the epithelial remnants of tooth-forming organs. Hereby, we present a case of a 13-year-old young female patient presenting with DC that was treated successfully by marsupialization. The patient's chief complaint was the crowding of the anterior teeth. Clinical examination showed that the patient had all her permanent teeth present with a retained mandibular left second primary molar that was previously treated by pulpectomy. The radiographic examination revealed a unilocular radiolucent lesion with well-defined margins associated with a mesially-tipped unerupted mandibular left second premolar. The differential diagnosis confirmed that the lesion was a DC. The treatment consisted of surgical removal of the DC to allow proper eruption of the permanent tooth and to prevent the lesion from becoming an aggressive one causing gross expansion of bone with subsequent facial asymmetry, pain, displacement of teeth, and root resorption. A removable acrylic obturator was delivered to the patient keeping the path clear and guiding the eruption of the premolar until fully erupted.

1. Introduction

Odontogenic cysts are a group of common lesions occurring in the maxilla and mandible and are of the main causes of the destruction of these bones [1]. A dentigerous cyst (DC) is a cyst that is characterized by the attachment to the crown of an unerupted tooth [2]. The exact pathogenesis of DC is obscure; however, most authors believe that this cyst is of a developmental origin from tooth follicles.

The DCs are seldom discovered in young individuals since they frequently occur in individuals between 20 and 40 years of age. These cysts are discovered unexpectedly on routine radiographic examination since DCs are asymptomatic unless after an infection [3, 4].

The aim of the present study is to present a clinical case of a DC in a young female patient that was successfully treated by marsupialization.

2. Case Presentation

A 13-year-old female patient was presented for consultation to the Department of Orthodontics and Dentofacial Orthopedics, School of Dentistry, Lebanese University. Her chief complaint was the crowding of her anterior teeth. Her medical and dental histories were noncontributory, and the patient did not mention any previous or recent habit. On physical examination, no swelling or tenderness was documented.

Upon clinical examination, the patient had all her permanent teeth and a retained mandibular left second primary molar. Radiographic records consisted of an orthopantomogram, a lateral cephalogram, a posteroanterior cephalogram, and a hand wrist radiograph. The orthopantomogram revealed a well-defined radiolucent lesion on the mandibular left side surrounding the unerupted mandibular left second premolar which appeared to be mesially tipped below the retained primary second molar. The root of the adjacent premolar was included in the lesion but did not reveal any root resorption (Figures 1 and 2).

Going back to the old orthopantomogram (OPG) of the patient collected by the Pediatrics Department, it was noted that no lesion was visible at that time (Figure 3). The patient was referred to the Oral Pathology Department in order to obtain a meticulous diagnosis concerning the radiolucent lesion that was detected on the orthopantomogram during the initial diagnosis. The differential diagnosis for the lesion included a DC, an odontogenic keratocyst, and an ameloblastoma. Histologically, a thick epithelial lining with rete ridges was present. Moreover, chronic inflammatory cellular infiltration appeared in the capsule of the cyst. All these findings confirmed that the diagnosed cyst is a DC. The major objective of initiating the treatment as early as possible in this patient was to hinder the progression of the DC prohibiting its destructive consequences. Moreover, the aim of initiating a nonaggressive (marsupialization) treatment was to save the involved tooth, allowing its healthy eruption.

Several treatment modalities of a DC have been reported in the literature ranging from marsupialization to enucleation. The common treatment for DC is enucleation followed by extraction of the involved tooth. When the cyst is large, the first approach is marsupialization to decrease the size of the osseous defect and then enucleation and tooth extraction are performed afterwards [5–8].

Enucleation is the chosen treatment plan whenever the cyst is small and saving the involved tooth is impossible. This treatment modality should be avoided in large cysts since it is usually accompanied by facial, esthetic, and functional defects [9].

Other approaches are considered when the cyst is small and when the patient is young. In cases of enlarged follicles of impacted canines, exposing the affected tooth surgically and the traction of the tooth by orthodontic means leads to the cessation of the cystic lesion and the preservation of the affected tooth [10].

Taking into consideration that the diagnosed cyst can potentially become an aggressive lesion with a bone destructive ability that might lead to loss of the involved teeth, root resorption, pain, and facial asymmetry, and considering the age of the patient, a primary approach by marsupialization was initiated (Figure 4).

After the surgery, the patient was instructed to wear the acrylic resin obturator that was previously fabricated to maintain the surgical opening during healing and assure success of the surgery (Figure 5). The patient was asked to eat with the obturator in place and remove it only for cleaning. Follow-up appointments were scheduled every three

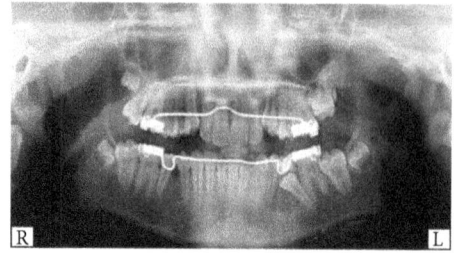

FIGURE 1: Orthopantomogram (OPG) showing a radiolucent lesion at the mandibular left side (second premolar region).

months postsurgery to assure the eruption of the second premolar and the absence of any recurrence.

The postsurgical orthopantomogram (OPG) that was taken 6 months after the surgery revealed the absence of any radiolucent lesion and the successful eruption of the mandibular left second premolar (Figures 6 and 7).

3. Discussion

Dentigerous cysts (DCs) have been reported extensively in the literature. The exact cause of this cyst is still unknown, but many theories are proposed. The "intrafollicular theory" suggests that a DC is a consequence of fluid accumulation between the outer and inner surfaces of the epithelium. This accumulation occurs during the formation of the crown. The second theory is the "enamel hypoplasia theory". It suggests the development of the cyst after stellate reticulum degeneration. "Main's theory" suggests that the cyst is a result of the hydrostatic pressure exerted by an impacted tooth on the follicle which results in the separation of the impacted crown from the surrounding follicle.

Some authors believe that a DC is more likely to occur as a result of an inflamed nonvital deciduous tooth during the maturation of the permanent successor. In 1928, Bloch-Jorgensen reported 22 cases of DCs with the cystic wall being in a direct contact with an affected deciduous tooth. Azaz and Shteyer [11], Shaw et al. [12], and many others also pointed out the same inflammatory cause of the cyst.

In the case described in this report, the most probable cause of the DC could be the nonvital deciduous second molar. After a thorough inspection of the radiographic file of the patient, one can notice the absence of radiolucency in the initial orthopantomogram that was taken when the patient was 9 years and 6 months old (Figure 3). Later, after root resorption of the treated root canal of the deciduous molar, the cyst started developing (Figure 2(b)). One explanation is that the nonresorbable material that was used in the pulpectomy of the previously infected deciduous molar acted as a stimulus for the development of the cyst. Pulpectomy, by definition, is the elimination of infected pulp tissues by chemical and mechanical means. After removing the pulp, the canals are filled with a material that supposedly should resorb along with the resorption of the associated root [13].

The incidence of DCs is highest in the second and third decades of life [1, 14]. This cyst is usually rare in the first

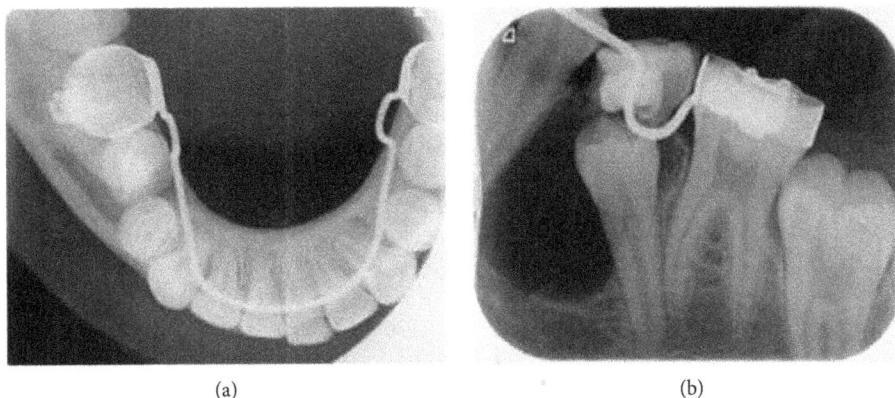

(a)   (b)

FIGURE 2: (a) Occlusal radiograph to further investigate the well-defined radiolucent lesion. (b) Periapical radiograph to further investigate the well-defined radiolucent lesion.

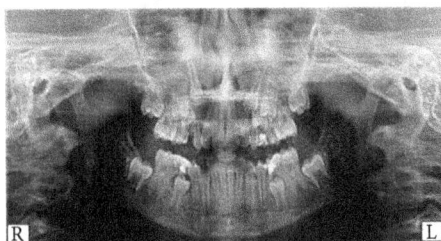

FIGURE 3: Older orthopantomogram (OPG) showing the absence of any radiolucent lesion at the mandibular left side (second premolar region).

decade. For this reason, when it comes to diagnosis in young patients, it is usually difficult to state a definitive diagnosis without a pathological and radiographic diagnosis. In the reported case, the definitive diagnosis was confirmed by the Pathology Department at the Lebanese University. The report we received from the Pathology Department included not only the definitive diagnosis of the cyst, but also the differential diagnosis. The differential diagnosis of DCs included odontogenic keratocyst, primordial cyst, ameloblastoma, and ameloblastic fibroma. A comprehensive and meticulous report interpreted the reason for the final diagnosis.

Dentigerous cysts are detected by chance after the patient/dentist realizes that some of his/her primary teeth are still retained. This cyst, because it is usually asymptomatic, is sometimes recognized after it has expanded into the alveolar bone and has led to destruction. Berden et al. found that it is important to choose a safe treatment in young individuals and avoid surgical approaches that lead to esthetic, functional, and psychological problems if facial defects occur. The decompression of large cysts was outweighed when the cyst is large to avoid the previously mentioned drawbacks of enucleation [9]. Whenever these cysts are detected in a late stage, they are usually treated by enucleation followed by the extraction of the involved tooth [15].

Several factors predicting the spontaneous eruption of premolars following marsupialization have been extensively discussed in the literature. For this purpose, many angular and linear values were measured on an orthopantomogram.

Hyomoto et al. measured the cusp depth of the impacted tooth, angle formed between the long axis of the impacted tooth and the bisector of the long axis of adjacent teeth. He also measured the root maturity, the cyst area, and the eruption space available. He found that the smaller the patient, the greater the chance of eruption. A depth of inclusion of 4.4 mm and an angulation of tooth of $20.4° \pm 21.8°$, 1/2 root formation were associated with spontaneous eruption of impacted teeth. Moreover, he concluded that the space present for eruption did not influence the eruption. In his study, he found that spontaneous eruption of premolars following marsupialization occurred in 72.4% of the cases [16].

Fujii et al. in 2008 analyzed similar factors as Hyomoto et al. [16, 17]. They concluded that spontaneous eruption of impacted teeth associated with DCs after marsupialization is possible in patients less than 10 years old. He added that the depth of inclusion should be smaller than 5.1 mm and that tooth angulation must be smaller than 25°. The space present for eruption should be larger than 1 cm, and the root should be incompletely formed [17].

Yahara et al., in attempt to measure the same factors, found that spontaneous eruption occurred when the mean age was 9.8 years. They also explained that the smaller the depth of inclusion, the better chance of eruption. The angulation that was measured by the abovementioned authors was also measured by Yahara et al. This angle should be close to 60° for the tooth to erupt without any traction [18].

Trying to find the possibility of spontaneous eruption of the affected premolar in this reported case, the same factors were measured. The patient was 13 years old, and depth of inclusion was 3.6 mm. The angle formed between the long axis of the tooth and the bisector of the long axis of both adjacent teeth was 40°. Moreover, three-quarters of the root was formed on the final panoramic radiograph.

Although the age of the patient and the stage of rhizogenesis (root formation) were discouraging, we preferred the conservative approach hoping for the spontaneous eruption of the second premolar.

Conservative treatment of a DC was reported in some cases [19]. The primary objective of such a treatment was to save the involved tooth especially in young patients. This cautious therapy is adopted in children due to the bone

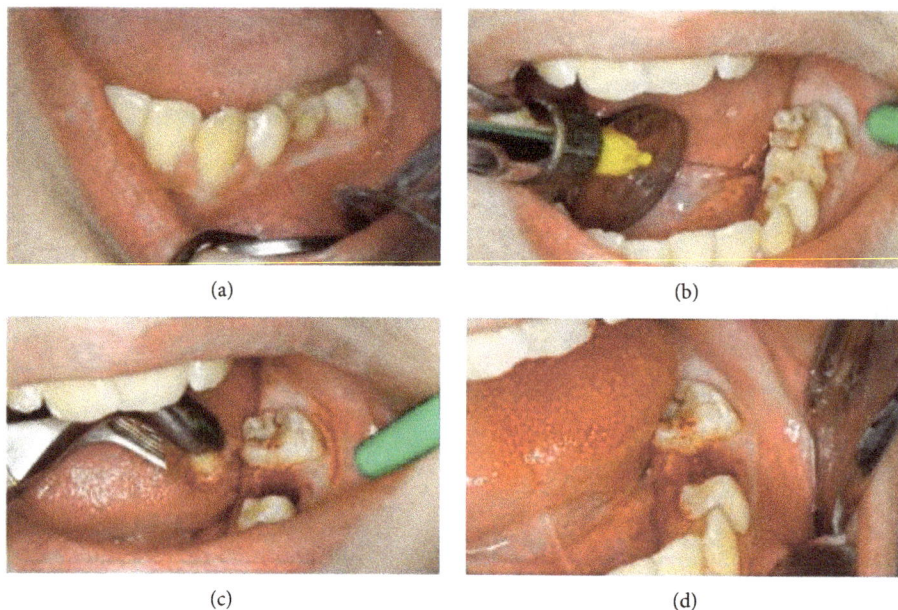

(a)

(b)

(c)

(d)

FIGURE 4: Marsupialization of the cystic lesion after extraction of the deciduous second molar, revealing retraction to visualize the surgical site at first (a), then anesthetizing the site (b), followed by extraction of the primary second molar and drainage (c), and finally opening of the surgical site after marsupialization (d).

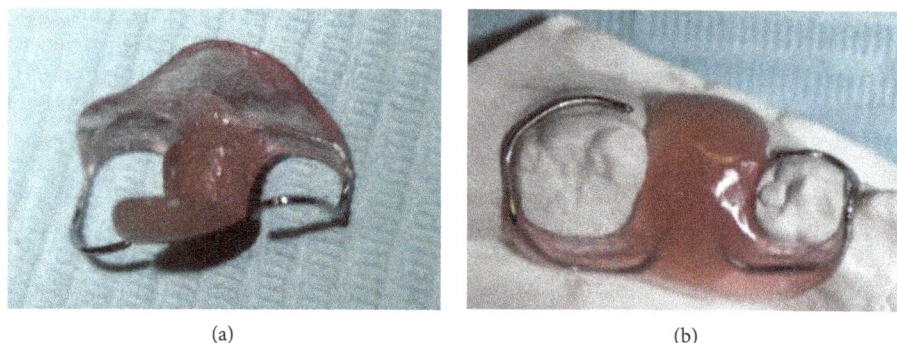

(a)

(b)

FIGURE 5: The acrylic resin obturator to maintain the surgical opening during healing.

reparative capacity in these patients and the potential of teeth with open apices to erupt after the removal of the cyst. When this treatment approach is rendered, the cyst is left opened allowing the cystic drainage and a stent or a removable appliance is placed afterwards. This removable obturator facilitated the drainage of the cyst into the oral cavity, thus relieving the pressure and allowing the tooth to erupt spontaneously. Moreover, being a removable appliance, the oral hygiene was not affected and unwanted inflammation did not occur. In the case reported in the following article, the advocated first line of treatment was a conservative marsupialization that was initiated in attempt to save the premolar. After performing the marsupialization and leaving the surgical site open to the oral cavity, the involved tooth successfully erupted into the dental arch.

4. Concluding Remarks

Dentigerous cysts are the most prevalent developmental odontogenic cysts that occur in middle-aged individuals

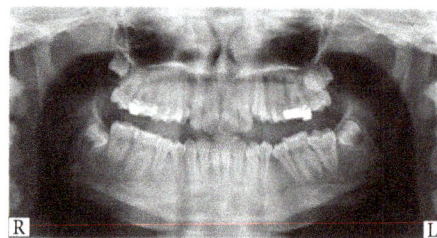

FIGURE 6: Orthopantomogram (OPG) showing the absence of any radiolucent lesion and the successful eruption of the mandibular left second premolar.

[20]. Although abundant theories had been suggested concerning the cause of this cyst, the precise cause is still unidentified.

Most reported cases of DCs in young individuals were due to infected nonvital deciduous primary molars. The pulpectomy treatment of these nonvital teeth did not cease the enlargement of the cyst. Such a treatment in an attempt to

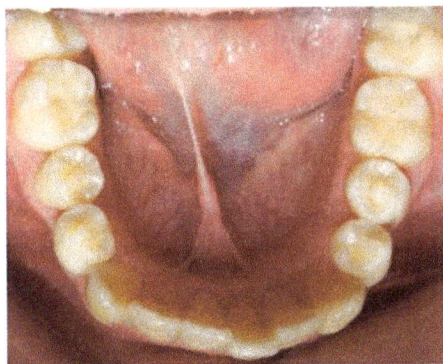

FIGURE 7: Intraoral photo postmarsupialization with the mandibular left second premolar completely erupted on the arch.

save a primary tooth has led to the extraction of the permanent successor after the cyst has spread and was discovered by chance.

The material used in pulpectomy and the procedure itself should be further studied, and the benefit-to-risk ratio before performing such a treatment should be considered. Moreover, if the practitioner chooses this option, he should insist on the importance of regular checkup appointments. In this way, early detection of abnormal pathological cysts would be possible.

Numerous treatment procedures were discussed in the literature depending on the age of the patient, severity and size of the cyst, and the objectives behind the treatment. A conservative approach should be the first line of treatment whenever possible. The predicting factors for the spontaneous eruption of the permanent successor following marsupialization that were reported in the literature should not be taken as strict guidelines and should not guide the choice of the treatment plan. In the case reported in this paper, marsupialization was performed in order to save the affected tooth. Successful eruption of the mandibular left second premolar was reported.

Ethical Approval

This study was carried out in accordance with the recommendations of the Institutional Review Board (IRB) of the Lebanese University (LU) with written informed consent from the parents of the included subject.

Consent

Parents of the patient gave written informed consent in accordance with the Declaration of Helsinki. Written informed consent was obtained from the parents of the patient for the publication of this case report and accompanying images and for the participation in this case report study.

Authors' Contributions

Samar Bou-Assi, Layal Ghandour, and Hisham F. Bahmad worked on the case study conception and design. Layal Ghandour was responsible for getting the clinical data from medical records. Samar Bou-Assi provided other authors with explanations about the case reported. Layal Ghandour and Hisham F. Bahmad were responsible for writing the introduction, case presentation, and discussion and editing the whole manuscript, in addition to proofreading. Samar Bou-Assi was responsible for the study supervision and conduction of the whole project. All authors contributed to the drafting of the manuscript and critically revised and edited the manuscript prior to approving the final draft. All authors approved the final draft of the manuscript.

Acknowledgments

The authors would like to thank the family of the patient whose case is presented here for granting us their permission to publish this case report and the Department of Oral and Maxillofacial Surgery, Faculty of Dentistry, for their permission to disclose this information.

References

[1] G. Ochsenius, E. Escobar, L. Godoy, and C. Peñafiel, "Odontogenic cysts: analysis of 2,944 cases in Chile," *Medicina Oral, Patología Oral y Cirugía Bucal*, vol. 12, no. 2, pp. E85–E91, 2007.

[2] B. G. Koseoglu, B. Atalay, and M. A. Erdem, "Odontogenic cysts: a clinical study of 90 cases," *Journal of Oral Science* vol. 46, no. 4, pp. 253–257, 2004.

[3] L. T. Friedlander, H. Hussani, M. P. Cullinan et al., "VEGF and VEGFR2 in dentigerous cysts associated with impacted third molars," *Pathology*, vol. 47, no. 5, pp. 446–451, 2015.

[4] D. W. Anderson and D. Evans, "Dentigerous cyst of mandible presenting as sepsis," *The American Journal of Emergency Medicine*, vol. 32, no. 12, pp. 1561.e3–1561.e4, 2014.

[5] I. Reynoso Obregon, "Clinical evaluation of cases of cysts treated by permanent drainage," *Acta Odontológica Venezolana*, vol. 5, no. 3, pp. 350–364, 1967.

[6] B. W. Fickling, "Cysts of the jaw: a long-term survey of types and treatment," *Proceedings of the Royal Society of Medicine* vol. 58, 11, Part 1, pp. 847–854, 1965.

[7] J. Eyre and J. M. Zakrzewska, "The conservative management of large odontogenic keratocysts," *The British Journal of Oral & Maxillofacial Surgery*, vol. 23, no. 3, pp. 195–203, 1985.

[8] R. Dammer, H. Niederdellmann, P. Danuner, and M. Nuebler-Moritz, "Conservative or radical treatment of keratocysts: a retrospective review," *The British Journal of Oral & Maxillofacial Surgery*, vol. 35, no. 1, pp. 46–48, 1997.

[9] J. Berden, G. Koch, and C. Ullbro, "Case series: treatment of large dentigerous cysts in children," *European Archives of Paediatric Dentistry*, vol. 11, no. 3, pp. 140–145, 2010.

[10] A. Becker, "In defense of the guidance theory of palatal canine displacement," *The Angle Orthodontist*, vol. 65, no. 2, pp. 95–98, 1995.

[11] B. Azaz and A. Shteyer, "Dentigerous cysts associated with second mandibular bicuspids in children: report of five cases," *ASDC Journal of Dentistry for Children*, vol. 40, no. 1, pp. 29–31, 1973.

[12] W. Shaw, M. Smith, and F. Hill, "Inflammatory follicular cysts," *ASDC Journal of Dentistry for Children*, vol. 47, no. 2, pp. 97–101, 1980.

[13] Y. Machida, "Root canal obturation in deciduous teeth," *Japan Dental Association*, vol. 36, no. 7, pp. 796–802, 1983.

[14] T. D. Daley, G. P. Wysocki, and G. A. Pringle, "Relative incidence of odontogenic tumors and oral and jaw cysts in a Canadian population," *Oral Surgery, Oral Medicine, and Oral Pathology*, vol. 77, no. 3, pp. 276–280, 1994.

[15] L. B. Kaban and M. J. Troulis, *Pediatric Oral and Maxillofacial Surgery*, WB Saunders Company, 2004.

[16] M. Hyomoto, M. Kawakami, M. Inoue, and T. Kirita, "Clinical conditions for eruption of maxillary canines and mandibular premolars associated with dentigerous cysts," *American Journal of Orthodontics and Dentofacial Orthopedics*, vol. 124, no. 5, pp. 515–520, 2003.

[17] R. Fujii, M. Kawakami, M. Hyomoto, J. Ishida, and T. Kirita, "Panoramic findings for predicting eruption of mandibular premolars associated with dentigerous cyst after marsupialization," *Journal of Oral and Maxillofacial Surgery*, vol. 66, no. 2, pp. 272–276, 2008.

[18] Y. Yahara, Y. Kubota, T. Yamashiro, and K. Shirasuna, "Eruption prediction of mandibular premolars associated with dentigerous cysts," *Oral Surgery, Oral Medicine, Oral Pathology, Oral Radiology, and Endodontics*, vol. 108, no. 1, pp. 28–31, 2009.

[19] S. Takagi and S. Koyama, "Guided eruption of an impacted second premolar associated with a dentigerous cyst in the maxillary sinus of a 6-year-old child," *Journal of Oral and Maxillofacial Surgery*, vol. 56, no. 2, pp. 237–239, 1998.

[20] J. M. V. Reyes, J. A. E. Bermúdez, and Y. E. G. Ruisánchez, "Dentigerous cysts: case report," *Journal of Advanced Oral Research*, vol. 7, no. 1, 2016.

23

Endo-Perio Lesion and Uncontrolled Diabetes

Sara Dhoum ⓘD, Kaoutar Laslami, Fatimazahraa Rouggani, Amal El Ouazzani, and Mouna Jabri

Department of Conservative Dentistry and Endodontics, School of Dentistry of Casablanca, Casablanca, Morocco

Correspondence should be addressed to Sara Dhoum; saradhoum@hotmail.com

Academic Editor: Jose López-López

This work is to discuss the management of an endo-perio lesion, which represents a challenge to clinicians when it comes to diagnosis and prognosis of the involved teeth and especially with an altered general condition. A 50-year-old female patient with uncontrolled diabetes type 2 is suffering from a purulent discharge coming from the upper right canine. Endodontic and periodontal treatments were realized with 36 months radiological and clinical follow-up with the collaboration of her internist doctor.

1. Introduction

The term "endo-perio" lesion emerged decades ago to designate a specific disease condition affecting the pulp and the periodontal tissues simultaneously [1, 2].

Diabetic patients are more exposed to oral infections and periradicular lesions caused by the changes of their immune system, qualitative and quantitative changes in normal flora of their oral cavity, and poor peripheral blood supply.

The pulp properties are changing with the aging process; moreover, uncontrolled diabetes can cause changes of the dental pulp tissue and reduce its activity by reducing the collateral blood flow. Since diabetes damages the blood circulation or causes ischemia, sometimes necrosis of the pulp may occur [3, 4].

The possible connection between chronical oral inflammatory processes, such as apical periodontitis, endodontic state, and systemic health, is one of the most interesting aspects faced by medical and dental scientific community, by monitoring the potential of healing after stabilization of all the parameters, in the present case, the inflammation and the infection states in a diabetic ground.

2. Case Report

A 50-year-old female patient, with uncontrolled type 2 diabetes, is suffering from a purulent discharge coming from number 13 sulcus, with dental mobility (grade 3) and no apparent decay, fracture, or fissure (Figure 1).

Initial periodontal treatment: nonresponsive (Figure 2).

The sensitivity tests: all negative.

Radiography: severe bone loss related to a periapical lesion (Figure 3).

3. Diagnosis

Diagnoses of the patient were primary periodontal disease with secondary endodontic involvement and chronic generalized periodontitis as a manifestation of systemic diseases (diabetes) (American Academy of Periodontology Classification, 1999).

3.1. Therapeutic Decision. Therapeutic decision was made after management of periodontal disease with scaling and root planning, patient education, and a program of periodontal hygiene maintenance (the protocol followed is the one recommended by Abbott [1]).

Endodontic treatment was administrated in two visits:

(1) First appointment

  (i) Patient under amoxicillin medication two days before the RCT treatment and the week following the procedure (collaboration with her internist doctor)

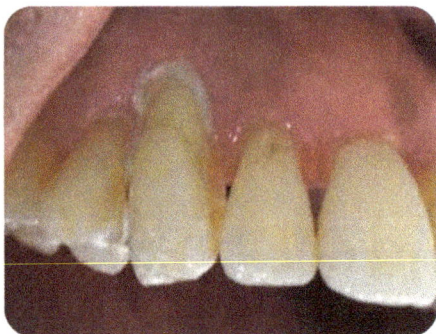

FIGURE 1: Purulent discharge related to number 13.

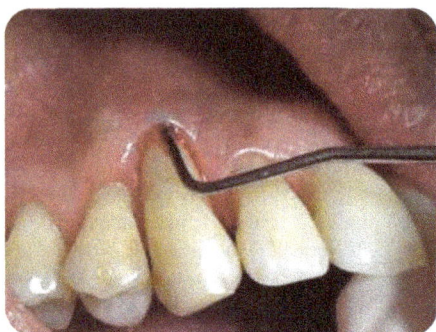

FIGURE 2: Punctual periodontal probing, 12 mm periodontal pocket.

(ii) Realization of the access cavity under a dental dam and without local anesthesia

(iii) Mechanical preparation of the root canal system using ProTaper Universal® rotary system (Dentsply International)

(iv) Chemical disinfection using 2,5% sodium hypochlorite

(v) Temporary filling of the root canal with calcium hydroxide

(vi) Placement of an adequate temporary coronal filling (Cavit™ 3M ESPE)

(2) Second appointment

(i) Adequate mechanical debridement of the root canal using stainless steel K-files combined to ProTaper Universal rotary files

(ii) Irrigation using 2,5% sodium hypochlorite

(iii) Proper drying of the root canal using sterile paper cones

(iv) Tridimensional root canal obturation using Thermafil® (Dentsply Maillefer) (Figure 4)

During the preparation of the root canal system since the first appointment, there was no exudation coming from the root canal.

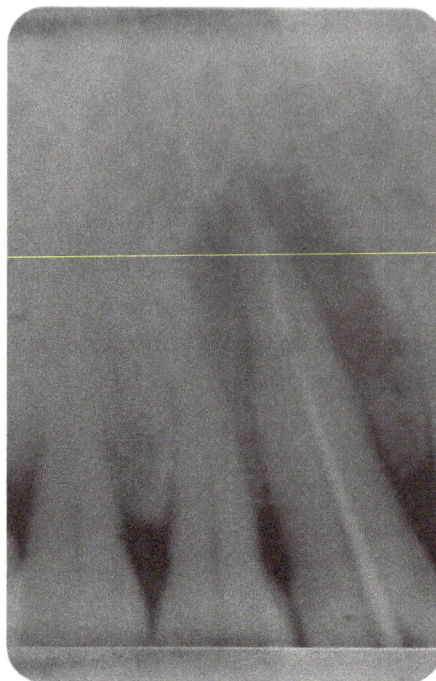

FIGURE 3: Initial state of the periodontal area.

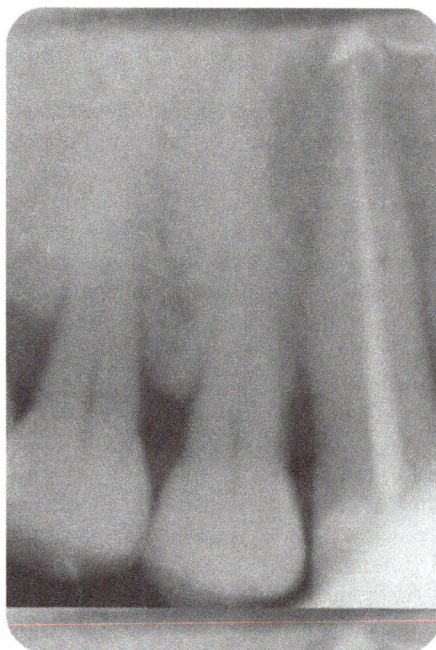

FIGURE 4: RCT and tridimensional filling with Thermafil—suspicion of lateral canal.

3.2. Two-Week Follow-Up (Figure 5).

(i) Beginning of bone reorganization

(ii) Decrease but without disappearance of the purulent discharge

(iii) Decrease of dental mobility

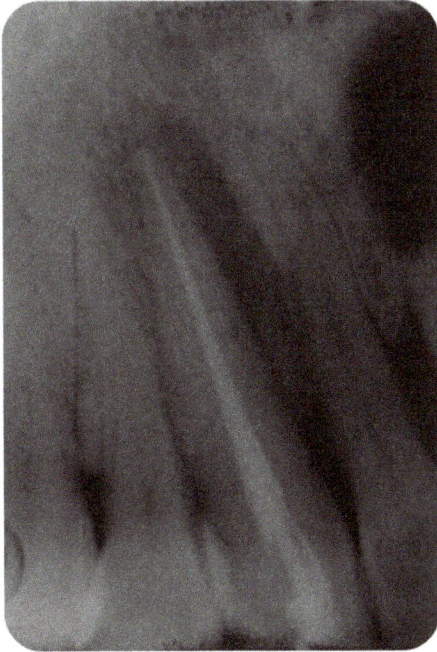

FIGURE 5: Disappearance of sealer puff two weeks after the endodontic therapy.

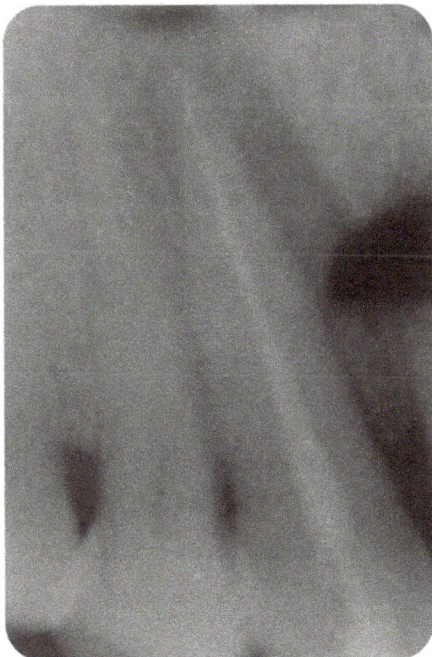

FIGURE 6: Two months' recall radiograph showing a continuous bone reorganization.

(iv) Stabilization of the patient's blood sugar level with the collaboration of the internist doctor

3.3. Two-Month Follow-Up (Figure 6).

(i) Stabilization of the radiolucent image revealed by radiographic examination

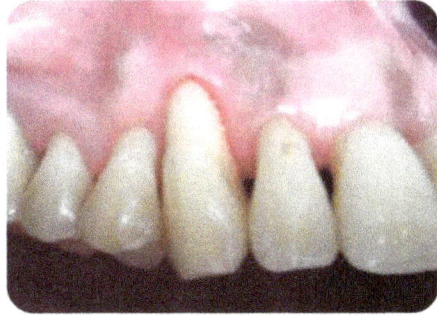

FIGURE 7: Beginning of soft tissue healing.

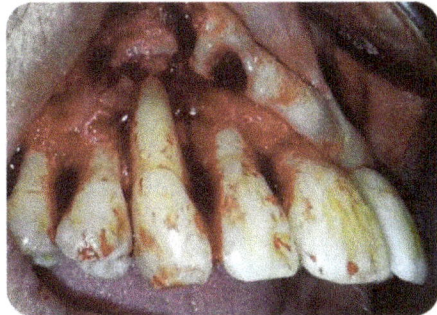

FIGURE 8: Open flap of upper right quadrant.

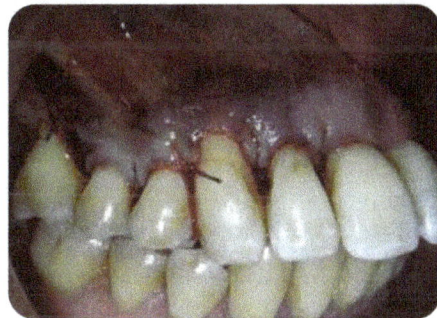

FIGURE 9: Operative site after suturing.

(ii) Beginning of bone reorganization

(iii) Decrease but without disappearance of the purulent discharge (Figure 7)

3.4. Six-Month Follow-Up

(i) Persistence of the purulent discharge from the sulcus was noted.

(ii) An open flap for periodontal cleaning was realized with a debridement of the root surface, and a full periodontal therapy was established to complete the treatment and to obtain a periodontal attachment repair (Figures 8 and 9).

(iii) Periodontal splinting was used to reinforce and improve the healing potential of the tooth in question (Figure 10).

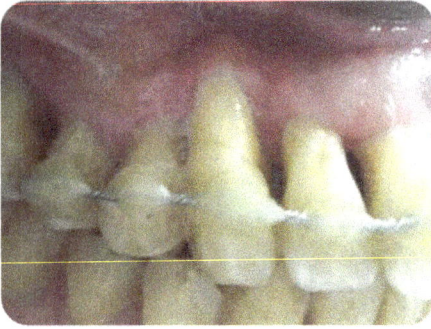

FIGURE 10: Soft tissue healing and periodontal splinting.

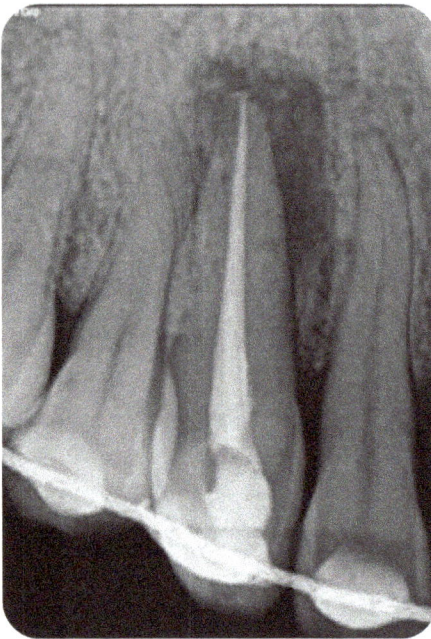

FIGURE 12: 18 months' recall radiograph.

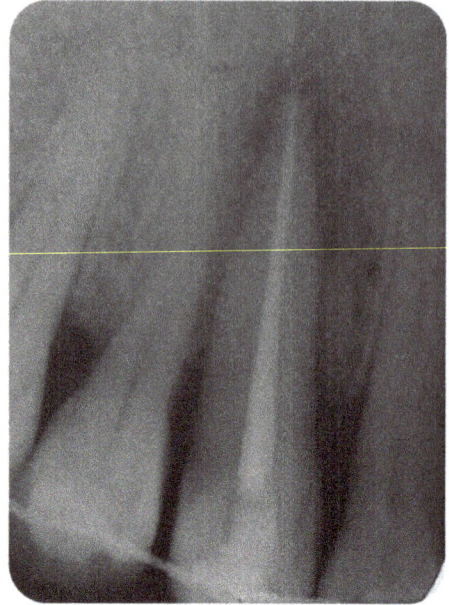

FIGURE 11: Six months' recall radiograph.

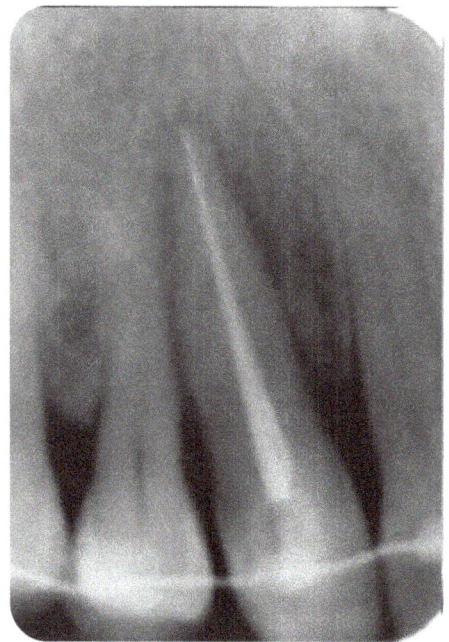

FIGURE 13: 39 months' recall radiograph showing a bone reorganization.

3.4.1. The Six Months' Recall Revealed

(i) Soft tissue healing with gingival recession located on number 13 (Figure 10);

(ii) A complete disappearance of the purulent production;

(iii) Partial bone regeneration with apparent bone trabeculations in the former radiolucency (Figure 11).

3.4.2. At 18 Months and 39 Months' Recall

(i) A progressive bone healing after 18 months was observed, then 39 months with a disappearance of the former radiolucency (Figures 12, 13, and 14).

This glycosylated hemoglobin curve demonstrates that the patient has an imbalanced diabetes (the treatment was established on February 2015.) (Figure 15).

4. Discussion

Diagnosis of primary endodontic disease and primary periodontal disease usually represents no clinical difficulty [2, 5]. Many classifications of endo-perio lesion are found in the literature; Simon et al. (1972) used a classification to separate lesions involving both periodontal and pulpal tissues into the following groups:

(i) Primary endodontic lesions with secondary periodontal involvement

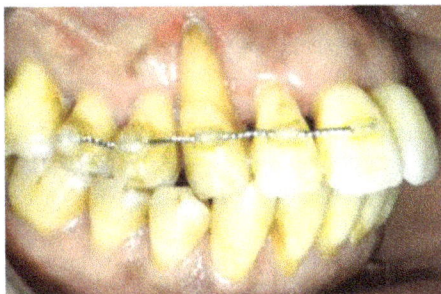

FIGURE 14: 39 months' recall check-up showing a complete disappearance of the purulent discharge with a buccal bone loss and gingival recession regarding number 13.

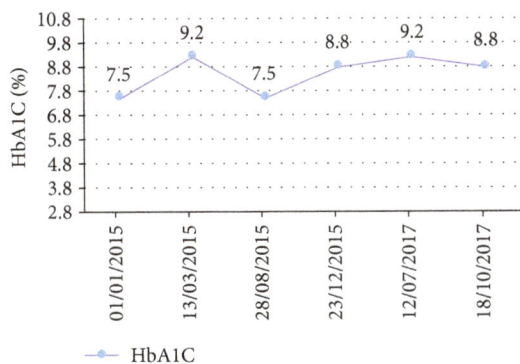

FIGURE 15: HbA1C follow-up from 2015 to October 2017.

(ii) Primary periodontal lesions with secondary endodontic involvement

(iii) True combined lesions

Many researches have reported substantial pathological change and frequent necrosis in the pulp tissue due to periodontal disease, especially with the presence of accessory canals [3, 6]. Other studies have stated that pulps in periodontally affected teeth remain within normal limits regardless of the severity of the periodontal pathosis and suggested that the systemic condition of the patient may have a big influence on the condition of the pulp than the status of the periodontal tissue or his chronologic age [4, 7].

Langeland et al. [8] have demonstrated that pathologic changes do occur in the pulp when periodontal disease is present; however, the pulp does not succumb as long as the apical foramen is not involved. It therefore seems evident that periodontal disease rarely jeopardizes the vital functions of the pulp unless the disease process has reached a terminal stage and involves the main pulpal blood supply, the apical area [9–11].

In diabetic patients, aging changes of pulp due to limited collateral blood flow are faster than nondiabetics. Since diabetes damages the blood circulation or ischemia, sometimes necrosis of pulp may occur [5, 12].

The prognosis depends on the differential diagnosis, the general state of the patient, the endodontic involvement, and the lesion age.

Diabetes mellitus (DM) is a significant and increasing global health problem. In 2013, the International Diabetes Federation estimated that there were 382 million people worldwide with diabetes increasing to 592 million in 2015 with the major part of this population is living in low- and middle-income countries [13, 14].

It is defined as a group of metabolic disorders characterized by chronic hyperglycaemia with disturbances in carbohydrates, fat, and protein metabolism resulting from defects in insulin secretion, insulin action on the target tissues, or both, and it is frequently associated with an increased susceptibility to infection [15–17].

Both diabetes mellitus type 1 (DM1) and type 2 (DM2) present numerous possible long-term complications. Epidemiological studies indicate that the severity of diabetic complications is generally proportional to the degree and duration of the hyperglycaemia.

Among the oral manifestations related to DM described are dry mouth, tooth decay, periodontal disease and gingivitis, oral candidiasis, burning mouth syndrome (BMS), taste disorders, rhinocerebral zygomycosis (mucormycosis), aspergillosis, oral lichen planus, geographic tongue and fissured tongue, delayed wound healing and increased incidence of infection, salivary dysfunction, altered taste and other neurosensory disorders, impaired tooth eruption, and benign parotid hypertrophy. Similar to the periodontium, the dentin-pulp complex is also affected by diabetes. Zehnder et al. [10] reported that angiopathy represented by a thickened basement membrane was observed in the dental pulp of diabetics. But still no systematic studies about the direct effect of the diabetes on the pulp tissue.

Periodontal healing after a proper RCT depends on the biological constants including the rate of blood sugar levels. Clinical and radiological follow-up must be completed with glycemic control which reveals in our case a chronic uncontrolled diabetes with regular visit controls with the internist doctor [18–20].

Lesion's age makes the prognosis of an endo-perio lesion much more uncertain, in periodontal pocket, complicated the lesion management. Bacterial ecosystem of chronic lesion adapts itself and becomes more resistant to endodontic and periodontal treatments [19, 21, 22].

Healing potential of an endodontic lesion is very high if the lesion is surrounded with 5 or 6 bone walls (Machtou and Cohen, 1988). According to Ng et al., Kambale et al., and Rudranaik et al. "the larger is the part caused by pulpal infection, the better the prognosis of attachment regeneration" [23–25].

5. Conclusion

The primary goal of all treatment must be to rid the patient of the infection.

Endodontic treatment success criteria were established in 1994 by the European Society of Endodontology and included the following:

(i) Absence of pain, swelling, and fistula

(ii) Maintenance of tooth function

(iii) Presence of radiological evidence of a normal periodontal ligament space

(iv) Absence of apical periodontitis or radicular resorption

It can be stated that, in the majority of the endo-perio lesions, the bacterial etiology dictates the clinical course of the disease and therefore the treatment plan.

Changes in the immune system defense in diabetic patients against infection and pathological changes in pulp and periradicular tissue, lack of awareness of patients about the effect of diabetes on oral health, asymptomatic dental infections, poor dental and oral health, and lack of regular visit to dentists because of its high costs all may have influence.

Other factors, such as patient cooperation, restorability, and economics, will influence treatment decisions.

Neither periodontic nor endodontic treatment can be considered in isolation; clinically, they are closely related, and this must influence the diagnosis and treatment.

The clinical burden of diabetes is high in Morocco, and the majority of patients do not achieve the recommended glycaemia target, suggesting that there is a huge gap between evidence-based diabetic management and real-life practice. Better education of patients and improved compliance with international recommendations are necessary to deliver a better quality of diabetic care [14].

Disclosure

The manuscript has been presented as a poster in the Biennial Congress of the European Society of Endodontology, September 2015, Barcelona, Spain.

References

[1] P. Abbott, "Endodontic management of combined endodontic-periodontal lesions," *Journal of the New Zealand Society of Periodontology*, vol. 83, pp. 15–28, 1998.

[2] K. S. Al-Fouzan, "A new classification of endodontic-periodontal lesions," *International Journal of Dentistry*, vol. 2014, Article ID 919173, 5 pages, 2014.

[3] W. C. Rubach and D. F. Mitchell, "Periodontal disease, accessory canals and pulp pathosis," *Journal of Periodontology*, vol. 36, no. 1, pp. 34–38, 1965.

[4] R. T. Czarnecki and H. Schilder, "A histological evaluation of the human pulp in teeth with varying degrees of periodontal disease," *Journal of Endodontics*, vol. 5, no. 8, pp. 242–253, 1979.

[5] H. Sasaki, K. Hirai, C. M. Martins, H. Furusho, R. Battaglino, and K. Hashimoto, "Interrelationship between periapical lesion and systemic metabolic disorders," *Current Pharmaceutical Design*, vol. 22, no. 15, pp. 2204–2215, 2016.

[6] S. Seltzer, I. B. Bender, and M. Ziontz, "The dynamics of pulp inflammation: correlations between diagnostic data and actual histologic findings in the pulp," *Oral Surgery, Oral Medicine, Oral Pathology*, vol. 16, no. 7, pp. 846–871, 1963.

[7] B. Mazur and M. Massler, "Influence of periodontal disease on the dental pulp," *Oral Surgery, Oral Medicine, Oral Pathology*, vol. 17, no. 5, pp. 592–603, 1964.

[8] K. Langeland, H. Rodrigues, and W. Dowden, "Periodontal disease, bacteria, and pulpal histopathology," *Oral Surgery, Oral Medicine, Oral Pathology*, vol. 37, no. 2, pp. 257–270, 1974.

[9] E. Foce, *Endo-Periodontal Lesions*, Quintessence publishing, London, 2011.

[10] M. Zehnder, S. I. Gold, and G. Hasselgren, "Pathologic interactions in pulpal and periodontal tissues," *Journal of Clinical Periodontology*, vol. 29, no. 8, pp. 663–671, 2002.

[11] H. Aksel and A. Serper, "A case series associated with different kinds of endo-perio lesions," *Journal of Clinical and Experimental Dentistry*, vol. 6, no. 1, pp. e91–e95, 2014.

[12] M. M. Ferreira, E. Carrilho, and F. Carrilho, "Diabetes mellitus and its influence on the success of endodontic treatment: a retrospective clinical study," *Acta Médica Portuguesa*, vol. 27, no. 1, pp. 15–22, 2014.

[13] L. Guariguata, D. R. Whiting, I. Hambleton, J. Beagley, U. Linnenkamp, and J. E. Shaw, "Global estimates of diabetes prevalence for 2013 and projections for 2035," *Diabetes Research and Clinical Practice*, vol. 103, no. 2, pp. 137–149, 2014.

[14] A. Chadli, S. El Aziz, N. El Ansari et al., "Management of diabetes in Morocco: results of the International Diabetes Management Practices Study (IDMPS) – wave 5," *Therapeutic Advances in Endocrinology and Metabolism*, vol. 7, no. 3, pp. 101–109, 2016.

[15] E. Mauri-Obradors, A. Estrugo-Devesa, E. Jane-Salas, M. Vinas, and J. Lopez-Lopez, "Oral manifestations of diabetes mellitus. A systematic review," *Medicina Oral Patología Oral y Cirugía Bucal*, vol. 22, no. 5, pp. e586–e594, 2017.

[16] J. López-López, E. Jané-Salas, A. Estrugo-Devesa, E. Velasco-Ortega, J. Martín-González, and J. J. Segura-Egea, "Periapical and endodontic status of type 2 diabetic patients in Catalonia, Spain: a cross-sectional study," *Journal of Endodontics*, vol. 37, no. 5, pp. 598–601, 2011.

[17] E. Mauri-Obradors, A. Merlos, A. Estrugo-Devesa, E. Jané-Salas, J. López-López, and M. Viñas, "Benefits of nonsurgical periodontal treatment in patients with type 2 diabetes mellitus and chronic periodontitis: a randomized controlled trial," *Journal of Clinical Periodontology*, vol. 45, no. 3, pp. 345–353, 2018.

[18] A. Mesgarani, S. Haghanifar, N. Eshkevari et al., "Frequency of odontogenic periradicular lesions in diabetic patients," *Caspian Journal of Internal Medicine*, vol. 5, no. 1, pp. 22–25, 2014.

[19] B. Sánchez-Domínguez, J. López-López, E. Jané-Salas, L. Castellanos-Cosano, E. Velasco-Ortega, and J. J. Segura-Egea, "Glycated hemoglobin levels and prevalence of apical periodontitis in type 2 diabetic patients," *Journal of Endodontics*, vol. 41, no. 5, pp. 601–606, 2015.

[20] R. T. Demmer, B. Holtfreter, M. Desvarieux et al., "The influence of type 1 and type 2 diabetes on periodontal disease progression: prospective results from the Study of Health in Pomerania (SHIP)," *Diabetes Care*, vol. 35, no. 10, pp. 2036–2042, 2012.

[21] Y.-Y. Wu, E. Xiao, and D. T. Graves, "Diabetes mellitus related bone metabolism and periodontal disease," *International Journal of Oral Science*, vol. 7, no. 2, pp. 63–72, 2015.

[22] P. Carrotte, "Endodontics: part 9 calcium hydroxide, root resorption, endo-perio lesions," *British Dental Journal*, vol. 197, no. 12, pp. 735–743, 2004.

[23] Y.-L. Ng, V. Mann, and K. Gulabivala, "A prospective study of the factors affecting outcomes of nonsurgical root canal treatment: part 1: periapical health," *International Endodontic Journal*, vol. 44, no. 7, pp. 583–609, 2011.

[24] S. Kambale, N. Aspalli, A. Munavalli, N. Ajgaonkar, and R. Babannavar, "A sequential approach in treatment of endo-perio lesion a case report," *Journal of Clinical and Diagnostic Research*, vol. 8, no. 8, pp. ZD22–ZD24, 2014.

[25] S. Rudranaik, M. Nayak, and M. Babshet, "Periapical healing outcome following single visit endodontic treatment in patients with type 2 diabetes mellitus," *Journal of Clinical and Experimental Dentistry*, vol. 8, no. 5, pp. e498–e504, 2016.

24

Spontaneous and Excellent Healing of Bilateral Brown Tumors in Mandible after Endocrinal Therapy and Subtotal Parathyroidectomy: Case Report with 4-Year Follow-Up

Turker Yucesoy[ID],[1] Erdem Kilic,[1] Fatma Dogruel,[2] Fahri Bayram,[3] Alper Alkan,[1] Alper Celal Akcan,[4] and Figen Ozturk[5]

[1]Oral and Maxillofacial Surgery Department, Dentistry Faculty, Bezmialem Vakif University, Istanbul, Turkey
[2]Oral and Maxillofacial Surgery Department, Dentistry Faculty, Erciyes University, Kayseri, Turkey
[3]Endocrinology Department, Medicine Faculty, Erciyes University, Kayseri, Turkey
[4]General Surgery Department, Medicine Faculty, Erciyes University, Kayseri, Turkey
[5]Pathology Department, Medicine Faculty, Erciyes University, Kayseri, Turkey

Correspondence should be addressed to Turker Yucesoy; dt.yucesoy@hotmail.com

Academic Editor: John H. Campbell

Primary hyperparathyroidism is an endocrine disorder occurring due to increased secretion of parathormone resulting in a complex of clinical, anatomical, and biochemical alterations. On the other hand, excision of a parathyroid adenoma can normalize the metabolic status. A 24-year-old man was referred to the hospital with bilateral swelling and spontaneous gingival bleeding from posterior of the mandible also with radiolucent well-demarcated lesions bilaterally in the mandibular third molar regions. After consultations, the patient was hospitalized in the endocrinology department where further tests were performed due to highly increased PTH level as 714 pg/ml. Bilateral brown tumors started to regress spontaneously, and no additional surgery was required after subtotal parathyroidectomy was performed. The presented case is the first patient whose bilateral brown tumors in the jaws spontaneously and totally healed after subtotal parathyroidectomy and endocrinal therapy who was strictly followed up for 4 years even though the lesions were associated with impacted third molars.

1. Introduction

The giant cell lesions associated with primary hyperparathyroidism (PHPT) are referred to as brown tumors in the jaws. PHPT is an endocrine disorder occurring due to increased secretion of parathormone resulting in a complex of clinical, anatomical, and biochemical alterations. Parathormone (PTH) controls the calcium (Ca) level in the plasma and extracellular fluid. Increased production of PTH usually causes high levels of serum Ca and alkaline phosphatase (ALP) levels while P levels are decreased [1].

Increased PTH level can cause an imbalance of osteoblastic and osteoclastic activities. This imbalance is characterized by the resorption of the bone, leaving sinusoidal vascular spaces and fibrous connective tissue [2]. One of the skeletal lesions observed in PHPT is the brown tumor also termed

as Von Recklinghausen's disease of the bone or osteitis cystica fibrosa. Brown tumors have been associated with primary hyperparathyroidism which is mostly asymptomatic; a painful exophytic mass may be observed. Radiographically, it appears as a unilocular or multilocular lesion with an irregular periphery. Histologically, it is a focal giant cell lesion which demonstrates multinucleated giant cells within a fibrovascular stroma admixed with areas of hemorrhage and hemosiderin deposits [3].

Histological findings include dilated blood vessels, fibromuscular proliferation, and macrophages. Deposits of hemosiderin cause the "brown" appearance of this tumor [4]. HPT is categorized into 4 types: primary HPT is caused by parathyroid adenomas (85%), hyperplasias (10%), and carcinomas (5%); secondary HPT occurs as a compensatory increase in parathormone levels due to hypocalcemia or

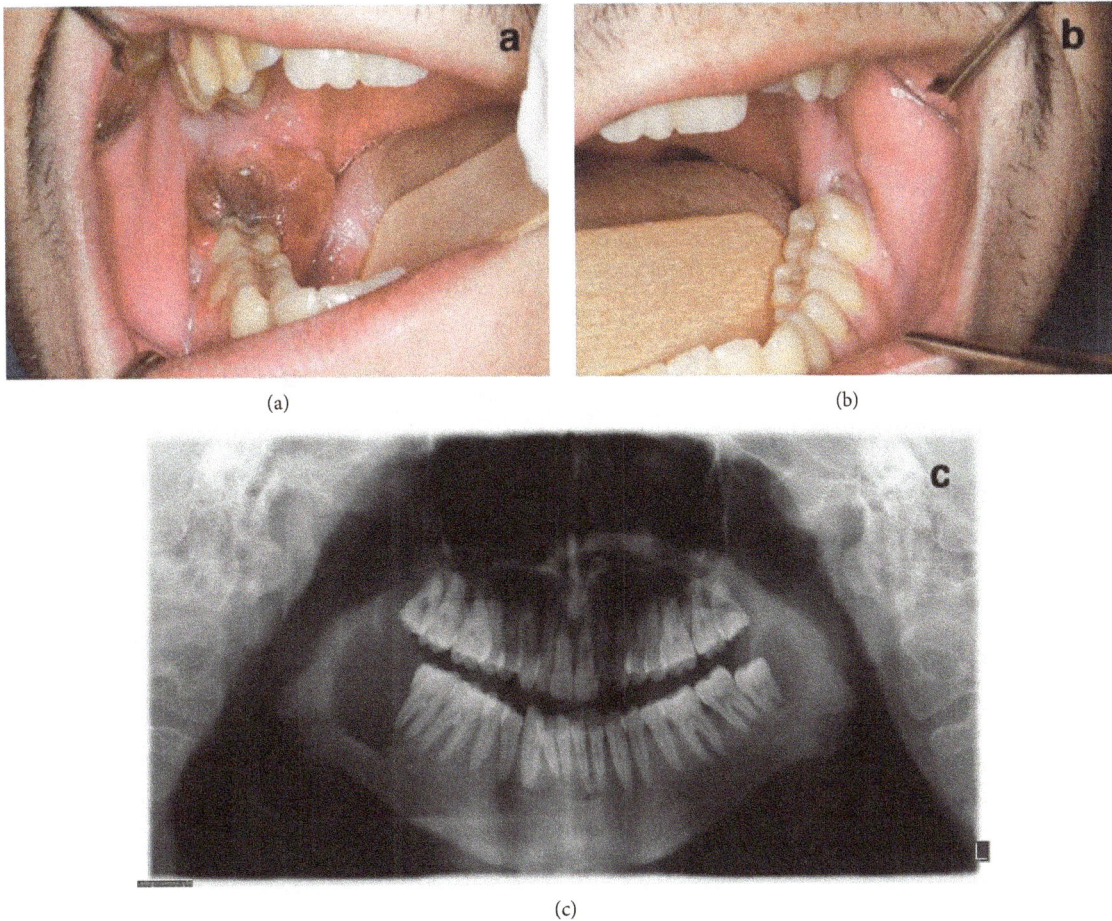

FIGURE 1: (a) Initial intraoral appearance of the brown tumor (right side). (b) Initial intraoral appearance of the brown tumor (left side). (c) Diagnostic panoramic radiography of bilateral brown tumors.

vitamin D deficiency; tertiary HPT presents in patients with long-standing secondary HPT resulting in autonomous functioning of parathyroid gland; the fourth type is an ectopic variant seen in patients with other malignancies [5]. PHPT is sporadic in the vast majority of the cases. However, it is essential for the surgeon managing PHPT to know that it may occur in familial settings. The commonly associated conditions are MEN (multiple endocrinal neoplasias) syndromes (MEN1, MEN2A), FIHP (familial isolated hyperparathyroidism), HPT-jaw tumor syndrome, autosomal dominant mild hyperparathyroidism (ADMH), and neonatal severe hyperparathyroidism (NSHPT) [6].

After the endocrine treatment, these lesions can regress spontaneously in other bones [7, 8], but to our knowledge, the presented case is the first patient whose bilateral brown tumors in the jaws spontaneously and totally healed after endocrinal therapy and who was followed up for 4 years.

2. Case Report

A 24-year-old man was referred to Erciyes University Faculty of Dentistry, Oral and Maxillofacial Surgery Department Clinic, Kayseri, Turkey, with bilateral swelling and spontaneous gingival bleeding from the posterior of the mandible. His medical history was noncontributory. There was no visible swelling, tenderness, or pus discharge. Skin color and temperature were normal. Intraoral examination revealed pericoronitis and spontaneous bleeding from the periodontal pocket of the right mandibular second molar and swelling in the bilateral retromolar regions (Figures 1(a) and 1(b)). In the radiographic examination, bilateral not well-demarcated radiolucent lesions in the posterior regions of the mandible, measuring $4 \times 3 \times 3$ cm on the right and $2.5 \times 1.5 \times 1.5$ cm on the left, were observed (Figure 1(c)).

After questioning the patient's family history, the patient stated that his father had a serious endocrinal disease 30 years ago and he received endocrine treatment because of a problem in his parathyroid glands. Therefore, we suspected of brown tumor for the presented case, because of his family's history of endocrine disorders and the panoramic radiography, so the patient was offered to receive some specific blood tests. Biochemical tests demonstrated extremely high PTH level and high level of serum Ca (12.8 mg/dl) and ALP (220 U/L). PTH level was 714 pg/ml which was conspicuously higher from the normal levels (15–65 pg/ml).

After consulting with Erciyes University Medicine Faculty Endocrinology Department, the patient was hospitalized in the endocrinology clinic and further tests were performed.

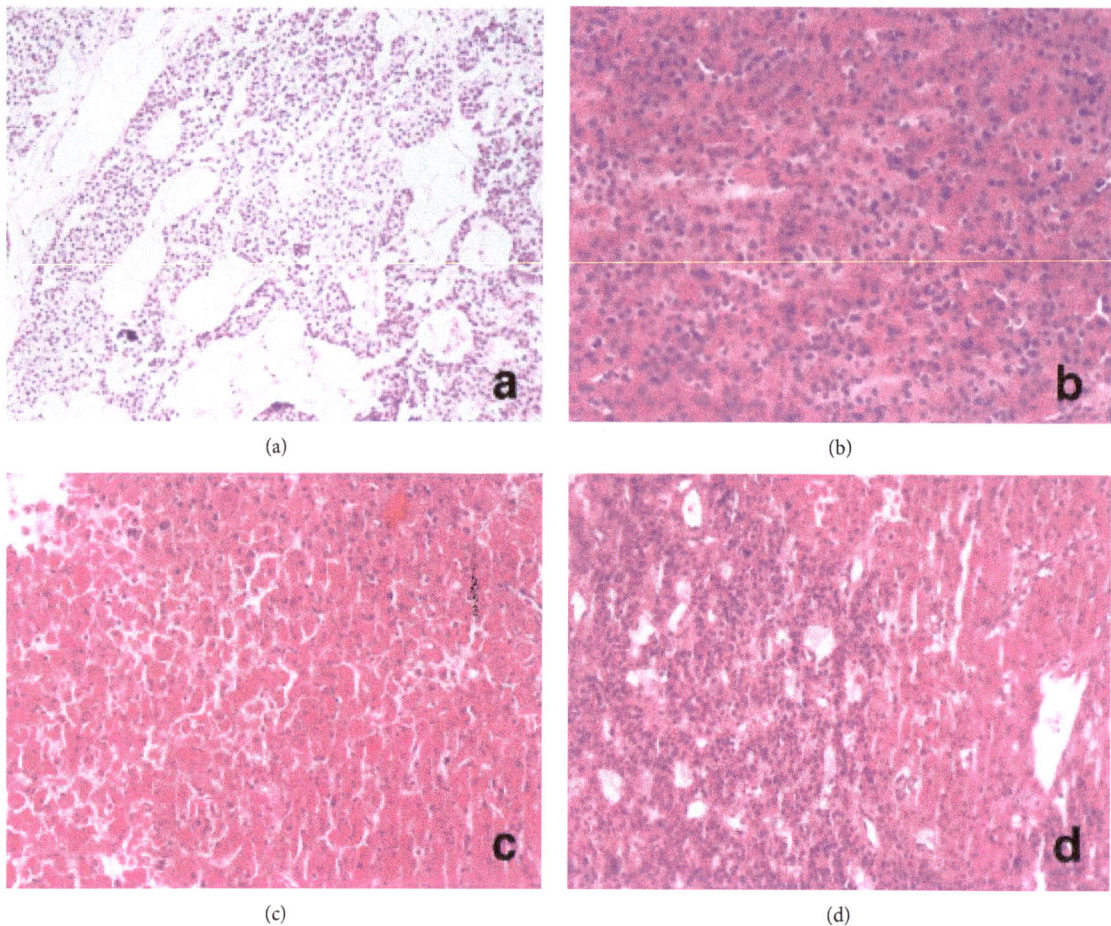

FIGURE 2: Microscopic finding from the parathyroid glands. (a) Right inferior paratiroid hyperplasia (H&E stain). (b) Right superior paratiroid hyperplasia (H&E stain). (c) Left inferior paratiroid hyperplasia (H&E stain). (d) Left superior paratiroid hyperplasia (H&E stain).

As mentioned earlier, because of the familial tendency of the patient and hyperplasia in the parathyroid gland, endocrinologists suspected of MEN syndrome. For that, the patient and some relatives received several examinations and genetic tests for MEN syndrome but the results were negative for MEN. So the endocrinologists consulted the patient to the General Surgery Department in Erciyes University Medicine Faculty for surgical treatment of hyperplastic parathyroid gland. After radiographical and clinical examinations by general surgeons, parathyroidectomy was decided to perform a surgical procedure as soon as possible. The general surgeons gained access to the thyroid gland under general anesthesia. After mobilizing of the left thyroid lobe, parathyroid glands were exposed with measurements: 4 cm in the inferior pole and 2 cm in the superior pole where the glands were measured as 3.5 cm in the superior pole and 2 cm in the inferior pole after mobilization of the right thyroid lobe, respectively. The surgeons performed subtotal parathyroidectomy for the lesions. All the pathological glands were removed, but only one small portion of the right inferior lobe was remained and signed with metallic clips. The recurrent laryngeal nerves were protected during the operation.

Four different-sized macroscopic biopsy specimens from parathyroid glands were sent to the Pathology Department of

the Erciyes University Medicine Faculty. According to the results, no adipose tissue was observed in the whole specimen which was covered with a thin fibrous capsule macroscopically. Mostly, main cells of parathyroid gland but rarely oxyphilic cells were observed in the tissue. The cells showed a diffuse lining; however, trabecular or acinar structures were also seen. None of those atypical tissues were in the neighborhood of a normal parathyroid tissue. Some of the giant cells had a hyperchromatic nucleus. As a result, parathyroid hyperplasia was diagnosed pathologically because of morphological and clinical evidence (Figure 2).

After surgical treatment of parathyroid glands and successful endocrinal therapy by Erciyes University Medicine Faculty, the patient was hospitalized for almost 3 months. After being discharged from the hospital, the patient applied to our clinic for his follow-ups and bilateral regression of the lesions on the left side of mandible occurred spontaneously (Figures 3(a) and 3(b)).

However, even though lesion-related molars were indicated for extraction as soon as possible, the patient insisted that he did now want any surgical procedures because he felt no disturbance at all. Because the patient rejected all the alternative treatments for his lesions in the mandible, frequent follow-ups were considered for him and we did it for 4 years.

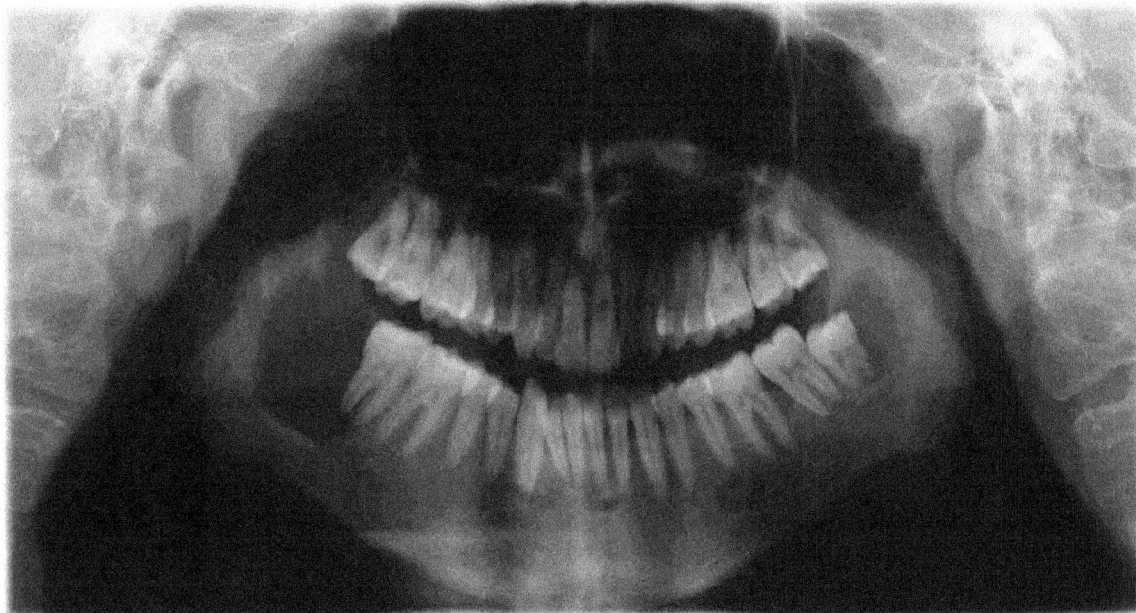

(a)

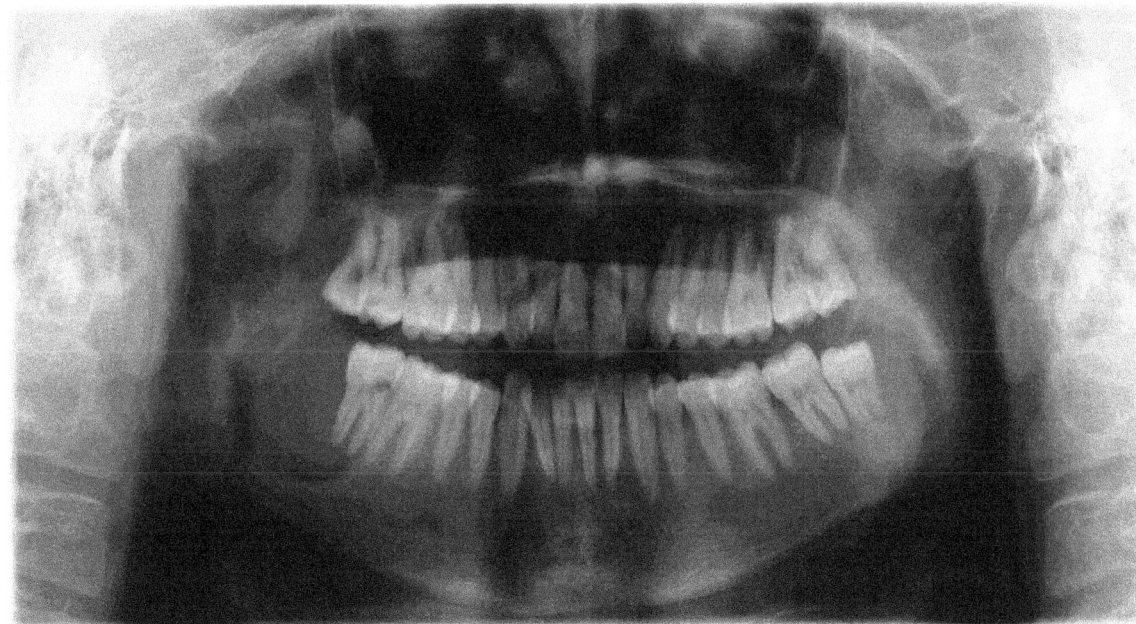

(b)

FIGURE 3: (a) Three months of follow-up: panoramic radiography of bilateral brown tumors. Notice to decreased radiolucency for the brown tumor in the left side of the mandible. (b) First year of follow up: panoramic radiography of bilateral brown tumors. Notice to decreased radiopacity for the brown tumor in the bilateral sides of the mandible.

In the radiographic examination, partial calcification of the lesions was observed after 6 months (Figure 4(a)). Also, after intraoral examination, spontaneous periodontal healing was uneventful (Figures 4(b) and 4(c)). Radiological and intraoral examinations were performed carefully in follow-ups for first and second years. (Figures 4(d)–4(f)). There was no evidence of recurrence at a 4-year follow-up, either radiographically or intraorally (Figures 4(g)–4(i)).

3. Discussion

Brown tumors arise in the jaws and they may be misdiagnosed with giant cell tumors, giant cell reparative granuloma, and cherubism. Because it is difficult to distinguish brown tumor from other giant cell lesions histopathologically, the clinical diagnosis should be made based on the association with HPT [7].

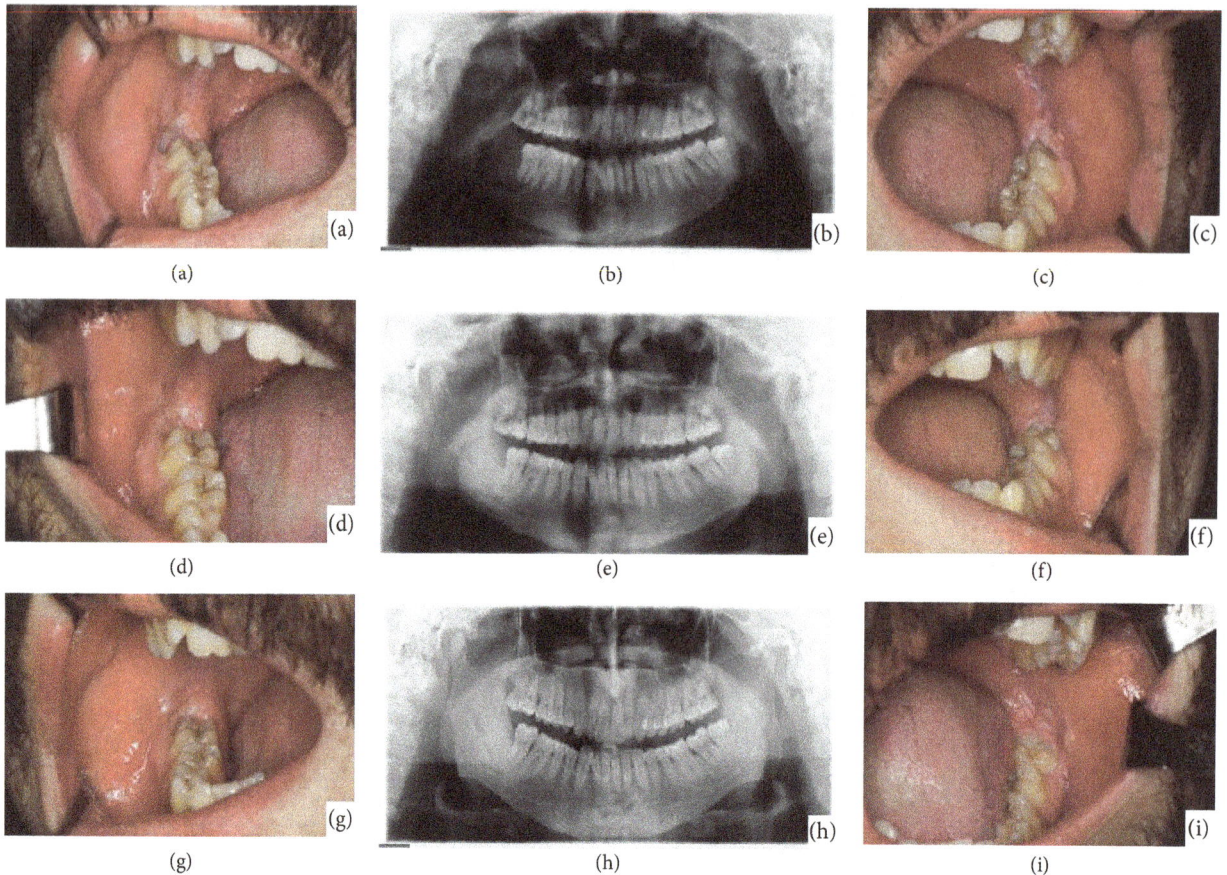

FIGURE 4: (a) Six months of follow-up: panoramic radiography of bilateral brown tumors. Notice to decreased radiolucency for the brown tumor in the bilateral sides of the mandible. (b) Six months of follow-up: intraoral appearance of the brown tumor (right side). (c) Six months of follow-up: intraoral appearance of the brown tumor (left side). (d) Second year of follow-up: panoramic radiography of bilateral brown tumors. Notice not to observe recurrence for brown tumors in the bilateral sides of the mandible. (e) Second year of follow-up: intraoral appearance of the brown tumor (right side). (f) Second year of follow-up: intraoral appearance of the brown tumor (left side). (g) Fourth year of follow-up: panoramic radiography of bilateral brown tumors. (h) Fourth year of follow-up: intraoral appearance of the brown tumor (right side). (i) Fourth year of follow-up: intraoral appearance of the brown tumor (left side). Notice to the left mandibular third molar eruption is almost completed.

Radiographically, the lesions appear as well-demarcated monocular or multilocular osteolytic radiolucencies resembling cystic lesions. Other radiographic findings are the loss of lamina dura surrounding roots of teeth and reduced bone density [9, 10]. Our patient had similar radiographic features as mentioned previously (Figure 1).

The diagnosis of a brown tumor can be made through the use of biochemical tests such as serum calcium, alkaline phosphatase (ALP), phosphorus (P), sodium (Na), potassium (K), calcium (Ca), and parathyroid hormone (PTH) levels in the presence of giant cell lesions [11]. Uhluhizarci et al. revealed that complicated hyperparathyroidism is an important health problem in our region, and primary hyperparathyroidism should be kept in mind in all patients with bone and joint complaints [12]. However, hyperparathyroidism is discovered coincidentally on routine biochemical and radiological investigations [13].

Ameloblastoma, osteomyelitis, and odontogenic cysts are considered for differential diagnosis of these tumors [14, 15]. Mostly, brown tumor is a sporadic disease but may also occur in a familial pattern as an autosomal dominant condition like hyperparathyroidism-jaw tumor syndrome (HPT-JT syndrome) and multiple endocrine neoplasia (MEN) syndrome [10]. About 1 in 10 cases of primary hyperparathyroidism is hereditary, occurring as an isolated form or associated with other abnormalities. If sporadic, individuals should be advised that there is a nonnegligible recurrence risk since there is a small but significant genetic component to this multifactorial disease but it can be difficult to exclude a hereditary syndrome [16]. For this reason, not only our patients but also some of his relatives were examined very carefully by the Endocrinology Department of Erciyes University after our patient's blood test revealed extremely high PTH level as 714 pg/ml and serum calcium was 12.8 mg/dl. But even though the genetical results were negative for MEN syndrome, the patient and the family were also recommended to be controlled for life-long time in the endocrinology department to avoid recurrence.

There are many options for treatment of the brown tumor. Before the medical or surgical treatment of the lytic bone lesions, hormonal regulation is necessary. Bony lesions tend to regress spontaneously if the calcium and PTH levels normalize [9]. Silverman et al. [2] reported that excising a brown tumor was not necessary when HPT resolved whereas Steinbach et al. [17] reported that brown tumors could be treated by local radiotherapy or curettage. However, many authors have reported that they resected any remaining brown tumors after HPT was resolved [18–21].

The surgical treatment for a brown tumor in the jaws includes enucleation and curettage and radical resection and reconstruction [4, 22]. Some authors initially treat this lesion with systemic or intralesional corticosteroids and when size was reduced, then surgical excision can be performed [21]. However, some authors reported that the osteitis fibrosa cyctica in the bone is a kind of PTH-related tumor which is possible to heal spontaneously [7, 8]. In the present case, although it is widely spread into the posterior mandible in the right side and possible to be the same on the left side, no surgical procedure was needed after endocrine therapy because of patient's tumors in both sides of the mandible reduced instantly during the follow-ups.

In the first year of his follow-up, we also were expecting to have a decrease in radiolucency and perform a more conservative surgery, but surprisingly, brown tumors in both sides were totally healed uneventfully. With the coordination of his endocrinal therapy controls, radiographical and oral examinations were also done in Erciyes University, Dentistry Faculty for 4 years as shown in Figure 4.

Because it is difficult to distinguish brown tumor from other giant cell lesions histopathologically, a clinical decision should be made with considering the underlying systemic event. In their study, Guney et al. aimed to remind endocrinologists and maxillofacial surgeons that these tumors have to be taken into account [23]. The clinicians should question their patients' medical and family history very carefully not to miss any clue for the diagnosis and proper treatment approach.

We report an unusual case of brown tumor in the mandible that completely recovered spontaneously after endocrine therapy. Thankfully, to the follow-ups which we performed carefully and patiently, the second molar in the right mandible was protected and the extraction of this tooth was not needed. Also, we want to encourage the clinicians not to perform the surgery so emergently and recommend them to follow their patients as long as possible for further tests or surgeries, because surgical excision of a brown tumor is not always necessary if the endocrinal disorder is treated and controlled properly via normalizing the PHPT markers.

References

[1] O. Goshen, S. Aviel-Ronen, S. Dori, and Y. P. Talmi, "Brown tumour of hyperparathyroidism in the mandible associated with atypical parathyroid adenoma," *The Journal of Laryngology & Otology*, vol. 114, no. 4, pp. 302–304, 2000.

[2] S. Silverman Jr., W. H. Ware, and C. Gillooly Jr., "Dental aspects of hyperparathyroidism," *Oral Surgery, Oral Medicine, Oral Pathology*, vol. 26, no. 2, pp. 184 189, 1968.

[3] M. M. Lessa, F. A. Sakae, R. K. Tsuji, B. C. Araújo Filho, R. L. Voegels, and O. Butugan, "Brown tumor of the facial bones: case report and literature review," *Ear, Nose, & Throat Journal*, vol. 84, no. 7, pp. 432–434, 2005.

[4] H. R. Vikram, A. Petito, B. F. Bower, and M. H. Goldberg, "Parathyroid carcinoma diagnosed on the basis of a giant cell lesion of the maxilla," *Journal of Oral and Maxillofacial Surgery*, vol. 58, no. 5, pp. 567–569, 2000.

[5] A. L. S. Guimarães, L. Marques-Silva, C. C. Gomes, W. H. Castro, R. A. Mesquita, and R. S. Gomez, "Peripheral brown tumour of hyperparathyroidism in the oral cavity," *Oral Oncology Extra*, vol. 42, no. 3, pp. 91–93, 2006.

[6] P. Stålberg and T. Carling, "Familial parathyroid tumors: diagnosis and management," *World Journal of Surgery*, vol. 33, no. 11, pp. 2234–2243, 2009.

[7] C. J. Gibbs, J. G. Millar, and J. Smith, "Spontaneous healing of osteitis fibrosa cystica in primary hyperparathyroidism," *Postgraduate Medical Journal*, vol. 72, no. 854, pp. 754–757, 1996.

[8] C. T. Wootten and E. A. Orzeck, "Spontaneous remission of primary hyperparathyroidism: a case report and meta-analysis of the literature," *Head & Neck*, vol. 28, no. 1, pp. 81–88, 2006.

[9] D. K. Kar, S. K. Gupta, A. Agarwal, and S. K. Mishra, "Brown tumor of the palate and mandible in association with primary hyperparathyroidism," *Journal of Oral and Maxillofacial Surgery*, vol. 59, no. 11, pp. 1352–1354, 2001.

[10] J. S. M. Daniels, "Primary hyperparathyroidism presenting as a palatal brown tumor," *Oral Surgery, Oral Medicine, Oral Pathology, Oral Radiology, and Endodontology*, vol. 98, no. 4, pp. 409–413, 2004.

[11] M. Mohan, R. S. Neelakandan, D. Siddharth, and R. Sharma, "An unusual case of brown tumor of hyperparathyroidism associated with ectopic parathyroid adenoma," *European Journal of Dentistry*, vol. 7, no. 4, pp. 500–503, 2013.

[12] K. Uhluhizarci, R. Çolak, and M. Kula, "Evaluation of sixteen patients with hyperparathyroidism," *Turkish Journal of Endocrinology and Metabolism*, vol. 4, no. 4, pp. 139–142, 2000.

[13] S. Mittal, D. Gupta, S. Sekhri, and S. Goyal, "Oral manifestations of parathyroid disorders and its dental management," *Journal of Dental and Allied Sciences*, vol. 3, no. 1, p. 34, 2014.

[14] S. N. Scott, Y. Sato, S. M. Graham, and R. A. Robinson, "Brown tumor of the palate in a patient with primary hyperparathyroidism," *The Annals of Otology, Rhinology, and Laryngology*, vol. 108, no. 1, pp. 91–94, 1999.

[15] J. Fernández-Sanromán, I. Anton-Badiola, and A. Costas-López, "Brown tumor of the mandible as first manifestation of primary hyperparathyroidism: diagnosis and treatment," *Medicina Oral, Patología Oral y Cirugía Bucal*, vol. 10, no. 2, pp. 169–172, 2004.

[16] G. N. Hendy and D. E. C. Cole, "Genetic defects associated with familial and sporadic hyperparathyroidism," in *Endocrine Tumor Syndromes and Their Genetics*, vol. 41, pp. 149–165, Karger Publishers, 2013.

[17] H. Steinbach, G. Gordan, J. Crane, L. Goldman, S. Silverman, and E. Eisenberg, "Primary hyperparathyroidism-a correlation of roentgen, clinical, and pathologic features," *American Journal of Roentgenology Radium Therapy and Nuclear Medicine*, vol. 86, no. 2, p. 329, 1961.

[18] R. Düsünsel, E. Güney, Z. de Gündüz, M. Poyrazoglu, O. Yigitbasi, and O. Kontas, "Maxillary brown tumor caused

by secondary hyperparathyroidism in a boy," *Pediatric Nephrology*, vol. 14, no. 6, pp. 529-530, 2000.

[19] I. Krause, B. Eisenstein, M. Davidovits, R. Cleper, A. Tobar, and S. Calderon, "Maxillomandibular brown tumor–a rare complication of chronic renal failure," *Pediatric Nephrology*, vol. 14, no. 6, pp. 499–501, 2000.

[20] C. H. Bedard and R. D. Nichols, "Osteitis fibrosa (brown tumor) of the maxilla," *The Laryngoscope*, vol. 84, no. 12, pp. 2093–2100, 1974.

[21] E. M. Martínez-Gavidia, J. V. Bagán, M. A. Milián-Masanet, E. Lloria de Miguel, and A. Pérez-Vallés, "Highly aggressive brown tumour of the maxilla as first manifestation of primary hyperparathyroidism," *International Journal of Oral and Maxillofacial Surgery*, vol. 29, no. 6, pp. 447–449, 2000.

[22] F. Alvarado, S. G. Waguespack, J. H. Campbell, and T. P. Williams, "Expansile intraosseus lesion of the mandible," *Journal of Oral and Maxillofacial Surgery*, vol. 61, no. 11, pp. 1318–1323, 2003.

[23] E. Guney, O. G. Yigitbasi, F. Bayram, V. Ozer, and Ö. Canoz, "Brown tumor of the maxilla associated with primary hyperparathyroidism," *Auris, Nasus, Larynx*, vol. 28, no. 4, pp. 369–372, 2001.

25

Mandibular Osteitis Fibrosa Cystica as First Sign of Vitamin D Deficiency

Nour Mellouli ⓘ,[1,2] Raouaa Belkacem Chebil,[1,2] Marwa Darej,[1,2] Yosra Hasni,[3] Lamia Oualha,[1,2] and Nabiha Douki[2,4]

[1]Oral Medicine and Oral Surgery, Dental Department, University Hospital Sahloul, Sousse, Tunisia
[2]Oral Health and Oro-Facial Rehabilitation Laboratory Research (LR12ES11), Faculty of Dental Medicine, University of Monastir, Avenue Avicenne, 5019 Monastir, Tunisia
[3]Endocrinology Department, University Hospital Farhat Hached, Sousse, Tunisia
[4]Endodontics, Dental Department, University Hospital Sahloul, Sousse, Tunisia

Correspondence should be addressed to Nour Mellouli; mellouli.nour@gmail.com

Academic Editor: Luis M. J. Gutierrez

Introduction. Brown tumors of hyperparathyroidism are locally destructive bone lesions. They are the late clinical consequence of the disease. They can occur in primary, secondary, and rarely tertiary forms. They affect usually long bones and less frequently those of the maxilla. *Case Report.* Our 45-year-old female patient presented with a mandibular tumor next to the first right lower molar. At first, we have chosen tooth extraction and tumor excision. When the histological report showed the giant cell tumor we suspected a metabolic bone disorder. Biochemical tests screened hyperparathyroidism and severe vitamin D deficiency, and parathyroid scintiscan revealed parathyroid adenoma. *Discussion.* The association of hyperparathyroidism and vitamin D deficiency leads to diagnostic uncertainty. First, secondary hyperparathyroidism can be due vitamin D deficiency. Second, data available show that vitamin D deficiency is more prevalent in patients with primary hyperparathyroidism than in general population. Hyperparathyroidism management is based on correct and precise diagnosis. Furthermore, the resolution of brown tumors depends on the cure of hyperparathyroidism. In fact, bone lesions should regress after biological tests' normalization. *Conclusion.* Clinicians should be aware of such rare and complicated presentation. They must consider the diagnosis of the brown tumor to avoid extensive surgical excision and teeth extractions.

1. Introduction

Hyperparathyroidism (HPT) is a prevailing endocrine disease. Determined by the cause of PTH production, HPT can be characterized into primary, secondary, and tertiary form(s). Primary hyperparathyroidism (PHPT) is a disorder of calcium, phosphate, and thus bone metabolism. The main cause of PHPT is adenoma in about 80% of cases followed by glandular hyperplasia (15%) and more rarely due to the presence of parathyroid carcinoma. In primary HPT, hypercalcemia and hypophosphatemia are omnipresent in laboratory tests [1]. Secondary hyperparathyroidism (SHPT) is caused by defective phosphate excretion and failure to activate vitamin D. Elevated phosphate level, decreased calcium level, and reduced serum vitamin D lead to continuous stimulation of the parathyroid glands that increases PTH release [1].

Tertiary hyperparathyroidism is a state of excessive secretion of PTH after a long period of SHPT. It leads to autonomous parathyroid glands that induce hypercalcemia [1].

HPT leads to bone involvement that includes generalized osteoporosis, multiple focal skull areas of demineralization, and brown tumors.

Brown tumors affect usually clavicles, ribs, and pelvis. Head and neck involvement is rare, and the mandible is affected more often than the maxilla.

The aim of this paper was to describe a case of the brown tumor in the mandible which was the first sign of hyperparathyroidism.

2. Case Report

A female patient aged 45 years with no known comorbidities came to our department at the university hospital Sahloul Sousse with the chief complaint of a right-sided swelling in the mandible. This swelling has caused slight asymmetry of the face since 6 months, which gradually enlarged up to the present size (Figure 1).

The patient gave a history of generalized weakness, lethargy, and weight loss noticed since past few months. Her family history and past medical history were nonsignificant.

Intraoral examination revealed a 4.0 × 4.0 cm bulbous mass hard to palpation arising from the mandible and extending from the distal aspect of the lower right first premolar (44) to the second right molar (47) (Figure 2). She had no associated bleeding or superficial ulceration of the mass. The patient denied pain but mentioned difficulty in eating. Positive response to sensitivity testing was found in the lower right premolars and molars. Neither mobility nor teeth dislocation were noticed.

Radiographic examination with orthopantamogram showed unilocular radiolucency close to the mandibular first right molar's roots, without involving the mandibular canal. Roots erosion of the relative tooth was noted (Figure 3).

A computed tomography (CT) scan showed multiloculated ground-glass ossification of the lesion (Figure 4).

After the first molar extraction (46) and the surgical excision of the lesion, the histological report was akin to the giant cell tumor (Figure 5).

So, serum parathormone level was advised to rule out metabolic bone disease. Laboratory investigations were done: serum PTH level was slightly high, and serum calcium and phosphorus levels were normal (Table 1).

The lesion was identified as a brown tumor of hyperparathyroidism, and the patient was referred to the endocrinology department.

Kidney function blood tests were done. Serum creatinine and blood urea nitrogen were normal. Chronic renal failure could not be considered the cause of hyperparathyroidism. However, we noted severe vitamin D deficiency (Table 1). The initial impression was of secondary hyperparathyroidism due to this vitamin D deficiency.

It was decided that vitamin D supplementation was the best therapeutic option. The patient was started on vitamin D 100,000 IU per fortnight for 6 weeks which is the equivalent of half an ampoule of 200,000 IU/1 ml. Thereafter, the patient was kept on 200,000 IU every 6 months. Her PTH levels decreased after 6 months on vitamin D therapy, and her calcium and phosphorus levels remained in the standards.

The patient underwent ultrasound scan of the neck, which showed a left lower lobe parathyroid solid nodule. The lesion had irregular hypoechoic component and was suggestive of parathyroid adenoma. Parathyroid technetium scintiscan (99mTc Sestamibi; Technetium-99 MIBI; methoxy-isobutyl-isonitrile) was requisite and revealed left lower parathyroid adenoma (Figure 6). Skeleton exploration was done by technetium 99 scintigraphy and did not reveal any abnormally high uptake.

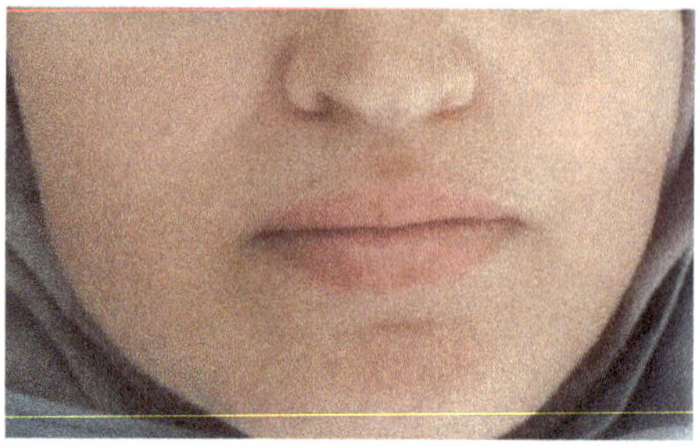

Figure 1: Clinical picture: slight asymmetry with swelling on the right side of the face.

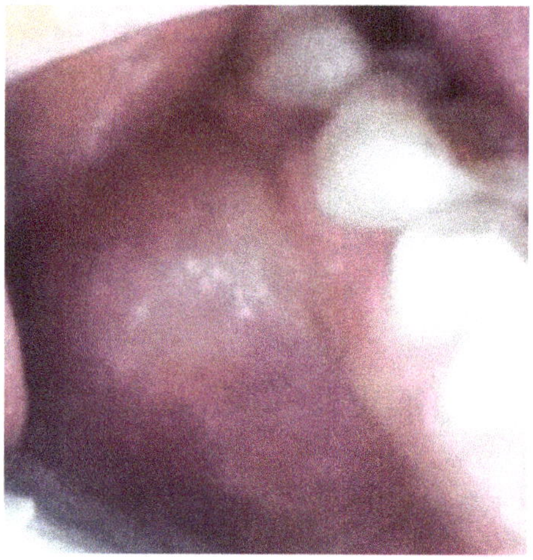

Figure 2: Clinical picture: a bulbous mass of 4 × 4 cm in the vestibule on the right side, extending from the distal aspect of 44 to the 47.

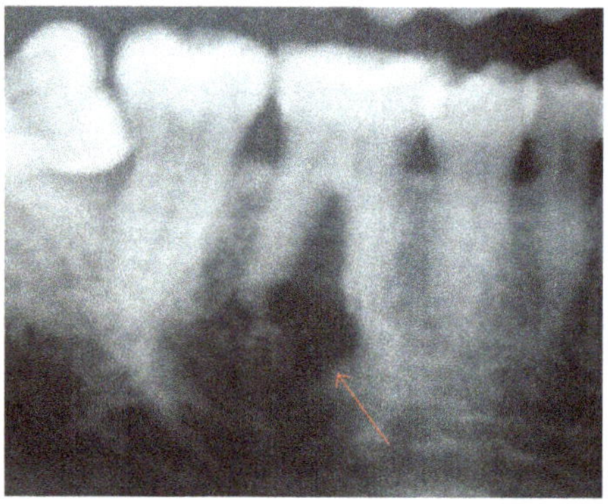

Figure 3: Panoramic radiography showing unilocular radiolucency close to the 46.

Accordingly, we retained the diagnosis of primary hyperparathyroidism masked by vitamin D deficiency and caused by parathyroid adenoma.

There was a normalization of calcium, PTH, and vitamin D serum levels. The bone mineral density test was not lower than normal which excludes osteopenia and osteoporosis. So, surgical treatment of the adenoma was not indicated. The patient was compliant and presented a favorable evolution (Figure 7).

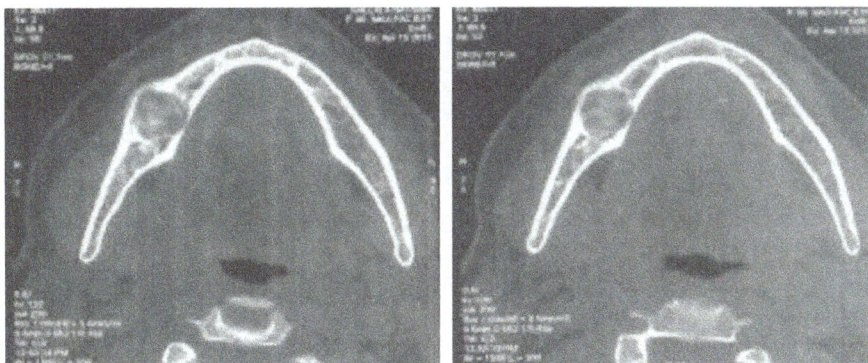

FIGURE 4: Computed tomography scan: axial views showing multiloculated ground-glass ossification of the lesion.

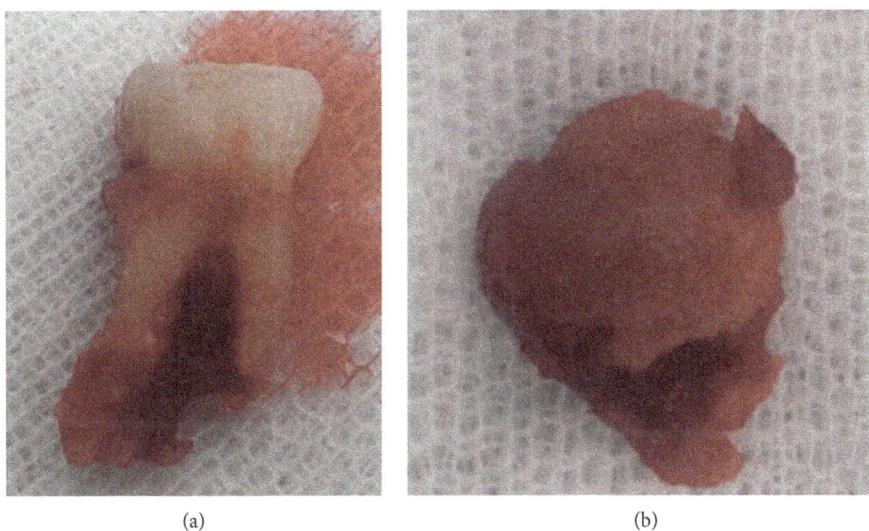

(a)

(b)

FIGURE 5: Biopsy specimen.

TABLE 1: Blood tests of the patient before and after vitamin D supplementation.

Serum level	Normal range	Initial values	After vitamin D therapy (6 months)
PTH (pg/ml)	15–65	81.5	56.3
Calcium (mmol/l)	2.15–2.5	2.3	2.4
Phosphorus (mmol/l)	0.87–1.45	1.3	1.1
25-hydroxyvitamin D (ng/ml)	>(20–30)	9.5	17.9

3. Discussion

Before the 1970s, the presentation of HPT was characterized by recurrent nephrolithiasis, brown tumors, neuromuscular dysfunction, symptomatic hypercalcemia, peptic ulcer disease, psychosis, and pancreatitis [2]. After then, with the introduction of the automated biochemistry analyzer, HPT could be diagnosed in the early and asymptomatic period of this disease [3]. Patients with profound symptoms became rare besides those apparently asymptomatic emerged. For these patients, elevated serum PTH level was discovered incidentally.

The brown tumor also known as osteitis fibrosa cystica or Von Recklinghausen's disease of bone is a reactive nonneoplastic giant cell lesion associated with hyperparathyroidism.

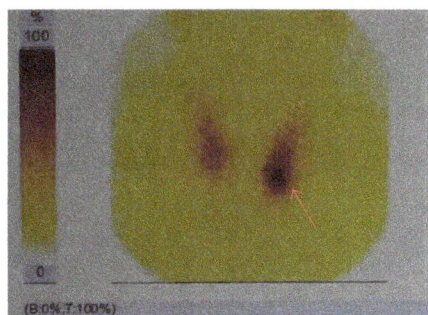

FIGURE 6: Parathyroid technetium scintiscan (99mTc Sestamibi; Technetium-99 MIBI; methoxy-isobutyl-isonitrile) showed increased uptake of the radiocontrast agent observed in the left lower parathyroid.

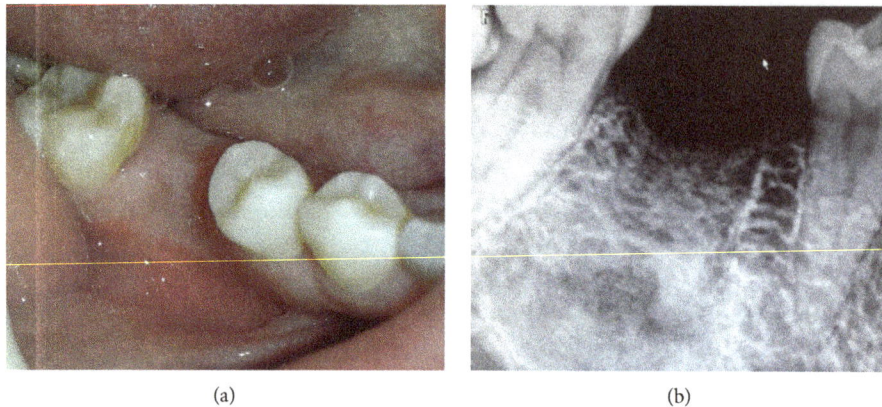

(a)   (b)

FIGURE 7: Clinical and radiological control at the 6 month with good mucosal and bone healing.

Products from microbleeding like hemosiderin assign the brown color to the lesion [4, 5]. The lesion is more prevalent in patients older than 50 years and three times more frequent in women [6]. The female preponderance is speculated to be due to women's lower body mass that would lead to an earlier clinical manifestation of the disease [7].

The preferential location of brown tumors is ribs, clavicle, and pelvic girdle. When they arise in the maxillofacial region, the mandible is so far the most frequent localization [8]. However, both mandible and maxilla affected individually or simultaneously were reported [7].

The physical examination usually reveals painful and hard bone swelling which may produce disfiguring deformities. However, our patient denied any ache. Asymptomatic brown tumors are also described by several authors. Therefore, their discovery is fortuitous following a radiological examination.

On radiographic and computed tomography exams, well-defined radiolucent or hypodense image are described, usually not demonstrating cortical disruptions and periosteal reactions or inflammatory signs [6]. This typical cyst-like radiographic appearance can be replaced by a multiloculated lesion with a "ground-glass opacification" which was found in our case [4].

Clinical and radiological presentation of the brown tumor can mimic other diseases, the most likely diagnoses include odontogenic and nonodontogenic cysts and tumors (radicular cyst, lateral periodontal cyst, ameloblastoma, keratocyst, eosinophilic granuloma, giant cell lesions, myxoma, and fibroosseous lesions), infectious diseases (bone abscess and localized osteomyelitis), and metastasis from a known or an unknown primary site (lung, breast, kidney, and prostate) [9, 10].

The usefulness of the tumor biopsy is controversial. When biological disorder guides to brown tumor diagnosis, it is useless. Histologically, the presence of diffuse giant cells is characteristic, but there is no pathognomonic sign [4].

Brown tumors occur in 4.5% of patients with PHPT and between 1.5% and 1.7% in cases of SHPT [5, 8] with an overall prevalence of 0.1% [4, 6]. The treatment of brown tumors is the cure of the underlying hyperparathyroidism. When hypersecretion of PTH is corrected, spontaneous regression of the lesion is expected. In our case, precipitated surgery led to loosing tooth and wide bone defect. Then, a proper diagnosis could have avoided inadequate excision and teeth extractions. Surgical therapy is required in a second step if the lesion persists or if bone healing is compromised, but only after HPT is controlled [4].

To correct hyperparathyroidism, it is worthwhile to know its form. Secondary HPT results when hypersecretion of PTH is a response to decreased calcium. It is generally associated with serum hypocalcemia and hyperphosphatemia. This condition is found in patients with chronic kidney disease or vitamin D deficiency [11].

The main cause of primary HPT is parathyroid adenoma. Glandular hyperplasia and parathyroid carcinomas are more rare etiologies. Primary HPT is characterized by elevated or inappropriately normal PTH levels and the persistent elevation of total serum calcium levels [12]. Normocalcemic primary HPT is a variant newly acknowledged. That clinical entity is poorly known and develops with high PTH levels and normal serum calcium levels [12].

The American Association of Endocrine Surgeons recommends the biochemical evaluation of serum total calcium, PTH, creatinine, and vitamin D levels if primary HPT is suspected (strong recommendation and moderate quality evidence) [12].

Low levels of vitamin D are found more often in primary HPT than in the general population. This observation is dyed in the wool [13] and is based upon measurement of the serum 25-hydroxyvitamin D level. Vitamin D deficiency's definition is controversial. Many experts define two groups: "insufficiency" in which the level of serum 25-hydroxyvitamin D is between 20 and 30 ng/mL and the other "deficiency" in which the level is <20 ng/mL [14]. The pathophysiological mechanism explaining the association between vitamin D deficiency and primary HPT is not clear. But chronic vitamin D deficiency seems to incite events leading to parathyroid gland hyperplasia and subsequent adenomatous changes [13].

In our case report, biological findings could go along not only with the secondary HPT but also with the normocalcemic variant of primary HPT. To fix on the diagnosis, neck scintiscan revealed parathyroid adenoma. So, diagnosis of primary HPT was retained.

The supplementation for vitamin D deficiency is required, and maintaining vitamin D to levels beyond 30 ng/ml is recommended. The endocrine society supported vitamin D2 or D3 supplementation of 50,000 IU once a week for 8 weeks or its daily equivalent followed by 1,500 to 2,000 IU daily use maintenance. In our case, the protocol has been modified since only pharmaceutical form of 200,000 IU/1 ml is available [15].

Parathyroidectomy should be considered for most patients with primary HPT and is more worthwhile than observation or pharmacologic therapy. It is the definitive treatment option for all patients with symptomatic primary HPT or associated with osteoporosis. Surgical treatment is also indicated when the serum calcium level is higher than 1 mg/dL (0.25 mmol/l) above normal, even if there are no symptoms. Patients, younger than 50 years, and those unable or unwilling to comply with observation protocols, are rather candidates for surgery [12, 13, 16].

4. Conclusion

The incidence of primary hyperparathyroidism is increasing. Surprisingly, it tripled between 1995 and 2010, and clinicians from all specialties will likely encounter patients with this disorder. There is some evidence to suggest that vitamin D deficiency may increase the likelihood of a more symptomatic presentation of PHPT. The exact influence of vitamin D status upon the modern presentation of PHPT is yet to be fully defined.

The treatment of brown tumors is the cure of the underlying hyperparathyroidism. When hypersecretion of PTH is corrected, spontaneous regression of the lesion is expected. A typical radiological presentation of the giant cell tumor should be completed by measurement of calcium, phosphorus, and PTH serum levels. Then, a proper diagnosis avoids inadequate surgical excision and teeth extractions.

References

[1] F. Selvi, S. Cakarer, R. Tanakol, S. D. Guler, and C. Keskin, "Brown tumour of the maxilla and mandible: a rare complication of tertiary hyperparathyroidism," *Dentomaxillofacial Radiology*, vol. 38, no. 1, pp. 53–58, 2009.

[2] P. J. Mazzaglia, E. Berber, A. Kovach, M. Milas, C. Esselstyn, and A. E. Siperstein, "The changing presentation of hyperparathyroidism over 3 decades," *Archives of Surgery*, vol. 143, no. 3, pp. 260–266, 2008.

[3] R. Pyram, G. Mahajan, and A. Gliwa, "Primary hyperparathyroidism: skeletal and non-skeletal effects, diagnosis and management," *Maturitas*, vol. 70, no. 3, pp. 246–255, 2011.

[4] P. Brabyn, A. Capote, M. Belloti, and I. Zylberberg, "Hyperparathyroidism diagnosed due to brown tumors of the jaw: a case report and literature review," *Journal of Oral and Maxillofacial Surgery*, vol. 75, no. 10, pp. 2162–2169, 2017.

[5] A. Guerrouani, A. Rzin, and K. El Khatib, "Hyperparathyroidism-jaw tumour syndrome detected by aggressive generalized osteitis fibrosa cystica," *Clinical Cases in Mineral and Bone Metabolism*, vol. 10, no. 1, pp. 65–67, 2013.

[6] A. D. Shetty, J. Namitha, and L. James, "Brown tumor of mandible in association with primary hyperparathyroidism: a case report," *Journal of International Oral Health*, vol. 7, no. 2, pp. 50–52, 2015.

[7] F. S. C. Pontes, M. A. Lopes, L. L. de Souza et al., "Oral and maxillofacial manifestations of chronic kidney disease-mineral and bone disorder: a multicenter retrospective study," *Oral Surgery, Oral Medicine, Oral Pathology and Oral Radiology*, vol. 125, no. 1, pp. 31–43, 2018.

[8] J. S. Keyser and G. N. Postma, "Brown tumor of the mandible," *American Journal of Otolaryngology*, vol. 17, no. 6, pp. 407–410, 1996.

[9] M. Hussain and M. Hammam, "Management challenges with brown tumor of primary hyperparathyroidism masked by severe vitamin D deficiency: a case report," *Journal of Medical Case Reports*, vol. 10, no. 1, p. 166, 2016.

[10] E. Proimos, T. S. Chimona, D. Tamiolakis, M. G. Tzanakakis, and C. E. Papadakis, "Brown tumor of the maxillary sinus in a patient with primary hyperparathyroidism: a case report," *Journal of Medical Case Reports*, vol. 3, no. 1, p. 7495, 2009.

[11] M. Qaisi, M. Loeb, L. Montague, and R. Caloss, "Mandibular brown tumor of secondary hyperparathyroidism requiring extensive resection: a forgotten entity in the developed world?," *Case Reports in Medicine*, vol. 2015, Article ID 567543, 10 pages, 2015.

[12] S. M. Wilhelm, T. S. Wang, D. T. Ruan et al., "The American Association of Endocrine Surgeons Guidelines for definitive management of primary hyperparathyroidism," *JAMA Surgery*, vol. 151, no. 10, pp. 959–968, 2016.

[13] M. D. Walker and J. P. Bilezikian, "Vitamin D and primary hyperparathyroidism: more insights into a complex relationship," *Endocrine*, vol. 55, no. 1, pp. 3–5, 2017.

[14] A. C. Ross, J. E. Manson, S. A. Abrams et al., "The 2011 report on dietary reference intakes for calcium and vitamin D from the Institute of Medicine: what clinicians need to know," *Journal of Clinical Endocrinology & Metabolism*, vol. 96, no. 1, pp. 53–58, 2011.

[15] M. F. Holick, N. C. Binkley, H. A. Bischoff-Ferrari et al., "Evaluation, treatment, and prevention of vitamin D deficiency: an Endocrine Society clinical practice guideline," *Journal of Clinical Endocrinology & Metabolism*, vol. 96, no. 7, pp. 1911–1930, 2011.

[16] M. W. Yeh, P. H. Ituarte, H. C. Zhou et al., "Incidence and prevalence of primary hyperparathyroidism in a racially mixed population," *Journal of Clinical Endocrinology & Metabolism*, vol. 98, no. 3, pp. 1122–1129, 2013.

26

Immediate Implant Placement by Interradicular Bone Drilling before Molar Extraction: Clinical Case Report with One-Year Follow-Up

Stuardo Valenzuela,[1] José M. Olivares (iD),[1] Nicolás Weiss,[1] and Dafna Benadof[2]

[1]Postgraduate Implant Dentistry Department, School of Dentistry, Universidad Andres Bello, Santiago, Chile
[2]School of Dentistry, Universidad Andres Bello, Santiago, Chile

Correspondence should be addressed to José M. Olivares; josemanuelolivaresr@gmail.com

Academic Editor: Gavriel Chaushu

The placement of immediate implants in the posterior sector is a widespread procedure where the success and survival rates are similar to those of traditional protocols. It has several anatomical challenges, such as the presence of interradicular bone septa that hinder a correct three-dimensional positioning of the implant and may compromise primary stability and/or cause damage of neighboring structures. The aim of this article is to present the treatment and the one-year clinical follow-up of a patient who received immediate implant placement using an interradicular bone-drilling technique before the molar extraction.

1. Introduction

Immediate implant placement has considerable advantages over the conventional approach. It has fewer numbers of surgical procedures, reduces overall treatment time, and therefore costs less. It also helps preserve the gingival architecture and increase the patient's comfort, acceptance, and satisfaction [1–5].

Immediate implant placement studies in the esthetic and premolar zone follow strict surgical protocols that have been established to optimize the three-dimensional positioning of the implant and its primary stability and the condition of the neighboring tissue [6–8]. However, there is less information on immediate implant placement in the posterior sector where the esthetical impact is lower, but the surgical difficulty of the tooth extraction, drilling, and implant placement is greater [9–11].

Despite the abovementioned issue, the cumulative survival rates reported for immediate implants placed in molar sites are similar to those placed in healed sites, which ranges from 93.9% to 99% [4–8, 10, 11]. An essential aspect to achieve this positive outcome is the primary stabilization of the implant in the apical and/or lateral bone, where anatomic conditions can hinder this goal. Therefore, a thorough implant surgery planning, skills, and clinical experience are relevant factors in the success of the surgical procedure [4, 12].

Modifications to the current surgical techniques are recommended to facilitate immediate implant placement in the posterior sector. Different authors propose implant drilling prior to tooth extraction in order to stabilize the interradicular bone septa through the remaining tooth roots [9, 13–15]. In 2017, a randomized pilot study of 22 patients compared the conventional technique of dental extraction, subsequent interradicular bone drilling, and immediate implant placement to the technique of interradicular bone drilling using ultrasound devices. The results were statistically higher for the implant positioning and primary stability using the proposed new technique [9].

The aim of this article is to present the treatment of a patient by means of immediate implant placement using an interradicular bone-drilling technique and its clinical follow-up one-year later.

2. Case Presentation

A 35-year-old patient with no significant medical history consulted the Implantology Department of Universidad Andres Bello in Santiago, Chile, for a complete evaluation and dental treatment. The dental team performed a clinical examination (Figure 1) and a radiographic study (Figures 2(a) and 2(b)) on the patient detecting decayed remaining roots in teeth 1.4 and 1.5 and performed an extensive restoration presenting deep, subgingival distal decay on tooth 1.6. Based on all the gathered information, the dental team decided to extract teeth 1.6, 1.5, and 1.4 and then perform immediate implant placement.

Before the surgery, the patient signed the informed consent. The surgical procedure for tooth 1.6 began with the infiltration of local anesthesia (standard Lignospan, Septodont) in the treatment zone. Then, the tooth was decoronated at the gingival margin level using a cylindrical AV-010 diamond burr (Beavers Dental, Kerr Corp). Once the roots were clinically visible, the drilling sequence recommended by the implant manufacturer was performed through the tooth, always corroborating the drilling direction with a paralleling pin (Figure 3). When the drilling sequence was completed, the remaining root fragments were carefully removed using desmotomes (Figure 4). This procedure was done with extreme care in order to preserve the alveolar walls and avoid bone deformation at the drilling path. The alveolus was carefully cleaned and washed surgically with a saline solution, and an Alpha Bio ICE 5.3×10 mm implant (Alpha Bio Tec.) was placed in the center of the interradicular bone, in a type B position according to the Tarnow classification (Figure 5). To promote a nonsubmerged healing approach, a standard healing abutment of 4.6 mm of diameter and 4 mm of length (Alpha Bio, Alpha Bio Tec.) was connected to the implant. The 3 mm horizontal gap between the implant and the bone walls was filled with a xenograft (Alpha Bio's Graft, Alpha Bio Tec.) Finally, platelet-rich fibrin (PRF) membranes were fixed through a monofilament nylon blue suture No. 5/0 (Tagum 2/0 HR25, Tagumedica S.A.). Additionally, Alpha Bio ICE $3.7 \text{ N} \times 10$ mm implants were placed in teeth 1.4 and 1.5 (Alpha Bio Tec.) (Figure 5).

3. Short- and Long-Term Follow-Ups

The patient received regular check-ups on days 3, 7, and 14 after the implant placement surgery, and no pain or infection was observed. On day 21, the suture was removed and the soft architecture preservation looked uneventful. At 6 months, an apical reposition flap was performed at implants placed in teeth 1.4 and 1.5, and healing abutments were placed (Alpha Bio, Alpha Bio Tec.). After the soft tissue healed, a rehabilitation based on fixed partial metal-ceramic denture screwed on UCLA Cr-Co abutments was installed. At this time, the gingival architecture remained stable with preservation of a functionally attached gingiva (Figure 6). At 6 months and 12 months follow-ups, clinical and radiological exams showed that the bone levels remained stable (Figures 7 and 8). In addition, the prosthetic structure

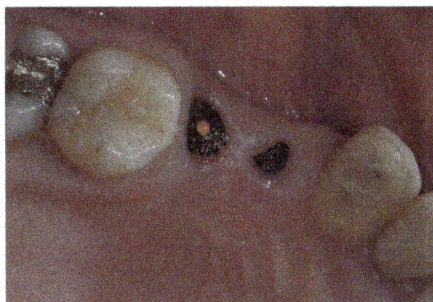

FIGURE 1: The remaining roots in teeth 1.4 and 1.5 presented decay and exposed endodontic treatment. Tooth 1.6 had an extensive crown restoration and deep, subgingival distal decay.

remained in optimal clinical condition, displaying optimal esthetic and functional results (Figure 9).

4. Discussion

The immediate placement of dental implants is a widely accepted procedure, achieving survival rates comparable to implants installed according to conventional treatment protocols [2, 9]. Although there are standardized protocols and numerous studies describing this technique in the esthetic zone, there is less information about the installation of immediate implants in the posterior sector where the esthetical impact is lower, but the surgical difficulty can be more challenging. For example, anatomical challenges, such as differences between the size of the implant and the alveolus postextraction, root length, height of root trunk, and divergence of roots make this surgical technique more difficult [10, 11].

To determine the possibility and prognosis of the implant placement in fresh extraction sockets prior to implant surgery, Smith and Tarnow [16] described a classification based on the morphology of the interradicular bone septa and its impact on the primary stability of the implant, permitting a more accurate presurgical planning. In 2016, Matsuda et al. [17] used a database of cone-beam imaging to evaluate the alveolar dimensions at molar sites and the possibility of immediate implant placement. The author reported that 46% of the sample ($n = 150$) had 5 mm of engaging apical bone below the apex of the buccal mesial and distal roots that is compatible with an immediate implant procedure. Of the analyzed molars, 32% had a 2 mm distance from the sinus floor to the furcation and 5 mm between buccolingual roots, preventing an immediate implant approach. The rest of the molars were in an intermediate situation, with bone width greater than 5 mm between the roots but lacking height, having 2 mm to 4 mm from the root apex to the sinus floor, making an immediate implant approach technically more challenging. In the case presented in this report, the patient presented a type B socket [16] with a distance of 9 mm from the apex to the maxillary sinus and 8 mm between roots, presenting enough interradicular bone height and width to perform an immediate implant procedure.

In this clinical report, a guided bone regeneration technique was performed, which combined bovine xenograft

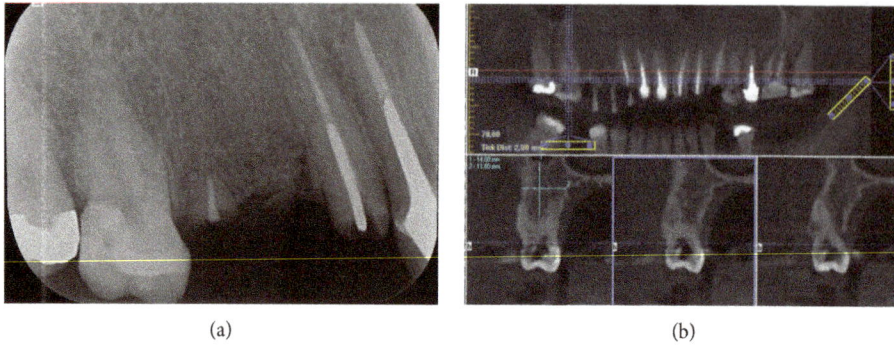

(a)   (b)

FIGURE 2: (a) Preoperative radiograph. (b) Upper maxillary CBCT of Tooth 1.6.

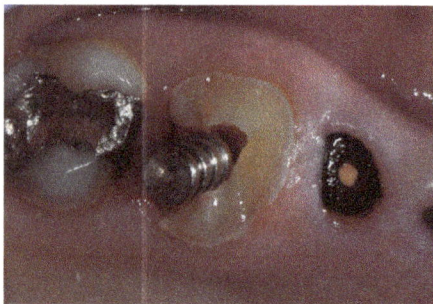

FIGURE 3: Implant paralleling pin inserted after interradicular bone drilling.

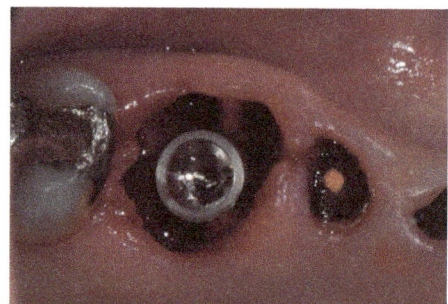

FIGURE 5: Immediate implant placement of an Alpha Bio ICE 5.3 × 10 mm implant in fresh extraction socket.

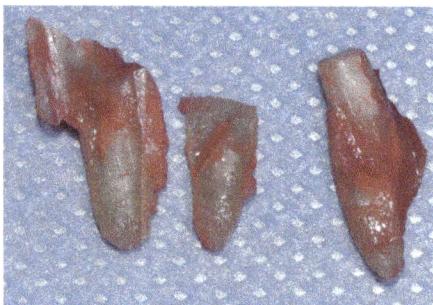

FIGURE 4: Remaining root aspects were carefully extracted using desmotomes.

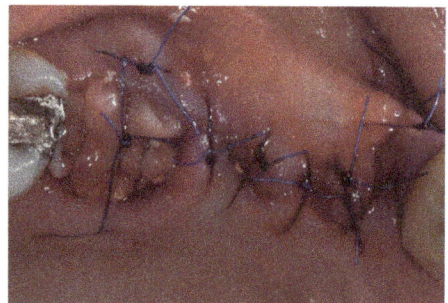

FIGURE 6: Closure using a 5.0 nylon suture.

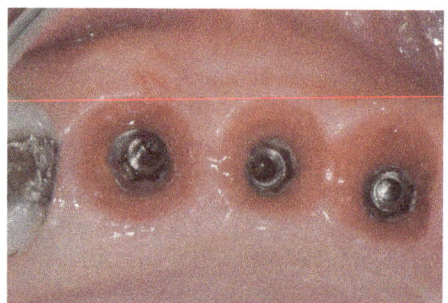

FIGURE 7: Follow-up at 6 months.

grafting and PRF membrane placement on top of the extraction socket [18–20]. The available literature does not mention any potential benefit of this type of membrane on bone formation. Nevertheless, the authors used this approach to promote prolonged and continued release of growth factors and proteins by the extracellular matrix during the first few days, to strengthen the proliferation of blood vessels and accelerate the healing of soft tissue [21].

Even though there are a few, but similar, reported cases using an interradicular drilling technique before the extraction procedure, this clinical report contributes to the literature by increasing the scientific data regarding this technique and by adding a one-year clinical and radiographical follow-up after the placement of the prosthetics [8, 9]. Most of the articles found in this topic reported follow-ups only until the prosthetic

delivery stage. This situation may be because the advantage of this technique is the surgical stage in which a primary stability and ideal three-dimensional positioning of the implants are

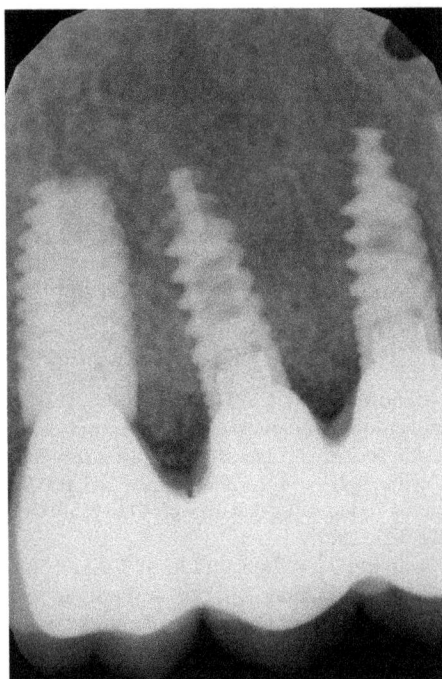

FIGURE 8: Prosthetic delivery radiograph.

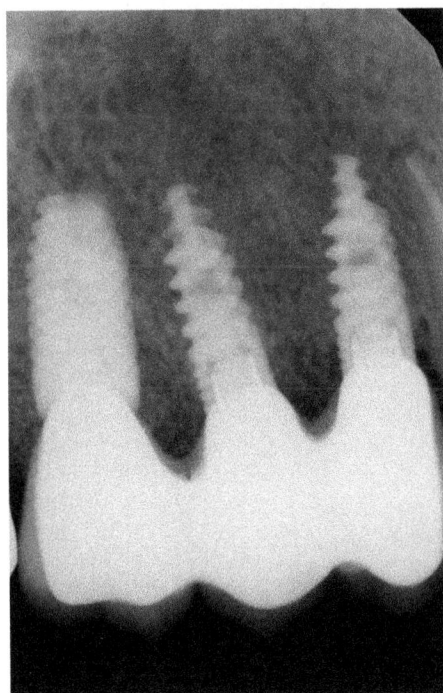

FIGURE 9: One-year follow-up.

attained. However, once osseointegration occurs, the behavior of peri-implant tissue should not differ from traditional procedures.

In Scarano's study [9], drilling in the interradicular bone septa before and after the extraction of molar roots was compared. The author concluded that using a guide on the position of the roots resulted in an ideal implant positioning ($p < 0.05$). Also, the primary stability of the implant based on

a resonance frequency analysis had significantly higher implant stability quotient values ($p < 0.05$) as compared to the traditional technique of extraction, subsequent drilling, and immediate implant placement. However, we do not know whether other variables may affect these results. For example, the use of the ultrasound device is comparable to drilling with conventional rotary instruments, so these results cannot be generalized. Moreover, the criteria for inclusion were only molar sites with interradicular septa that had crown dimensions above 2.5 mm and apical dimensions above 3.5 mm, which does not necessarily represent what most prevails in the population nor mean that these minimum measurements will suffice to attain a primary stability.

The interradicular bone-drilling technique prior to dental extraction could be considered a simple yet useful modification to the standard drilling procedure. Its indications are absence of active infection, integrity of the roots, and sufficient remaining bone to allow an immediate implant approach [15]. Contraindications are dental mobility, due to severe loss of periodontal insertion, unfavorable root position, such as fused roots, ankyloses, and active infections [13, 15]. The authors have described that even active infections such as apical periodontitis do not lead to an increased risk of complications, as long as they are asymptomatic [4].

This procedure has an increased risk to alter the socket wall's morphology during the extraction procedure, leading to a deficient implant insertion. Therefore, careful extraction using desmotomes or ultrasonic appliances is advised to avoid any deformation of the interradicular bone that could lead to a modification of the bone-drilling path and alter the final implant position.

Researchers have even stated that this technique could be suitable to nonexpert clinicians, making it simpler to obtain a correct tridimensional position of the implant and primary insertion torque. This is also supported by studies that show the traditional approach where the level of expertise is key factor in the success of the procedure [12].

Some limitations of this technique are increased hardness of the root tissue, which may result in longer clinical time and greater risk of increasing intrabone temperature and of altering the normal healing because of the remains of dental tissue from drilling. Regarding the latter point, Davarpanah and Szmukler-Moncler [22] made a case report on 5 patients; according to the results, dental waste did not seem to interfere with implant osseointegration, but there was little scientific evidence on this latter point, so caution is recommended, with an emphasis on meticulous irrigation and surgical cleaning.

Although this technique is promising and the clinical yield has been good for the authors during intraoperation management and post-op check-ups, controlled randomized clinical testing is required, using a comparative method, to evaluate the benefits and limitations of this technique in the long term.

References

[1] L. Schropp and F. Isidor, "Timing of implant placement relative to tooth extraction," *Journal of Oral Rehabilitation*, vol. 35, no. s1, pp. 33–43, 2008.

[2] A. Barone, P. Toti, A. Quaranta, G. Derchi, and U. Covani, "The clinical outcomes of immediate versus delayed restoration procedures on immediate implants: a comparative cohort study for single-tooth replacement," *Clinical Implant Dentistry and Related Research*, vol. 17, no. 6, pp. 1114–1126, 2015.

[3] R. J. Lazzara, "Immediate implant placement into extraction sites: surgical and restorative advantages," *International Journal of Periodontics & Restorative Dentistry*, vol. 9, no. 5, pp. 332–343, 1989.

[4] R. Crespi, P. Capparè, and E. Gherlone, "Fresh-socket implants in periapical infected sites in humans," *Journal of Periodontology*, vol. 81, no. 3, pp. 378–383, 2010.

[5] D. H. Lee, B. H. Choi, S. M. Jeong, F. Xuan, and H. R. Kim, "Effects of flapless implant surgery on soft tissue profiles: a prospective clinical study," *Clinical Implant Dentistry and Related Research*, vol. 13, no. 4, pp. 324–329, 2011.

[6] K.-G. Hwang and C.-J. Park, "Ideal implant positioning in an anterior maxillary extraction socket by creating an apico-palatal guiding slot: a technical note," *International Journal of Oral & Maxillofacial Implants*, vol. 23, no. 1, pp. 121-122, 2008.

[7] T. G. Wilson and D. Buser, "Timing of anterior implant placement postextraction: immediate versus early placement," *Clinical Advances in Periodontics*, vol. 1, no. 1, pp. 61–76, 2011.

[8] P. A. Fugazzotto, "Implant placement at the time of maxillary molar extraction: treatment protocols and report of results," *Journal of Periodontology*, vol. 79, no. 2, pp. 216–223, 2008.

[9] A. Scarano, "Traditional postextractive implant site preparation compared with pre-extractive interradicular implant bed preparation in the mandibular molar region, using an ultrasonic device: a randomized pilot study," *International Journal of Oral & Maxillofacial Implants*, vol. 32, no. 3, pp. 655–660, 2017.

[10] M. A. Atieh, A. G. T. Payne, W. J. Duncan, R. K. de Silva, and M. P. Cullinan, "Immediate placement or immediate restoration/loading of single implants for molar tooth replacement: a systematic review and meta-analysis," *International Journal of Oral & Maxillofacial Implants*, vol. 25, no. 2, pp. 401–415, 2009.

[11] M. Peñarrocha, R. Uribe, and J. Balaguer, "Immediate implants after extraction: a review of the current situation," *Medicina Oral*, vol. 9, no. 3, pp. 234–242, 2004.

[12] A. Barone, P. Toti, S. Marconcini, G. Derchi, M. Saverio, and U. Covani, "Esthetic outcome of implants placed in fresh extraction sockets by clinicians with or without experience: a medium-term retrospective evaluation," *International Journal of Oral & Maxillofacial Implants*, vol. 31, no. 6, pp. 1397–1406, 2016.

[13] S. F. Rebele, O. Zuhr, and M. B. Hürzeler, "Pre-extractive interradicular implant bed preparation: case presentations of a novel approach to immediate implant placement at multirooted molar sites," *International Journal of Periodontics and Restorative Dentistry*, vol. 33, no. 1, pp. 88–95, 2013.

[14] A. Scarano, F. Carinci, A. Quaranta, G. Iezzi, M. Piattelli, and A. Piattelli, "Correlation between implant stability quotient (ISQ) with clinical and histological aspects of dental implants removed for mobility," *International Journal of Immunopathology and Pharmacology*, vol. 20, no. 1, pp. 33–36, 2007.

[15] M. H. Tizcareño and C. Bravo-Flores, "Anatomically guided implant site preparation technique at molar sites," *Implant Dentistry*, vol. 18, no. 5, pp. 393–401, 2009.

[16] R. B. Smith and D. P. Tarnow, "Classification of molar extraction sites for immediate dental implant placement: technical note," *International Journal of Oral & Maxillofacial Implants*, vol. 28, no. 3, pp. 911–916, 2013.

[17] H. Matsuda, A. Borzabadi-Farahani, and B. T. Le, "Three-dimensional alveolar bone anatomy of the maxillary first molars," *Implant Dentistry*, vol. 25, no. 3, pp. 367–372, 2016.

[18] S. T. Chen, I. B. Darby, E. C. Reynolds, and J. G. Clement, "Immediate implant placement postextraction without flap elevation," *Journal of Periodontology*, vol. 80, no. 1, pp. 163–172, 2009.

[19] D. P. Tarnow and S. J. Chu, "Human histologic verification of osseointegration of an immediate implant placed into a fresh extraction socket with excessive gap distance without primary flap closure, graft, or membrane: a case report," *International Journal of Periodontics & Restorative Dentistry*, vol. 31, no. 5, pp. 515–521, 2011.

[20] K. R. Morjaria, R. Wilson, and R. M. Palmer, "Bone healing after tooth extraction with or without an intervention: a systematic review of randomized controlled trials," *Clinical Implant Dentistry and Related Research*, vol. 16, no. 1, pp. 1–20, 2012.

[21] D. M. Dohan Ehrenfest, L. Rasmusson, and T. Albrektsson, "Classification of platelet concentrates: from pure platelet-rich plasma (P-PRP) to leucocyte- and platelet-rich fibrin (L-PRF)," *Trends in Biotechnology*, vol. 27, no. 3, pp. 158–167, 2009.

[22] M. Davarpanah and S. Szmukler-Moncler, "Unconventional implant treatment: I. Implant placement in contact with ankylosed root fragments: a series of five case reports: case report," *Clinical Oral Implants Research*, vol. 20, no. 8, pp. 851–856, 2009.

27

Recurrent Ameloblastoma: A Surgical Challenge

Chithra Aramanadka ⓘ**, Abhay Taranath Kamath** ⓘ**, and Adarsh Kudva**

Department of Oral and Maxillofacial Surgery, Manipal College of Dental Sciences, Manipal, Karnataka, India

Correspondence should be addressed to Abhay Taranath Kamath; abhay.kamath@manipal.edu

Academic Editor: Giuseppe Colella

Ameloblastoma is locally aggressive benign odontogenic tumour with increased risk of recurrence rate. The choice of treatment depends on the histologic subtype. Radical therapy is the recommended modality for solid ameloblastomas. The possibilities of recurrence even after enbloc resection are still high. The author presents two case reports of recurrent ameloblastomas postradical resection. First case describes the recurrence of ameloblastoma in the bone graft which was used for reconstruction, and the second case depicts recurrence in the infratemporal fossa. Intraoperative radiography of the frozen section of the soft tissue margin plays an important role in the holistic management of these lesions.

1. Introduction

Ameloblastoma is the common locally aggressive benign epithelial odontogenic tumour of the oral cavity. It was first recognized by Cusack in 1827 and named in 1930 by Ivy and Churchill [1]. According to WHO classification in 2005, there are 5 subtypes of benign ameloblastoma documented, and they are (1) solid/multicystic type, (2) desmoplastic type, (3) unicystic type, and (4) extraosseous/peripheral type [2]. Histopathologically, the 6 subtypes are follicular, plexiform, acanthomatous, basal, unicystic, and desmoplastic ameloblastoma. It can be managed either by the conservative method or radical approach depending on the type, location, and size and age of the patient. A systematic review by Almaida et al. described that the 50% of recurrence is seen in follicular subtype and the recurrence rate is significantly low if a radical approach is used [3].

This paper describes two cases of recurrence of ameloblastoma in patients who underwent segmental resection of the jaw. These case reports can be added to the list of reported cases of recurrent ameloblastomas.

2. Case 1

A 46-year-old male patient referred by a private practitioner complained of swelling in the previously operated area of the right lower jaw since one month. He had a history of surgery in the same region. While going through the records of the patient, he had undergone segmental resection and reconstruction of the defect with rib graft 15 years ago. Histopathology reports of the previous pathology were not available in the records. Panoramic radiograph and CT scan revealed multilocular radiolucent lesion in the previously operated site (Figure 1). The clinical diagnosis at present was recurrent multicystic ameloblastoma involving the bone graft. The excision of the lesion with 1 cm uninvolved soft tissue margin was performed through the previous scar (Figures 2 and 3). The histopathology report of the specimen suggested follicular ameloblastoma with acanthomatous changes with tumour-free margins. A 1-year-follow-up showed no recurrence. He is planned for alloplastic reconstruction of the right hemimandible, considering the benign nature of the lesion.

3. Case 2

A 45-year-old male patient visited the Department of Oral and Maxillofacial Surgery with swelling over the right temple area of the face. He reported an asymptomatic swelling since 1 month which progressively increased in size. It was soft dumbbell shaped swelling in the right temporal region with no signs of infection.

Back in 2012, he had been referred to the same unit by general practitioner for gross swelling in the right jaw. Panoramic radiograph and CT scan showed multilocular

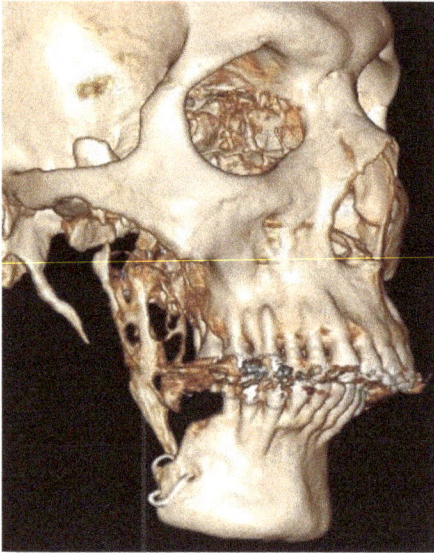

FIGURE 1: 3-Dimensional reconstruction of CT imaging shows recurrent tumour of the grafted bone and remnant coronoid process.

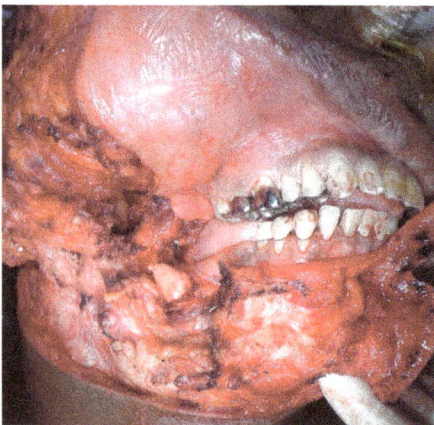

FIGURE 2: Surgical photograph shows the exposure of the lesion.

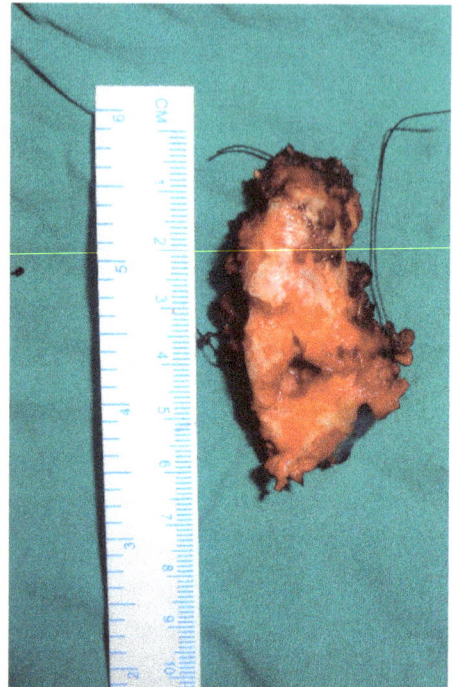

FIGURE 3: Surgical specimen.

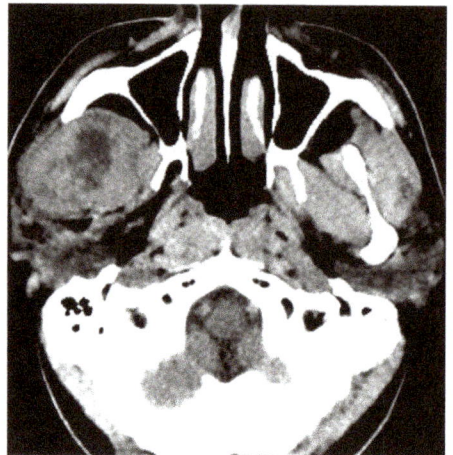

FIGURE 4: Preoperative CT scan shows the recurrent ameloblastoma in the infratemporal fossa.

radiolucency. The patient was subjected for biopsy and reported as ameloblastoma of the right mandible. He underwent right hemimandibulectomy. On table, the resected specimen was subjected for intraoperative radiography to understand the clearance of 1.5 cm safe radiologic margin. The histological report also revealed ameloblastoma with atypical features showing hypercellularity. Hence, he was kept on regular follow-up.

In 2016, he reported with a swelling on the right temple region. MR imaging studies showed heterogeneously enhancing altered signal intensity lesion (measures 4.4 cm × 3.7 cm × 4.6 cm) with tiny cystic areas noted in the right infratemporal fossa (Figure 4). The patient underwent tumour excision with a layer of overlying soft tissue through transzygomatic approach (Figures 5 and 6). The defect was packed with temporalis muscle flap. The specimen was sent for pathologic evaluation. Frozen sections confirmed the diagnosis of follicular ameloblastoma with a tumour-free

margin. His hospital stay was uneventful, and he is currently on regular follow-up.

4. Discussion

Ameloblastoma is a locally aggressive, anatomically benign tumour of the oral cavity which rarely undergoes malignant transformation. It is the second most common odontogenic tumour, the first being odontoma. Ameloblastoma is a common tumour in developed countries (70%) compared to developing countries, probability of unreported case in the latter [4].

WHO in 2005 classified ameloblastoma into four subtypes: multicystic/solid, unicystic, desmoplastic, and extraosseous

163

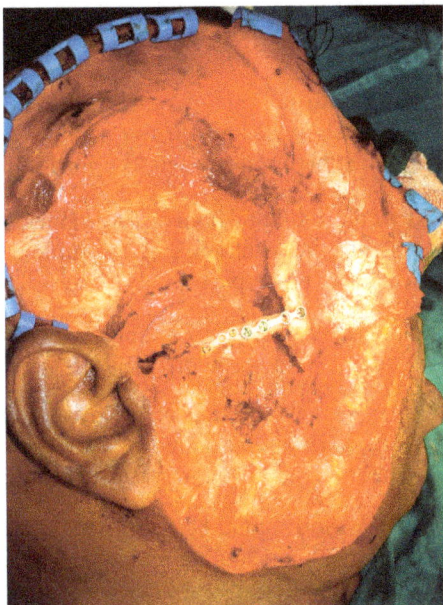

FIGURE 5: Intraoperative photograph shows the transzygomatic approach and the defect restored with temporalis muscle.

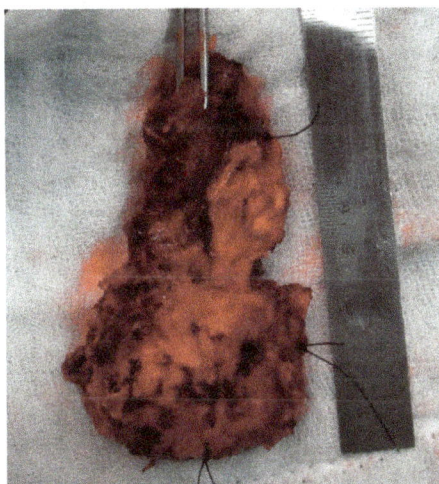

FIGURE 6: Excised specimen.

type. Solid/multicystic variant is the most common type, and it is highly aggressive and has a 90% recurrence after conservative management such as curettage and enucleation [5]. The high rate of recurrence is observed in mandibular ameloblastomas than maxillary ameloblastomas [6] and in follicular type than in plexiform or any other type [3].

Pathogenesis of the ameloblastoma is unclear. The genetic theory explains the involvement of the BRAF protein in the mitogen-activated protein kinase pathway (MAPK) that has been commonly found to be mutated, rendering the pathway constitutively active [7]. Ahlem et al. observed that the cell proliferation activity evaluated by Ki67 and CD10 was significantly higher in recurrent tumours [6].

More commonly, it affects the mandibular posterior region. The infiltration of the tumour cells occurs more predominantly in the cancellous portion of the cortical bone. Hence, CT scan is most promising in identifying the cortical destruction and soft tissue involvement [8].

The management involves either conservative or radical approach. The conservative method involves enucleation with adjunctive procedure either chemical cauterization or peripheral ostectomy of 1–1.5 cm normal margin. Conservative approach can be utilized for unicystic type. According to Pogrel and Montes, a unicystic variant can be best managed by enucleation with an application of Carnoy's solution or cryotherapy [9].

Radical approach is indicated for large ameloblastoma involving the inferior alveolar canal or below or for more aggressive variants like intramural ameloblastoma or multicystic type [10, 11]. It involves segmental or marginal resection with 1.5–2 cm normal bony margin beyond the radiologic margin. Use of intraoperative radiographs has been advocated for confirmation of bone margins.

The resection with 2-3 cm clear bone margin is indicated in cases of ameloblastic carcinoma [12].

Possible factors for recurrence after radical resection may be the histologic type and location of the tumour and solid type particularly follicular variety is the most aggressive type. The mandible posterior region is the common site of occurrence, and as it invades the cancellous portion beyond radiologic margin, over a time it can cause the cortical perforation. Invasion of the periosteum can lead to spread of the tumour cells to the soft tissue. Inadequate resection of the hard and soft tissues beyond a tumour would cause recurrence [13].

Several reports are available in literature related to the recurrence of ameloblastoma as shown in Table 1.

Recurrences are described in the study of radical treatment of ameloblastoma by Sehdev et al. [14], Shatkin and Hoffmeister [16], Mehlisch et al. [17], Muller and Slootweg [18], Olaitan et al. [19], Ueno et al. [20], Eckhardt et al. [10], and Nakamura et al. [21].

It is the known fact that the rate of recurrence with the conservative management is high (around 60%) compared to radical treatment (13%). The pattern of recurrences postresection has to be evaluated in a larger extent. Reports have been suggested that there are higher possibilities of retained soft tissue tumour islands during the surgical procedure in the complex regions like infratemporal fossa [34, 35].

In the first case report, the grafted tissue underwent tumorigenesis. This could be due to the remaining cells at the osteotomy site. It would be wise to wait for the histological report with the free margin before reconstruction in any case of the solid type to avoid donor site morbidities. The complication of primary reconstruction should be explained to the patient before surgery.

Lesions of infratemporal fossa remain asymptomatic, and the chief complaint of the patient is usually facial swelling or deformity.

Infratemporal fossa is pyramidal in shape that consists of complex structures, located on the lateral aspect of the cranial base, deep to the zygomatic arch, masseter, and mandibular ramus. The base formed by the medial aspect of the ramus and floor of the skull forms the upper surface of the pyramid. The anteromedial aspect corresponds to the posterior aspect of the

TABLE 1

Case Report	
Grafft et al. [22, 23]	Mandibular molar region; iliac graft
Carvalho et al. [24]	Iliac graft
Dolan et al. [25]	Rib graft
Marinelli et al. [26]	Iliac graft
Stea [27]	Iliac graft
Zacharides [28]	1 case of iliac graft; 2 cases of rib graft
Vasan [29]	Iliac graft
Bianchi et al. [30]	Iliac graft
Martins and Favaro [31]	Iliac graft
Su et al. [32]	Iliac graft
Choi et al. [33]	Iliac graft
Jian et al. [23]	1 case of iliac graft; 1 case of rib graft
Basat et al. [13]	1 case of free fibula flap

maxilla and the posteroinferior aspect to the pterygomaxillary fascia [36]. It is anatomically confined, making it relatively inaccessible and allowing undetected neoplastic growth. A close approximation to vital structures such as the calvaria, nasopharynx, and the maxillary artery add to its anatomic complexity. Diagnosis and treatment planning should follow CT scan and MRI to determine the extent of the lesion in such areas. Conventional radiography may not provide sufficient information.

Numerous surgical approaches have been employed to access the infratemporal region, some of them being the transoral, transanal, transpalatine, transzygomatic, transcervical, and extended maxillectomy approach [37]. We found that transzygomatic approach was appropriate to approach the lesion and to harvest the temporalis flap into the defect. The choice of surgical approach to each type of neoplasm depends on the clinical presentation and histologic subtype as well as its extent and location.

A possible explanation for recurrence in the second case would be retained periosteum over the coronoid process. Composite resection would eliminate the retention of a tumour infiltrated tissues.

Carlson and Marx described the technique of excising the next uninvolved anatomical structure to prevent recurrence of a tumour. We do agree with his opinion of scientific approach towards curative management with histopathologic free soft and hard tissue margin [11]. Similar cases of recurrence of reconstructed bone have been reported in the literature following 30 years of surgery [25–32, 38–40].

Laborde et al. and Becelli et al. reported no recurrence in his study of 7 patients' postsegmental resection [41, 8]. Similar reports are documented by Vayvada et al., Chaine et al., and Basat et al. on postresection and free flap reconstruction [13, 15, 34, 42].

Vaishampayan et al. suggested the possible cause for recurrence in the infratemporal region after segmental resection would be due to the retraction of pathologically weakened coronoid process fragment during temporal dissection [43].

Peacock et al. concluded that there no additional benefit in confirming the margin by performing frozen section in addition to intraoperative specimen radiograph in his study of 35 patients. However, this study did not include the soft tissue margin [44].

Though several reports suggest the radio resistant nature of ameloblastoma, I^{125} brachytherapy is tried to irradiate the recurrent lesion by delivering high prescribed doses of radiation (110 Gy) with satisfactory outcome [45].

We propose few guidelines in the management when dealing with ameloblastoma eroding the cortical borders:

(1) MRI study should be done in large ameloblastomas to evaluate the infiltration of the tumour into the adjacent soft tissue planes.

(2) Intraoperative radiography should be done to rule out positive hard tissue margin.

(3) Compartmental resection of the tumour should be performed to involve all positive margins and on table frozen section of the soft tissue margins [46].

(4) Reconstruction should be performed as staged surgery in giant ameloblastomas after the complete histopathology report is available.

(5) Long-term follow-up with MRI and CT imaging should be conducted after the primary surgery to evaluate any form of recurrence.

5. Conclusion

Our experience with two case reports suggests high local aggressiveness of the solid type of ameloblastoma. Tumour-free soft tissue margin in three dimensions should be considered when treating large lesions with an erosion of cortical outline. Clinical and histological study in larger extent will provide added information in the management.

Consent

Informed consent is taken from the patients.

References

[1] P. V. Angadi, "Head and neck: odontogenic tumor: ameloblastoma," *Atlas of Genetics and Cytogenetics in Oncology and Haematology*, vol. 15, pp. 223–229, 2011.

[2] L. Barnes, J. W. Eveson, P. A. Reichart, and D. Sidransky, *World Health Organization Classification of Tumours. Pathology & Genetics. Head and Neck Tumours. World Health Organization*, International Agency for Research on Cancer (IACR) Press, Lyon, France, 2005.

[3] R. A. C. Almeida, E. S. S. Andrade, J. C. Barbalho, A. Vajgel, and B. C. E. Vasconcelos, "Recurrence rate following treatment for primary multicystic ameloblastoma: systematic review and meta-analysis," *International Journal of Oral and Maxillofacial Surgery*, vol. 45, no. 3, pp. 359–367, 2016.

[4] C. K. J. Richard and P. M. Speigh, "Current concepts of odontogenic tumours," *Diagnostic Histopathology*, vol. 15, no. 6, pp. 303–310, 2009.

[5] A. C. McClary, R. B. West, A. C. McClary et al., "Ameloblastoma: a clinical review and trends in management," *European Archives of Oto-Rhino-Laryngology*, vol. 273, no. 7, pp. 1649–1661.

[6] B. Ahlema, A. Wideda, L. Amanib, Z. Nadiaa, A. Amiraa, and F. Fatena, "Study of Ki67 and CD10 expression as predictive factors of recurrence of ameloblastoma," *European Annals of Otorhinolaryngology, Head and Neck diseases*, vol. 132, no. 5, pp. 275–279, 2015.

[7] F. Faras, F. A. Alhassan, Y. Israël, B. Hersant, and J. P. Meningaud, "Multi-recurrent invasive ameloblastoma: a surgical challenge," *International Journal of Surgery Case Reports*, vol. 30, pp. 43–45, 2017.

[8] R. Becelli, A. Carboni, G. Cerulli, M. Perugini, and G. Iannetti, "Mandibular ameloblastoma: analysis of surgical treatment carried out in 60 patients between 1977 and 1998," *Journal of Craniofacial Surgery*, vol. 13, no. 3, pp. 395–400, 2002.

[9] M. A. Pogrel and D. M. Montes, "Is there a role for enucleation in the management of ameloblastoma?," *International Journal of Oral and Maxillofacial Surgery*, vol. 38, no. 8, pp. 807–812, 2009.

[10] A. M. Eckardt, H. Kokemuller, P. Flemming, and A. Schultze, "Recurrent ameloblastoma following osseous reconstruction: a review of twenty years," *Journal of Cranio-Maxillofacial Surgery*, vol. 37, no. 1, pp. 36–41, 2009.

[11] E. R. Carlson and R. E. Marx, "The ameloblastoma:primary surgical curative management," *Journal of Oral and Maxillofacial Surgery*, vol. 64, no. 3, pp. 484–494, 2006.

[12] J. Hong, P. Y. Yun, I. H. Chung et al., "Long-term follow up on recurrence of 305 ameloblastoma cases," *International Journal of Oral and Maxillofacial Surgery*, vol. 36, no. 4, pp. 283–288, 2007.

[13] S. O. Basat, A. R. Oreroglu, C. Orman, T. Aksan, I. U. Uscetin, and M. Akan, "Recurrent ameloblastoma in the free fibula flap: review of literature and an unusual case report," *Journal of Maxillofacial and Oral Surgery Journal of Maxillofacial and Oral Surgery*, vol. 14, no. 3, pp. 821–825, 2015.

[14] M. K. Sehdev, A. G. Huvos, E. W. Strong, F. P. Gerold, and G. W. Willis, "Ameloblastoma of maxilla and mandible," *Cancer*, vol. 33, no. 2, pp. 324–333, 1974.

[15] H. Vayvada, F. Mola, A. Menderes, and M. Yilmaz, "Surgical management of ameloblastoma in the mandible, segmental mandibulectomy and immediate reconstruction with free fibula or deep circumflex iliac artery flap (evaluation of the long-term esthetic and functional results)," *Journal of Oral and Maxillofacial Surgery*, vol. 64, no. 10, pp. 1532–1539, 2006.

[16] S. Shatkin and F. S. Hoffmeister, "Ameloblastoma: a rational approach to therapy," *Oral Surgery, Oral Medicine, Oral Pathology*, vol. 20, no. 4, pp. 421–435, 1965.

[17] D. R. Mehlisch, D. C. Dahlin, and J. K. Masson, "Ameloblastoma: a clinicopathologic report," *Journal of Oral Surgery*, vol. 30, no. 1, pp. 9–22, 1972.

[18] H. Muller and P. J. Slootweg, "The ameloblastoma, the controversial approach to therapy," *Journal of Maxillofacial Surgery*, vol. 13, no. 2, pp. 79–84, 1985.

[19] A. A. Olaitan, D. S. Adeola, and E. O. Adekeye, "Ameloblastoma: clinical features and management of 315 cases from Kaduna, Nigeria," *Journal of Cranio-Maxillofacial Surgery*, vol. 21, no. 8, pp. 351–355, 1993.

[20] S. Ueno, K. Mushimoto, and R. Shirasu, "Prognostic evaluation of ameloblastoma based on histologic and radiographic typing," *Journal of Oral and Maxillofacial Surgery*, vol. 47, no. 1, pp. 11–15, 1989.

[21] N. Nakamura, Y. Higuchi, T. Mitsuyasu, F. Sandra, and M. Ohishi, "Comparison of long-term results between different approaches to ameloblastoma," *Oral Surgery, Oral Medicine, Oral Pathology, Oral Radiology, and Endodontology*, vol. 93, no. 1, pp. 13–20, 2002.

[22] M. L. Grafft, H. J. Sazima, F. P. Parker, and I. Rappaport, "Ameloblastoma recurring in previously placed iliac crest autograft: report of case," *Journal of Oral Surgery*, vol. 28, pp. 285–291, 1970.

[23] X.-C. Jian, D.-Y. Liu, R. Zhu et al., "Recurrences of ameloblastoma in bone grafts: report of two cases and literature review," *Oral Health and Dental Management*, vol. 14, no. 5, 2015.

[24] F. S. Carvalho, G. A. Valadad, and C. E. Cespedes, "Ameloblastoma (recurrence after 21 months)," *Revista da Associação Médica Minas Gerais*, vol. 27, pp. 28–30, 1976.

[25] E. A. Dolan, J. C. Angelillo, and N. G. Georgiade, "Recurrent ameloblastoma in autogenous rib graft: report of case," *Oral Surgery, Oral Medicine, Oral Pathology, Oral Radiology and Endodontology*, vol. 51, no. 4, pp. 357–360, 1981.

[26] M. Marinelli, D. Badia, P. Vallogini et al., "Ameloblastoma recidivo in trapianto autogeno di cresta iliaca," in *Maxillofacial Surgery*, G. Giardino, Ed., pp. 94–96, Monduzzi Editore, Bologna, Italy, 1982.

[27] G. Stea, "Recurrence of an ameloblastoma in an autogenous iliac bone graft," *Journal of Oral and Maxillofacial Surgery*, vol. 43, no. 5, pp. 374–377, 1985.

[28] N. Zacharides, "Recurrences of ameloblastoma in bone grafts," *International Journal of Oral and Maxillofacial Surgery*, vol. 17, pp. 316–318, 1988.

[29] N. T. Vasan, "Recurrent ameloblastoma in an autogenous bone graft after 28 years: a case report," *The New Zealand Dental Journal*, vol. 91, pp. 12-13, 1995.

[30] S. D. Bianchi, F. Tarello, F. Polastri, and G. Valente, "Ameloblastoma of the mandible involving an autogenous bone graft," *Journal of Oral and Maxillofacial Surgery*, vol. 56, pp. 1187–1191, 1998.

[31] W. Martins and D. M. Favaro, "Recurrence of an ameloblastoma in an autogenous iliac bone graft," *Oral Surgery, Oral Medicine, Oral Pathology, Oral Radiology, and Endodontology*, vol. 98, no. 6, pp. 657–659, 2004.

[32] T. Su, B. Liu, X. M. Chen, M. Hisatomi, H. Konouchi, and K. Kishi, "Recurrence of ameloblastoma involving iliac bone graft after 16 years," *Oral Oncology Extra*, vol. 42, pp. 150–152, 2006.

[33] Y. S. Choi, J. Asaumi, Y. Yanagi et al., "A case of recurrent ameloblastoma developing in an autogenous iliac bone graft 20 years," vol. 35, no. 1, pp. 43–46, 2006.

[34] S. P. Xavier, A. C. Faria, F. V. de Mello Filho, E. R. Silva, and T. de Santana Santos, "Recurrence of ameloblastoma in soft tissue," *Journal of Craniofacial Surgery*, vol. 24, no. 5, pp. 1866-1867, 2013.

[35] R. Rauso, G. Tartaro, G. Gherardini, F. Puglia, M. Santagata, and G. Colella, "Recurrence of ameloblastoma in temporal area: primary treatment influences recurrence rate," *Journal of Craniofacial Surgery*, vol. 21, no. 3, pp. 887–891, 2010.

[36] W. H. Hollinshead, "Anatomy for surgeons," in *The Head and Neck*, vol. 1, pp. 335-336, Harper and Row, Philadelphia, PA, USA, 3rd edition, 1982.

[37] R. Tiwari, J. Quak, S. Egeler et al., "Tumors of the infratemporal fossa," *Skull Base Surgery*, vol. 10, no. 1, 2000.

[38] S. J. Collings and A. Harrison, "Recurrent ameloblastoma?: an historic case report and a review of the literature," *British Dental Journal*, vol. 174, no. 6, pp. 202–206, 1993.

[39] J. R. Hayward, "Recurrent ameloblastoma after 30 years after surgical treatment," *Journal of Oral Surgery*, vol. 31, pp. 368–370, 1973.

[40] D. G. Gardner, "A pathologist's approach to the treatment of ameloblastoma," *Journal of Oral and Maxillofacial Surgery*, vol. 42, no. 3, pp. 161–166, 1984.

[41] A. Labordea, R. Nicota, T. Wojcikc, J. Ferri, and G. Raoul, "Ameloblastoma of the jaws: management and recurrence rate," *European Annals of Otorhinolaryngology, Head and Neck diseases*, vol. 134, no. 1, pp. 7–11, 2017.

[42] A. Chaine, P. Pitak-Arnnop, K. Dhanuthai, B. Ruhin-Poncet, J. C. Bertrand, and C. Bertolus, "A treatment algorithm for managing giant mandibular ameloblastoma: 5-yearexperiences in a Paris university hospital," *European Journal of Surgical Oncology (EJSO)*, vol. 35, no. 9, pp. 999–1005, 2009.

[43] S. S. Vaishampayan, D. Nair, A. Patil, and P. Chaturvedi, "Recurrent ameloblastoma in temporal fossa: a diagnostic dilemma," *Contemporary Clinical Dentistry*, vol. 4, no. 2, pp. 220–222, 2013.

[44] Z. S. Peacock, Y. D. Ji, and W. C. Faquin, "What is important for confirming negative margins when resecting mandibular ameloblastomas?," *Journal of Oral and Maxillofacial Surgery*, vol. 75, no. 6, pp. 1185–1190, 2017.

[45] J.-Y. Liua, Q.-W. Mana, Y.-Q. Maa, and B. Liu, "I125 brachytherapy guided by individual three-dimensionalprinted plates for recurrent ameloblastoma of the skull base," *British Journal of Oral and Maxillofacial Surgery*, vol. 55, no. 7, pp. e38–e40, 2017.

[46] A. Kudva, A. T. Kamath, N. N. Rao, and J. Rajan, "Rare case of giant unicystic ameloblastoma: luminal variant," *Cranio*, vol. 36, no. 1, pp. 1–4, 2017.

28

The Use of a Hybrid Pillar and Its Importance for Aesthetic Rehabilitation and Tissue Stability: A Clinical Report

Guilherme da Gama Ramos ⓘ,[1] Danilo Lazzari Ciotti,[1] Samuel Rehder Wimmers Ferreira,[2] Maide Rehder Wimmers Ferreira Margarido,[2] Raquel Adriano Dantas,[1] and Marina Nottingham Guerreiro[1]

[1]São Leopoldo Mandic Institute and Research Center, R. José Rocha Junqueira 13, 13045-755 Campinas, SP, Brazil
[2]Paulista Association of Dental Surgeons, Rua José Nardon 177, 13419-000 Piracicaba, SP, Brazil

Correspondence should be addressed to Guilherme da Gama Ramos; gdagama@yahoo.com

Academic Editor: Mine Dündar

In the past, aesthetics had a secondary role in implant rehabilitation. Nowadays, the search for a perfect and harmonious aesthetic has stimulated the development of new materials and techniques. Due to this aesthetic requirement, the hybrid abutment (titanium link + zirconia) emerged as an alternative to metallic pillars. The hybrid abutment made a more favorable aesthetic possible, provided reliable mechanical properties, and increased biocompatibility to the surrounding tissues. Additionally, the individual zirconia abutment improves the emergency profile and the final white aesthetics. The objective of this paper is to report a clinical case with a manufactured individualized hybrid abutment for a metal-free indirect restoration, showing the applicability, mechanical properties, and biocompatibility of the hybrid abutment.

1. Introduction

Aesthetic demands led us to new concepts and prosthetic resources in dentistry. We now use new materials with optical, mechanical, and biological properties [1]. Zirconia abutment fabrication and metal-free-implant-supported prostheses favor a better aesthetic situation than the metal counterpart [2]. These methods allow translucency in dental restoration, provide gingival tissue shade reduction, and result in a very natural and healthy appearance [3].

Zirconia abutments not only allow light transmission in the same manner as natural teeth [2, 4, 5] but also present reliable mechanical properties and soft tissue biocompatibility.

The aesthetic success of implant-supported prostheses is strongly related to the surrounding soft tissue appearance. Unlike metal abutments, which cause an unpleasant appearance in a fine gingival biotype [6], the use of zirconia abutment allows light scattering and customization for each individual case. This creates an emergence profile that provides color, shape, and gingival symmetry similar to natural teeth [4, 5].

As observed in several studies, zirconia has shown satisfactory results in aesthetic of prosthetic crowns as well as in adjacent gingival tissues [2, 7–11]. Due to the increase of the use of aesthetic abutments and restorations, new technologies have appeared, such as CAD/CAM systems [12, 13].

The CAD/CAM system consists of a planning and production computerized system for crowns, facets, inlays, onlays, crown copings, implant abutments, and even zirconia structures for fixed and removable partial prostheses. Through this system, pieces are fabricated with quality, high accuracy, minimal human intervention, error reduction during production, and lowered manufacturing costs [13, 14].

The objective of this paper was to show the importance of aesthetic customized prosthetic abutment and its indications and advantages and disadvantages, along with a clinical case presentation.

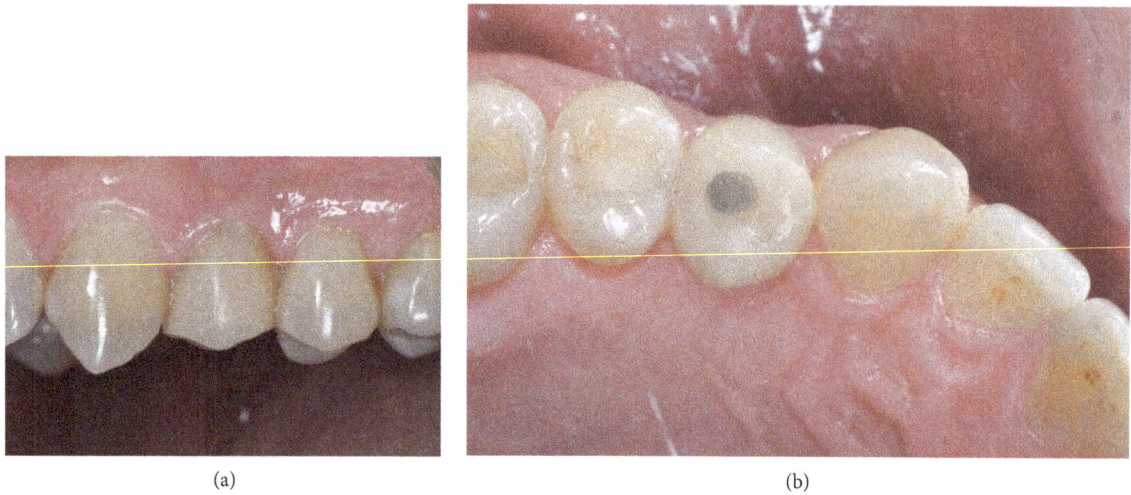

(a)   (b)

FIGURE 1: Provisional restauration properly prepared and screwed on the implant.

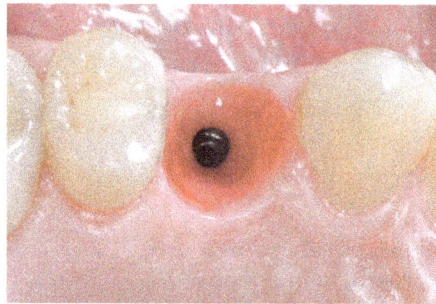

FIGURE 2: Gingival contour and emergence profile obtained by the provisional restauration.

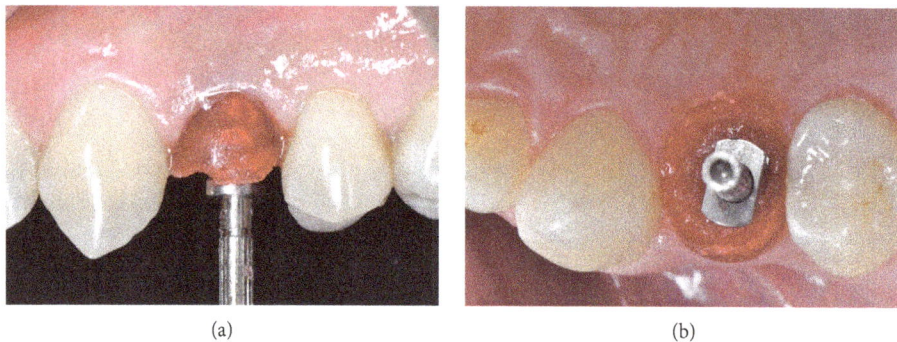

(a)   (b)

FIGURE 3: Molding with customized transfer in position, made with Pattern Resin.

2. Case Presentation

A 46-year-old male patient with absence of element 24 presents with a need for aesthetic rehabilitation. The patient had tooth extraction indicated due to root fracture. After Anthogyr PX 4.0 × 8 mm implant installation, a provisional restauration for gingival tissue maintenance was made, in respect of the ideal critical and subcritical contour, providing a more predictable and stable gingival emergence profile.

During the osseointegration period (120 days), the temporary customized crown did not have any occlusal contact. After this period, the acrylic temporary crown, previously prepared, was adjusted. For a better gingival tissue conditioning, we proceeded with temporary crown reassembly. Figures 1(a) and 1(b) display the temporary component properly prepared and screwed on the implant.

Figure 2 shows an excellent emergence profile and the quality of the soft tissue obtained by the provisional component that was made in respect of the gingival biotype, and a

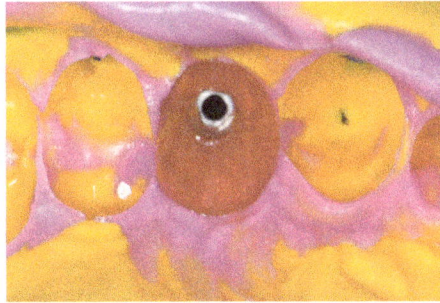

FIGURE 4: Transfer mold.

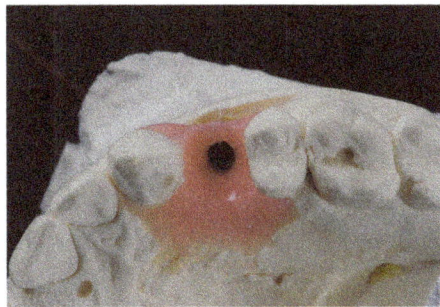

FIGURE 5: Working cast.

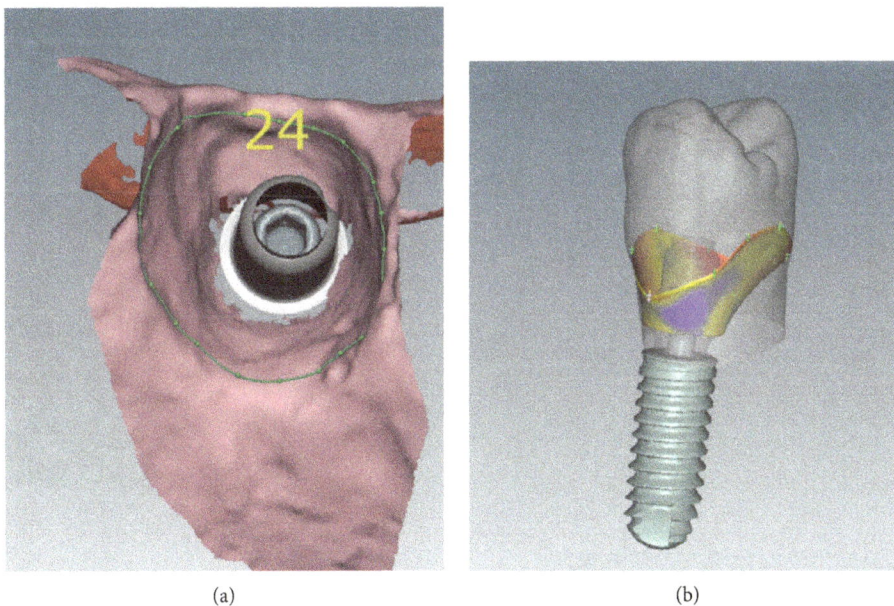

(a)   (b)

FIGURE 6: Gingival margin delimitation and abutment customization.

concave critical and subcritical transmucosal emergence profile ensured the soft tissue quality [15#x2013;17].

For the preparation of the working cast, customized transfer was used (Figures 3(a) and 3(b)) and molding was done with polyvinyl siloxane (Figure 4).

Even though the working cast reproduces the clinical situation faithfully (Figure 5), we proceeded with the rehabilitation using the CAD/CAM technology-customized zirconia (hybrid) for link abutment (FLEXIBASE®, Anthogyr) which offers advantages over prefabricated ones.

Figure 6(a) enables us to observe that through this technology, the gingival margin is delimitated in order to make the abutment emerge throughout the soft tissue as similar as a natural clinical crown (Figure 6(b)).

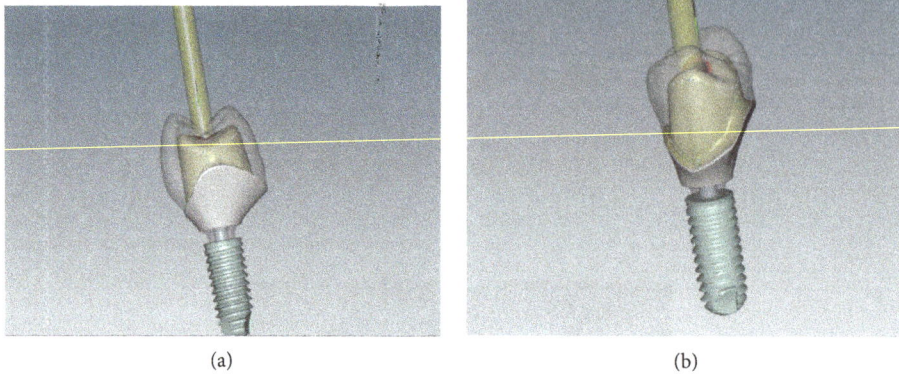

(a)

(b)

FIGURE 7: Divergent angle of implant trajectory and agglutination correction.

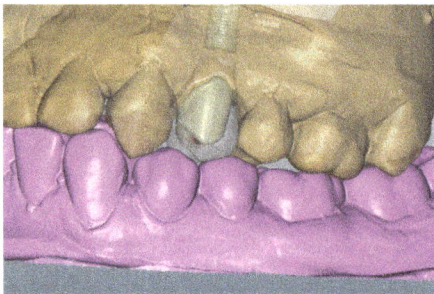

FIGURE 8: Adjustment of the proportion abutment/crown for ideal retention.

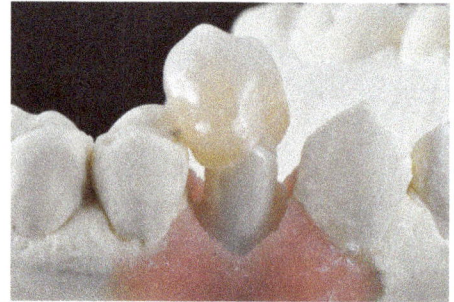

FIGURE 11: Zirconia of the hybrid abutment and E-max crown.

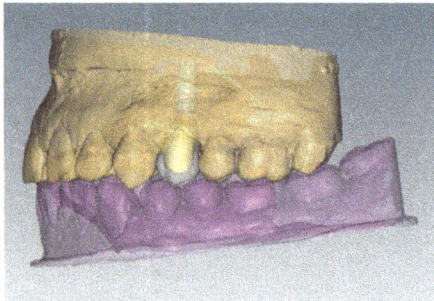

FIGURE 9: Interproximal adjustment and occlusal check.

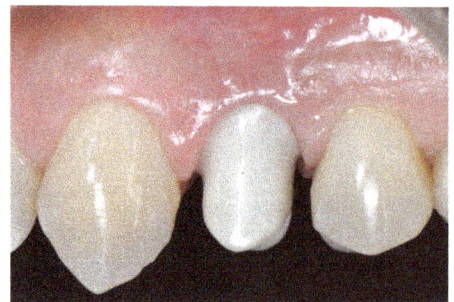

FIGURE 12: Abutment in position, manufactured in CAD/CAM technology.

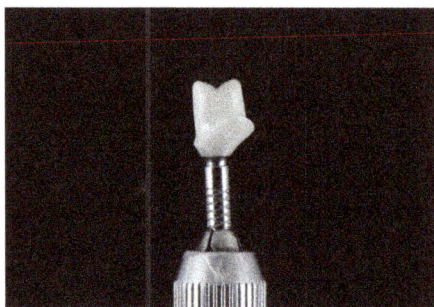

FIGURE 10: Zirconia of the hybrid abutment.

The zirconia project enables angular corrections in the trajectory position, in order to avoid or minimize differences between implant and crown position (Figures 7(a) and 7(b)).

Once the crown is designed, the outer part of the abutment is adjusted to create support and to provide retention which is achieved by planning an ideal proportion between the hybrid abutment and restorative crown, interocclusal space, and cementation line appropriated to the final restoration (Figures 8 and 9).

An E-max (ips-E-max, ivoclaire) pure crown final restoration was manufactured (Figures 10 and 11).

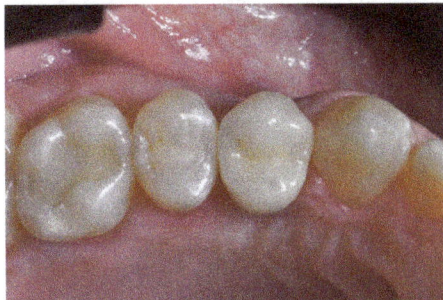

FIGURE 13: Cemented crown.

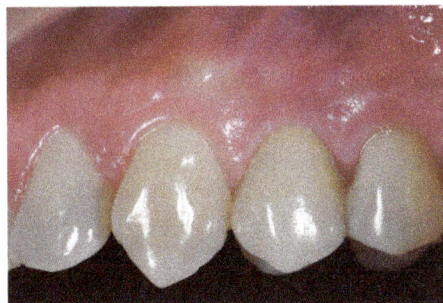

FIGURE 14: Crown as noticed by the color, shape, texture, and contour of the gingival tissue.

To cement the zirconia abutment in the link abutment, the flex base, the bonding surfaces of the titanium, and the zirconia ceramic were air-abraded with 50 mm aluminum oxide particles at 2.0 bars of pressure (0.25 MPa) for 20 seconds at a distance of 10 mm, after which they were cleaned in alcohol and then cemented using a resin luting (Relyx U200, 3M ESPE®) [18]. Excess resin was removed from the bonding margins before it became fully set and was light-cured per the manufacturer's recommendations.

The hybrid abutment was placed (Figure 12) with 25 N definitive torque, and the crown was cemented using a resin luting (Relyx U200, 3M ESPE).

The clinical results (Figures 13 and 14), one month after prosthesis installation, prove the component adaptation placement and the quality in the contour of the gingival tissues. The successful aesthetic can be noticed by the smile harmony, color, texture, and natural brightness in comparison to the adjacent teeth.

3. Discussion

Dental implant treatment for dental element replacement considering the maintenance of gingival architecture and restoration has occurred for some years. However, by pursuing better aesthetics, hybrid abutments have surpassed metal abutments and provide a more natural appearance to the ceramic restorations.

CAD/CAM systems enabled the fabrication of the customized zirconia for link abutments that are individualized for both the anterior region and posterior teeth. Nowadays, through the CAD/CAM technology, hybrid abutment can

be designed and manufactured ensuring mechanical characteristics of the materials [13, 19, 20].

CAD/CAM systems present several advantages, such as fast production, biocompatibility, aesthetics, and mechanical resistance with low fracture rate (because the blocks are industrially produced and have high homogeneity, without the need for refractory casts) [21, 22]. Furthermore, they enable excellent adaptation between margin restoration and soft tissues [23, 24].

There are several studies comparing metal and hybrid abutment characteristics [25]. Taking aesthetics into consideration, it was observed that hybrid abutments did not give grayish appearance to the gingival margin as noticed when metal abutments were used. This is a great advantage, especially to patients who have a high smile line and fine gingival genotype [3].

Studies have shown that the zirconia oxide presents mechanical resistance similar to titanium. This property combined with new automated techniques (CAD/CAM) made the use of hybrid abutment possible in rehabilitation both in the anterior region and in regions with higher masticatory load [13, 21, 24–28].

Material biocompatibility is very important for the longevity of implant-supported restorations. A great deal of studies observed that zirconia has presented low bacterial adherence, and hybrid abutments accumulate bacteria with lower pathogenic potential in relation to titanium abutments [6, 7].

Single hybrid abutments have aesthetics, mechanical resistance, and biocompatibility which enable metal components to be replaced in implanted supported prostheses. However, each case should be evaluated carefully as these components were recently introduced to the market and there are no long-term studies on their clinical use.

References

[1] R. Faria and M. A. Bottino, "Zircônia monolítica de alta translucidez na reabilitação sobre implantes," *PróteseNews*, vol. 3, no. 1, pp. 36–50, 2016.

[2] S. A. Gehrke, P. C. V. Dos Santos, N. T. A. Carvalho, R. M. De Mello, and M. J. Carbonari, "Abutment cerâmico para prótese individual metalfree sobre implante: parafusada ou cimentada - demonstração laboratorial e clínica," *Full Dentistry in Science*, vol. 1, no. 3, pp. 248–253, 2010.

[3] P. L. B. Tan and J. T. Dunne Jr., "An esthetic comparison of a metal ceramic crown and cast metal abutment with an all-ceramic crown and zirconia abutment: a clinical report," *The Journal of Prosthetic Dentistry*, vol. 91, no. 3, pp. 215–218, 2004.

[4] M. Anderson, M. E. Razzoog, A. Odén, E. A. Hegenbarth, and B. R. Lang, "Procera: a new way to achieve an all-ceramic crown," *Quintessence International*, vol. 29, no. 5, pp. 285–296, 1998.

[5] P. Odman and B. Andersson, "Procera AllCeram crowns followed for 5 to 10.5 years: a prospective clinical study," *The International Journal of Prosthodontics*, vol. 14, no. 6, pp. 504–509, 2001.

[6] V. M. Barros, B. F. de Oliveira, S. G. de Oliveira, and P. I. Seraidarian, "Intermediário de zircônia," *PróteseNews*, vol. 1, no. 1, pp. 52–64, 2014.

[7] L. Rimondini, L. Cerroni, A. Carrassi, and P. Torricelli, "Bacterial colonization of zirconia ceramic surfaces: an in vitro and in vivo study," *The International Journal of Oral & Maxillofacial Implants*, vol. 17, no. 6, pp. 793–798, 2002.

[8] A. Scarano, M. Piattelli, S. Caputi, G. A. Favero, and A. Piattelli, "Bacterial adhesion on commercially pure titanium and zirconium oxide disks: an in vivo human study," *Journal of Periodontology*, vol. 75, no. 2, pp. 292–296, 2004.

[9] R. Scotti, K. Zanini Kantorski, N. Scotti, C. Monaco, L. F. Valandro, and M. A. Bottino, "Early biofilm colonization on polished- and glazed-zirconium ceramic surface. Preliminary results," *Minerva Stomatologica*, vol. 55, no. 9, pp. 493–502, 2006.

[10] R. Scotti, K. Z. Kantorski, C. Monaco, L. F. Valandro, L. Ciocca, and M. A. Bottino, "SEM evaluation of in situ early bacterial colonization on a Y-TZP ceramic: a pilot study," *The International Journal of Prosthodontics*, vol. 20, no. 4, pp. 419–422, 2007.

[11] A. M. M. Mesquita, R. O. A. Souza, and E. Miyashita, "Restaurações cerâmicas metal free," in *Atualização em clínica Odontológica - Clínica do Dia-a-Dia*, pp. 679–719, Artes Médicas, São Paulo, Brazil, 2008.

[12] A. M. M. Mesquita, E. Miyashita, R. O. de Assunção e Souza, R. de Vasconcellos Moura, S. Watinaga, and J. A. Shibli, "A tecnologia CAD/CAM e a zircônia a serviço da prótese sobre implante," *PróteseNews*, vol. 2, no. 3, pp. 51–70, 2015.

[13] F. P. Pastor, F. Kfouri, and T. de Mello Rezende, "Confecção de pilares metal free com o uso do sistema CAD/CAM," *PróteseNews*, vol. 3, no. 2, pp. 174–183, 2016.

[14] R. Van Noort, "The future of dental devices is digital," *Dental Materials*, vol. 28, no. 1, pp. 3–12, 2012.

[15] H. Su, O. Gonzalez-Martin, A. Weisgold, and E. Lee, "Considerations of implant abutment and crown contour: critical contour and subcritical contour," *The International Journal of Periodontics & Restorative Dentistry*, vol. 30, p. 335, 2010.

[16] E. Rompen, N. Raepsaet, O. Domken, B. Touati, and E. van Dooren, "Soft tissue stability at the facial aspect of gingivally converging abutments in the esthetic zone: a pilot clinical study," *The Journal of Prosthetic Dentistry*, vol. 97, no. 6, pp. S119–S125, 2007.

[17] M. Katafuchi, B. F. Weinstein, B. G. Leroux, Y. W. Chen, and D. M. Daubert, "Restoration contour is a risk indicator for peri-implantitis: a cross-sectional radiographic analysis," *Journal of Clinical Periodontology*, vol. 45, no. 2, pp. 225–232, 2018.

[18] P. Gehrke, J. Alius, C. Fischer, K. J. Erdelt, and F. Beuer, "Retentive strength of two-piece CAD/CAM zirconia implant abutments," *Clinical Implant Dentistry and Related Research*, vol. 16, no. 6, pp. 920–925, 2014.

[19] I. Sailer, T. Sailer, B. Starwarczyk, R. E. Jung, and C. H. Hämmerle, "In vitro study of the influence of the type of connection on the fracture load of zirconia abutments with internal and external implant-abutment connections," *The International Journal of Oral & Maxillofacial Implants*, vol. 5, pp. 850–858, 2009.

[20] P. Magne, M. P. Paranhos, L. H. Burnett Jr., M. Magne, and U. C. Belser, "Fatigue resistance and failure mode of novel-design anterior single-tooth implant restorations: influence of material selection for type III veneers bonded to zirconia abutments," *Clinical Oral Implants Research*, vol. 22, no. 2, pp. 195–200, 2011.

[21] M. Morim, "CEREC: the power of technology," *Compendium of Continuing Education in Dentistry*, vol. 22, no. 6, pp. 27–29, 2001.

[22] A. Kurbad and K. Reichel, "Multicolored ceramic blocks as an esthetic solution for anterior restorations," *International Journal of Computerized Dentistry*, vol. 9, no. 1, pp. 69–82, 2006.

[23] P. F. Manicone, P. Rossi Iommetti, and L. Raffaelli, "An overview of zirconia ceramics: basic properties and clinical applications," *Journal of Dentistry*, vol. 35, no. 11, pp. 819–826, 2007.

[24] M. Yildrim, D. Edelhoff, O. Hanisch, and H. Spiekermann, "Ceramic abutments—a new era in achieving optimal esthetics in implant dentistry," *The International Journal of Periodontics & Restorative Dentistry*, vol. 20, no. 1, pp. 81–91, 2000.

[25] M. A. Bottino, R. Faria, and J. C. Dinato, "Pilares ceramicos em implantodontia: o estado da arte," in *Odontologia Estetica - O Estado da Arte*, E. Miyashita and A. S. Fonseca, Eds., vol. 1, pp. 591–633, Artes Medicas, Sao Paulo, Brazil, 2004.

[26] R. F. Sallenave, C. B. Vicari, and M. Borba, "Pilares cerâmicos na implantodontia: revisão de literatura," *Cerâmica*, vol. 62, no. 363, pp. 305–308, 2016.

[27] F. Butz, G. Heydecke, M. Okutan, and J. R. Strub, "Survival rate, fracture strength and failure mode of ceramic implant abutments after chewing simulation," *Journal of Oral Rehabilitation*, vol. 32, no. 11, pp. 838–843, 2005.

[28] M. A. Bottino, L. F. Valandro, R. Scotti, and L. Buso, "Effect of surface treatments on the resin bond to zirconium-based ceramic," *The International Journal of Prosthodontics*, vol. 18, no. 1, pp. 60–65, 2005.

29

Dislodged Bonded Molar Tube into Wound during Orthognathic Surgery

Tengku Aszraf Tengku Shaeran[1] and A. R. Samsudin ⓘ[1,2]

[1]Oral and Maxillofacial Surgery Unit, School of Dental Sciences, University of Science Malaysia (USM), 16150 Kubang Kerian, Kelantan, Malaysia
[2]Sharjah Institute for Medical Research (SIMR), University of Sharjah, Sharjah, UAE

Correspondence should be addressed to A. R. Samsudin; drabrani@sharjah.ac.ae

Academic Editor: Carla Evans

Introduction. Dislodgement of orthodontic appliance into operation wounds may occur while performing orthognathic surgery. Its occurrence is commonly associated with bonded upper molar tube. *Case Report.* A 25-year-old gentleman presented with recurrent upper right vestibular abscess three months following a bimaxillary orthognathic surgery. A bonded molar orthodontic tube had dislodged into the wound during the operation. The clinical presentation initially mimics an odontogenic infection until our investigations revealed that it originated from the dislodged appliance. The abscess was drained, the wound site was explored, and the molar tube and neighbouring rigid fixation plates and screws were removed. The patient recovered well following the procedure. *Conclusion.* Dislodged metal orthodontic appliance in oral wound acts as a foreign body that may exert allergic reactions, infection, or inflammation. Pre- and postoperative intraoral examination of fixed orthodontic appliances including its count should be recorded in orthognathic surgery protocol.

1. Introduction

Patients requiring orthognathic surgery for correction of their maxillo-mandibular disharmony will also have to undergo orthodontic treatment during both pre- and post-surgical treatment phases. Tooth alignment and preparation of the future predicted occlusion are required, so that the osteotomized jaws can be easily repositioned in the surgery in order to achieve stable results. This is followed by a period of fine-tuning and maintenance of the occlusion afterwards.

Among orthodontists, the use of bonded orthodontic molar tubes has gained popularity compared to the conventional molar banding because the former are easier to place, without the need for orthodontic separator, more friendly to the periodontium, and more comfortable to the patient [1].

Banks and Mcfarlane [2] revealed that failure rates and displacement of bonded molar and banded molar are in the range of 33.7% and 18.8%, respectively. This might contribute to the higher percentage of dislodged bonded appliance in orthognathic surgery as highlighted by Godoy et al. [3]. According to them, 76.3% of dislodged orthodontic appliance associated with orthognathic are related to involve the maxillary molars, and they were the bonded rather than banded-type appliance [2].

2. Case Report

A 25-year-old gentleman presented to our clinic with a complaint of recurrent pain and swelling on his right cheek of three-month duration. He visited a general practitioner each time, and the condition was resolved with analgesic and antibiotics. However, his symptoms got worse and he attended our Oral Surgery Clinic for consultation.

The patient is a fit and healthy young man with no relevant medical history and no known history of allergy. Past surgical history revealed that he had underwent bimaxillary orthognathic surgery one and half year earlier in a local hospital. Although the postoperative period was uneventful, the surgical team informed him that there was a dislodged orthodontic appliance in his right cheek that must have occurred during the operation. The team explained to the patient that this accident was realized later on the next day after the surgery when the molar tube from the right maxillary second molar was found missing, and its presence was confirmed high up in the right maxillary-zygomatic buttress area shown in the postoperative X-ray image taken on the next day following the surgery. A series of further postoperative radiographs confirmed its location, lying outside the right maxillary antrum. Due to the pronounced postoperative facial oedema at that time, no attempt was made to remove the appliance. The absence of sign and symptoms during further follow-up sessions confirmed the decision to leave it in-situ with continuous clinical observation.

On examination, there was no extraoral swelling noted. The mandible and maxilla seemed firm indicating good healing following previous mandibular saggital split and maxillary Le Fort I osteotomy sites and a stable class I dental occlusion. Intraorally, there was a sinus with slight pus discharge on the upper right buccal sulcus region adjacent to the upper right first premolar. All teeth in that quadrant were firm and vital. Tenderness was elicited upon palpation on the upper right vestibular region. We suspected the sinus track may originate from the dislodged appliance embedded in the cheek soft tissue. A periapical view was then taken with gutta-percha inserted into the sinus for foreign body localization purpose. The radiograph revealed the gutta-percha pointed towards the site of titanium plate and screws placed used for rigid fixation, and with the molar orthodontic tube appliance in its vicinity (Figure 1). A cone beam CT was performed to provide a 3D detailed location of the appliance (Figures 2(a) and 2(b)) and confirmed it to be located outside the maxillary antrum.

The presence of the molar orthodontic tube foreign body reaction was suspected as the most probable cause of the recurrent right cheek pain and swelling associated with an intraoral discharging sinus. Exploration of the site was performed through the sulcular incision under general anesthesia. The dislodged molar tube was identified lying on the zygomatic bone just beneath the raised flap. It was removed by dividing some surrounding fibrous tissue strands. Just below it, one titanium straight bone plate with four screws used for fixing the previous Le Fort I osteotomy site was inspected and found to be rigidly embedded in normal bone. However, a decision was made to remove them based on the fact that they are present in an infected area. (Figure 3). The Le Fort I osteotomy site showed good healing with new bone formation. Patient had an uneventful recovery thereafter, and the orthognathic surgical team who attended him previously was informed of his progress.

3. Discussion

The incidence of dislodged orthodontic appliance during orthognathic surgery is rare but been recognized as one of its surgical complications. Failed orthodonthic appliances frequently occur in double jaw surgery, as in our patient who had Le Fort I and bilateral sagittal split osteotomy. It has become an accepted practice to place the wire using the

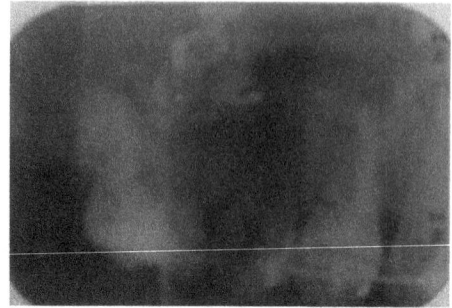

FIGURE 1: Periapical radiograph with gutta-percha (GP) in situ which had been inserted through the sinus. The GP pointing towards the area of plate and screws with the dislodged molar tube in its vicinity.

cleats and hooks of molar tube or band both intraoperative and postoperatively. Intraoral manipulations during placing and removing intermaxillary fixation wire with the interim splint contribute to the appliance failure during surgery [3]. Molar tubes or orthodontic brackets are indeed a very small appliance. Hence, its displacement during orthognathic surgery may or may not be identified intraoperatively [4].

Surgeons may have different opinion with regard to the management of a dislodged orthodontic appliance. When the event occurred and notified intraoperatively, a thorough search for the foreign body till it is found is the norm, due to the fact that the dislodged orthodontic appliance is "nonsterile" and the risk of metallic ion leach deep in the tissue. However, when the foreign body is identified postsurgically, commonly during the subsequent postoperative days following routine postoperative check X-rays, there is less urge by the surgical team to search for it due to the presence of postoperative oedema, the risk of further compromising patient's airway resulting from soft tissue dissections in the exploration site, and the already drop in postoperative hemoglobin concentration, thus increasing further morbidity. The surgeon in this case had opted to leave the molar band in situ with continuous observation to minimize those morbidities since experience has taught that searching for a 4 mm size foreign body in inflamed, oedematous, and blood oozing soft tissue may take several hours!

Lammers [5] in his surgical review claimed that removal of foreign body embedded in soft tissue can be difficult and time-consuming, and the potential damage to tissues caused by the procedure must be weighed against the risk posed by a particular foreign body. He further emphasized that not all foreign bodies are discovered during the initial patient encounter [5]. Yildirim et al. investigated the diagnosis and management of retained surgical foreign bodies and recommended removal of the foreign body when identified in a symptomatic patient. However, for asymptomatic and selected cases, he supported follow-up of the patient as the treatment of choice, particularly if exploring and removing the foreign body will bring more harm to the patient [6, 7].

Despite that, the actual location of the foreign body in the face or neck also determine whether to advocate an urgent exploration or a wait and see policy. Metallic foreign bodies that have impacted into the maxillary sinus or in close

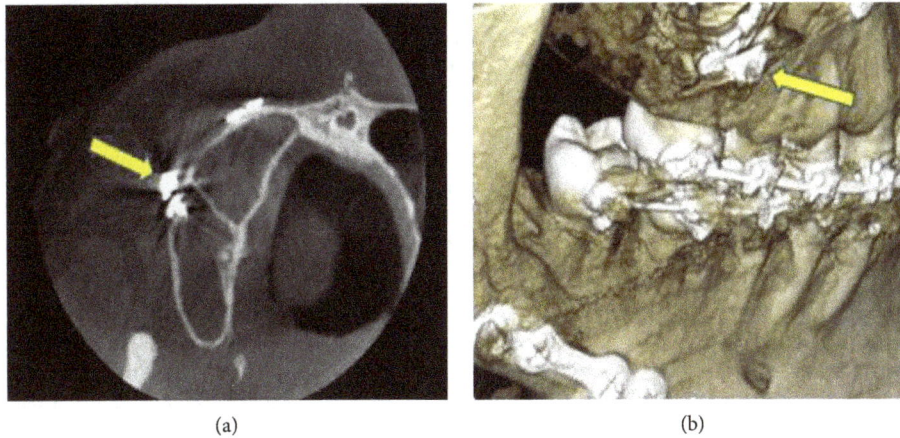

(a)

(b)

FIGURE 2: Cone Beam CT images showing the dislodged molar tube lying outside the right maxillary antrum, as indicated by the arrow in axial view (a), while its position in relation to the rigid plate and screws on the zygomatic buttress can be seen clearly in 3-D image (b).

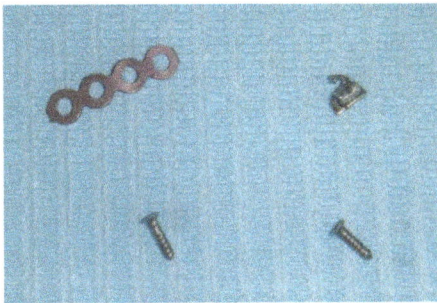

FIGURE 3: Titanium plate and screws and the stainless steel molar tube removed in the surgery.

proximity to major vessels or nerves or lying under the pharyngeal wall mucosa must be explored and removed in view of grave consequences. Such complications may end up with chronic maxillary sinusitis, risk of erosion and rupture of major arteries, nerve pain, and neck abscess. In the present case, the location of the molar tube high up at the zygomatic buttress, external to the maxillary sinus, seems to be less likely to cause life-threatening consequences, and it may preferably be left in situ. Reports by Teltzrow et al. and Wenger et al. supported this opinion. They found that displaced orthodontic brackets which were left in situ for longer periods had been without adverse sequelae [8, 9]. Others have reported dislodged brackets embedded into body tissues and were accidentally found later in the osseous tissue, which was theorized to be once an extraction socket [10] and in rare sites such as in the upper lip [11]. In the latter case, it was embedded following a dental trauma and remained silent for 10 years before the symptoms appeared.

On the other hand, de Queiroz et al. reported acute symptoms following loss of a bonded molar tube during orthognathic surgery [12]. The bonded maxillary second molar tube was found displaced to the inferior border of mandible in the postoperative period and a submandibular abscess developed afterwards. They advocated that the use of bonded molar tubes should be avoided in patients

undergoing orthognathic surgery, as the sequelae of dislodged appliance can result in grave consequences.

Most orthodontic metal appliances such as brackets and tubes are generally made of stainless steel. They contain a mixture of iron, chromium, nickel, and a small amount of molybdenum together with small traces of other metals [13]. Despite having molybdenum in its alloy, the molar tube may still undergo corrosion and induce an inflammatory response or foreign body reaction. This is evidenced in this case by the need to divide the fibrous tissue surrounding the tube during its removal.

Preexploration localization X-ray of the molar tube demonstrated that it is positioned close to the titanium bone plates and screws which were used for rigid fixation of the Le Fort I osteotomy site. This interesting situation recalled the manufacturer's advice on cautions against mixed metals in vivo [14]. Both the titanium implants and the molar tubes, each with its own corrosion potential, can react together and produce currents, if they are in contact together in an electrochemically conductive fluid such as body fluid. In turn, this can lead to accelerated corrosion of both metals, leaching metal ions into the surrounding area, and stimulate an inflammatory or hypersensitivity response, thus producing symptoms of recurrent pain and swelling at the operated site. Macro movements of the jaw and micromotion of titanium implants and dislodged molar tube may accelerate the corrosion process. This process may have been delayed in this case due to the routine intermaxillary fixation done for six weeks following the orthognathic operation with the aim of achieving adequate bony healing at the osteotomy site to achieve a stable occlusion. The patient continued on soft diet feeding for one month following release of the intermaxillary fixation which further explains the delay in producing the symptoms of inflammation and hypersensitivity secondary to the foreign body.

4. Conclusion

Intraoperative surgical manipulations carry the risk of dislodging fixed orthodontic appliances during orthognathic

TABLE 1: Safety measures to reduce risk of appliance failure and complications.

1	Thorough examination of orthodontic appliance in patient's mouth prior to surgery and before closure of the surgical wound (appliance count and its integrity)
2	Use of molar band rather than molar tube for orthodontic treatment of patients undergoing orthognathic surgery
3	Being vigilant and cautious handling of intermaxillary fixation intraoperatively
4	Good communication with orthodontist to help prepare the patient for the scheduled surgery

surgery, in particular the bonded molar tube. An immediate search for the loss metal foreign body is recommended. However, when the loss is discovered postoperatively, it may be retained in situ in the wound but the length of symptom-free period can never be ascertained. It is prudent for the surgeon to perform a thorough preoperative intraoral examination on the integrity of orthodontic appliances and its count in the patient's mouth at the beginning and at the end of the surgical operation. This mandatory practice should be part of the orthognathic surgery protocol (Table 1).

Consent

In this case report, the patient is sufficiently anonymized according to ICMJE guidelines.

References

[1] D. T. Millett, A. Hallgren, A. C. Fornell, and M. Robertson, "Bonded molar tubes: a retrospective evaluation of clinical performance," *American journal of orthodontics & dentofacial orthopedics*, vol. 115, no. 6, pp. 667–674, 1999.

[2] B. P and T. V. Macfarlane, "Bonded versus banded first molar attachments: a randomized controlled clinical trial," *Journal of Orthodontics*, vol. 34, no. 2, pp. 128–136, 2007.

[3] F. Godoy, J. R. Laureano Filho, A. Rosenblatt, and F. O'Ryan, "Prevalence of banding and bonding molar brackets in orthognathic surgery cases," *Journal of oral and maxillofacial surgery*, vol. 69, no. 3, pp. 911–916, 2011.

[4] J. R. Laureano Filho, F. Godoy, and F. O'Ryan, "Orthodontic bracket lost in the airway during orthognathic surgery," *American journal of orthodontics & dentofacial orthopedics*, vol. 134, no. 2, pp. 288–290, 2008.

[5] R. L. Lammers, "Soft tissue foreign bodies," *Annals of Emergency Medicine*, vol. 17, no. 12, pp. 1336–1347, 1988.

[6] T. Yildirim, A. Parlakgumus, and S. Yildirim, "Diagnosis and management of retained foreign objects," *Journal of the College of Surgeons and Physicians Pakistan*, vol. 25, no. 5, pp. 367–371, 2015.

[7] M. Zarenezhad, S. Gholamzadeh, A. Hedjazi et al., "Three years evaluation of retained foreign bodies after surgery in Iran," *Annals of Medicine and Surgery*, vol. 15, pp. 22–25, 2017.

[8] T. Teltzrow, F.-J. Kramer, A. Schulze, C. Baethge, and P. Brachvogel, "Perioperative complications following sagittal split osteotomy of the mandible," *Journal of Cranio-Maxillo-facial Surgery*, vol. 33, no. 5, pp. 307–313, 2005.

[9] N. A. Wenger, N. E. Atack, C. N. Mitchell, and A. J. Ireland, "Peri-operative second molar tube failure during orthognathic surgery: two case reports," *Journal of Orthodontics*, vol. 34, no. 2, pp. 75–79, 2007.

[10] R. V. Chandra, N. Anumala, and V. Vikrant, "An asymptomatic orthodontic bracket in the mandibular alveolar bone region," *BMJ case reports*, vol. 2013, 2013.

[11] G. Conti, M. Dolci, A. Borgonovo, and C. Maiorana, "Aesthetic restoration of upper lip after removal of post-trauma foreign body (orthodontic bracket)," *European journal of paediatric dentistry*, vol. 13, no. 3, pp. 239-240, 2012.

[12] S. B. de Queiroz, P. A. Curioso, F. S. Carvalho, and V. N. de Lima, "Submandibular-space abscess from loss of a bonded molar tube during orthognathic surgery," *American Journal of Orthodontics & Dentofacial Orthopedics*, vol. 143, no. 5, pp. 735–737, 2013.

[13] S. Steinemann, "Metal for craniomaxillofacial internal fixation implants and its physiologic implications," in *Craniomaxillofacial Reconstructive and Corrective Bone Surgery*, A. Greenberg and J. Prein, Eds., pp. 107–112, Springer, New York, NY, USA, 2006.

[14] DePuySynthes, "Technical specifications," 2017, http://sites.synthes.com.

30

Infant Oral Mutilation

Emily A. Pope ⓘ,[1] Michael W. Roberts ⓘ,[2] E. LaRee Johnson,[3] and Clark L. Morris[4]

[1]*University of North Carolina School of Dentistry, Chapel Hill, NC, USA*
[2]*Department of Pediatric Dentistry, University of North Carolina School of Dentistry, Chapel Hill, NC, USA*
[3]*Department of Pediatric Dentistry, Private Practice of Pediatric Dentistry, Raleigh, NC, USA*
[4]*Private Practice of Pediatric Dentistry, Raleigh, NC, USA*

Correspondence should be addressed to Emily A. Pope; emilyapope1@gmail.com

Academic Editor: Daniel Torrés-Lagares

Ebinyo refers to the practice of removing primary canine tooth follicles in infants without anesthetic by African traditional healers or elders using unsterilized instruments. This report describes a case of *ebinyo* or infant oral mutilation (IOM) and associated sequelae in a child adopted from a remote African tribe. The intraoral examination revealed that the patient was missing his primary maxillary and mandibular canines. The maxillary anterior periapical radiograph displayed a dysmorphic ectopic unerupted maxillary right primary canine positioned mesial to the maxillary right primary first molar. Periapical films taken confirmed partial or complete absence of the patient's primary mandibular left (73) and mandibular right (83) canines, and a bitewing and periapical film confirmed the absence of the patient's primary maxillary left (63) canine. The permanent canines will be monitored for possible hypoplasia secondary to trauma to the tooth buds during extirpation of the primary canines. Research presented in this report reveals that there are serious health implications involved with the practice of *ebinyo*.

1. Introduction

Celebrities like Madonna and Angelina Jolie have adopted children from Africa and apparently many others have also. Adoptions from Africa, as a whole, have risen worldwide from 5% in 2003 to 22% in 2009, with Ethiopia ranking second behind China in international adoptions [1]. This pattern of international adoptions, paired with unique cultural practices in the child's place of birth, will present novel challenges to healthcare professions involving customs and traditions with which they may not be familiar.

In Africa, traditional healers are part of a longstanding custom and tradition. These healers can be herbalists, faith healers, or diviners that are able to communicate with ancestral spirits for diagnostic assistance, but are not usually recognized by the government [2]. Thus, they have little interaction with the healthcare system, leading to practices that are often in conflict with western medicine [3].

Many Africans seek traditional healers for a variety of reasons, ranging from immunization against witchcraft to the treatment of sexually transmitted diseases. In fact, 80% of the African population utilizes traditional healers for medical advice and treatment [4]. Data from one study, collected from 30 traditional healers and 300 of their patients, revealed that 70% of patients turn to traditional healers as their first choice for medical advice [5].

With limited access to modern medical care, especially in remote tribal villages, traditional healers are often more affordable and easier to access. In South Africa, there are approximately 200,000 traditional healers compared to only 25,000 medically trained physicians. As this disparity pertains to dental medicine, the World Health Organization reports that, in Ethiopia, 93 dentists serve more than 77 million people [6]. This disproportion suggests that many people have few options but to rely on tribal elders and healers for dental as well as medical advice.

This report describes a case of infant oral mutilation (IOM) and associated sequelae in a child adopted from a remote African tribe and provides a context in which to understand the clinical findings.

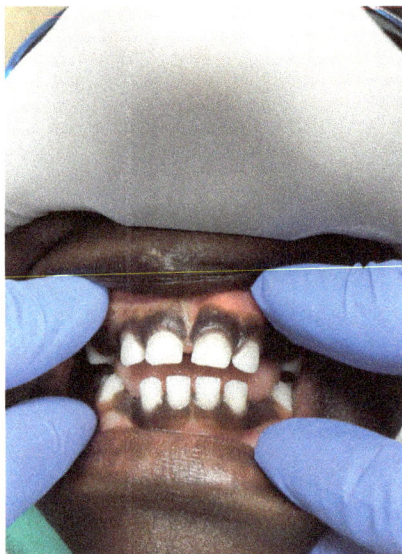

FIGURE 1: An intraoral photo of the 4-year-old male patient shows the missing maxillary and mandibular right and left primary canines.

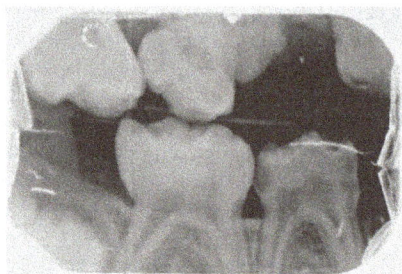

FIGURE 2: The right bitewing radiograph shows a suspicious area mesial to the maxillary right first primary molar. Caries are noted on the distal surface of the mandibular right first primary molar.

2. Case Report

A 4-year-old African male was referred to a private pediatric dental practice for an evaluation. The child was reported to have been adopted at nine months of age. By history, the patient's primary canines had been extracted prior to three months of age. According to the adoptive mother, the child had no outstanding health concerns. Beyond canine extirpation, all health history information prior to the time of the adoption, as well as family history, was unknown.

Upon evaluation, it was noted that the patient was missing the maxillary and mandibular right and left primary canines (Figure 1). Following the clinical evaluation, two bitewings in addition to maxillary and mandibular anterior periapical radiographs were obtained to evaluate proximal tooth surfaces for caries, investigate canine areas, and rule out other pathology.

Radiographs confirmed what clinically appeared to be the complete absence of the maxillary left and mandibular right primary canines (63 and 83). Additionally, the right bitewing radiograph showed a suspicious area mesial to the maxillary right first primary molar (Figure 2). A follow-up

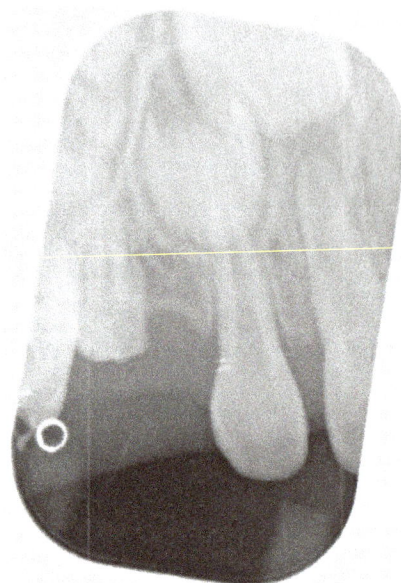

FIGURE 3: This radiograph demonstrates a dysmorphic maxillary right primary canine erupting ectopically into the mesial aspect of the maxillary right first primary molar. This is probably the result of incomplete extirpation by a tribal leader.

periapical radiograph of this region was obtained, which demonstrated an unerupted dysmorphic maxillary right primary canine tooth (53) positioned ectopically near the mesial aspect of the maxillary right first primary molar (Figure 3). Upper right and lower left periapical films have atypical presentation distal to the upper right lateral permanent incisors and between permanent lower left canines and lateral incisors. It appears that the tribal leader failed to completely extirpate the developing upper right maxillary primary canine (53), and probably the lower left primary canine (73) due to the continued development of the upper right maxillary primary canine (53) and what appears to be a developing tooth-like remnant on the lower left primary canine area (73) (Figure 4). Additional radiographs confirmed the absence of the maxillary and mandibular left primary canines (Figures 5 and 6). These areas will be followed for the possible formation of supernumerary teeth or odontomas.

Caries were also noted on the mandibular left first primary molar and the mandibular right first primary molar (Figure 2). All findings and a treatment plan to restore the carious lesions were presented to the caregiver. Regarding the missing primary canines, an orthodontic plan was developed to follow the patient's growth and development and refer the patient to an orthodontist for evaluation at age seven. The permanent canines, lateral incisors, and first premolars will be monitored for possible hypoplasia secondary to trauma caused by the extirpation of the primary canines.

3. Discussion

In parts of eastern Africa, specifically Ethiopia, Uganda, Tanzania, Somalia, and Sudan, infant oral mutilation (IOM) is commonly practiced among tribal healers [7]. This

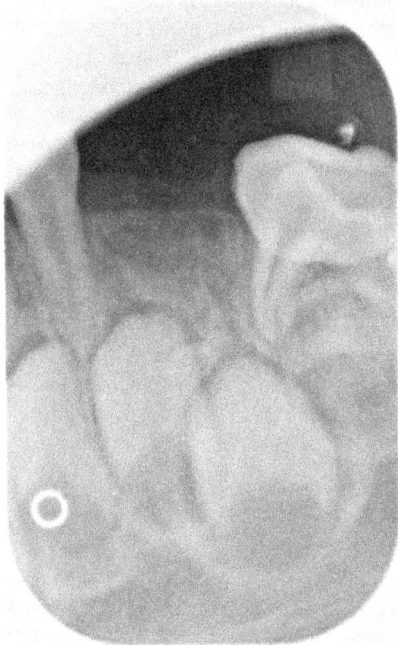

FIGURE 4: The tribal leader extirpated the lower left primary canine, but there appears to be a remaining tooth-like remnant.

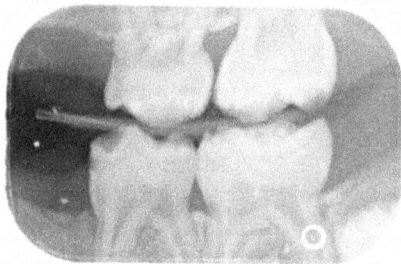

FIGURE 5: The radiograph demonstrates the absence of the maxillary and mandibular left primary canines.

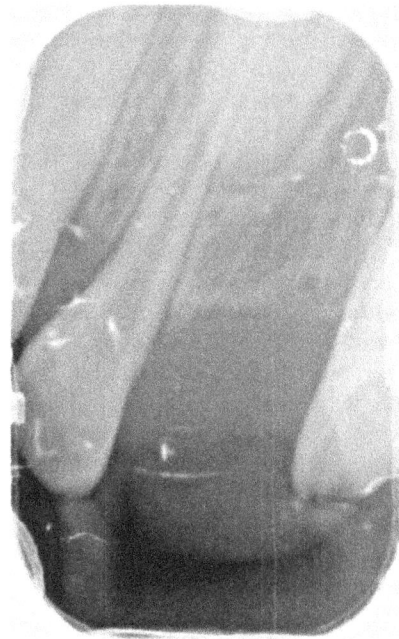

FIGURE 6: The periapical film confirms the absence of the primary maxillary left canine.

practice is known among traditional healers as *ebinyo*. *Ebinyo*, also called *ebino*, *lugbara*, and *nylon*, refers to a practice in which the primary canine tooth follicles of infants are extirpated, without anesthetic, by traditional healers or elders using unsterilized instruments [8]. These instruments include bicycle spokes, knives, razor blades, hot needles, and even fingernails. As one can imagine, the use of these instruments has the potential to result in medical complications and infections. Unlike tongue and lip piercings, the most common forms of oral mutilation in the United States, oral mutilations performed in these rural areas are for perceived medical benefit. It is believed that the canine tooth follicles are associated with headache, nausea, and vomiting—all common symptoms reported among African children. Upon removal, the canine tooth follicles have a worm-like appearance—further strengthening the belief that the canine tooth buds are symptom inducing and that *ebinyo* is of therapeutic value [9].

Research reveals that IOM is performed on infants with a median age of five months. Coincidentally, children are beginning to teeth and are often being weaned from breastfeeding at this age. The transition from breast milk to probably unclean water and food sources often leads to severe dehydration among African children. Common symptoms of dehydration include headache, nausea, and vomiting, while teething may also result in irritability and swollen gums. Moreover, primary canine follicles often appear larger in the mouths of dehydrated infants. Joseph Hurlock was a European surgeon who promoted incising the gingiva over erupting teeth to relieve pain [7]. This practice lost popularity in the 20th century, but it is possible that traditional healers adopted this practice from colonial dentists working in Africa.

In other studies involving IOM, sequelae that are consistent with the findings of this case and additional consequences of primary tooth bud extirpation are noted. In one analysis by Holan and Mamber [8], 59 children who were suspected to have had their primary canine tooth buds extirpated were examined clinically to assess the long-term consequences. Their findings indicated that common complications include missing mandibular primary lateral incisors, hypoplasia of adjacent primary and permanent teeth, dilacerations of primary canines, failure of development of the permanent canine, and early eruption of the permanent dentition. Another case involving three siblings from Uganda described by S. N. Dewhurst and C. Mason reports supernumerary teeth apical to the mandibular right permanent canine in one of the siblings [8]. In a study comparing Israeli children and those of Ethiopian immigrants living in the same community, an association was noted between the absence of canines and the prevalence of dental defects. The absence of canines and presence of dental defects occurred in 60% of the Ethiopian population compared to dental defects in only 7–12% of the Israeli population.

Only 10% of the Israeli children were missing canines [3]. Although it is challenging to study the long-term consequences associated with IOM due to limited cohorts of affected individuals, it should be noted that there are acute risks associated with the practice.

In a study conducted by Accorsi et al. [10], it was determined that one-fourth of the children in Northern Uganda who were hospitalized in 1999 died as a result of *ebinyo*. The most common complications leading to hospitalization are septicemia and severe anemia. In the same study, *ebinyo* ranked third behind meningitis and malnutrition in disease-specific case fatality rate. There have been several attempts to educate parents about the dangers associated with IOM, but the results are disappointing. In 1982, following a health program in Northern Uganda to prevent *ebinyo*, mothers began taking their children to the hospital immediately after IOM instead of avoiding the practice altogether. Even groups that immigrate, such as the Ethiopian community in Israel, continue the practice of *ebinyo* twenty years later, demonstrating a desire to preserve culture and reject western medicine [3]. Despite educational programs, *ebinyo* is still practiced in parts of Africa, and since most children survive the procedure, the false notion that there is medical benefit associated with IOM is, unfortunately, perpetuated.

References

[1] E. Rosman, "The downturn in international adoption. Adoptive Families Magazine," 2015, https://www.adoptivefamilies.com/how-to-adopt/international-adoption-statistics/.

[2] R. Kale, "Traditional healers in South Africa: a parallel health care system," *British Medical Journal*, vol. 310, no. 6988, pp. 1182–1185, 1993.

[3] E. Davidovich, E. Kooby, J. Shapira, and D. Ram, "The traditional practice of canine bud removal in the offspring of Ethiopian immigrants," *BMC Oral Health*, vol. 13, no. 1, p. 34, 2013.

[4] Health Systems-Traditional Healer Services, "The World Bank," 2016, http://web.worldbank.org/WBSITE/EXTERNAL/TOPICS/EXTHEALTHNUTRITIONANDPOPULATION/EXTHSD/0, contentMDK:20190826~menuPK:438812~pagePK:148956~piPK:216618~theSitePK:376793,00.html, Archived by WebCite at: http://www.webcitation.org/6gqQsxghY.

[5] P. Threethambal, M. Melody, M. Zama, and L. Johnson, "African traditional healers: what health care professionals need to know," *International Journal of Rehabilitation Research*, vol. 25, no. 4, pp. 247–251, 2002.

[6] P. C. Edwards, N. Levering, E. Wetzel, and T. Saini, "Extirpation of the primary canine tooth follicles," *Journal of the American Dental Association*, vol. 139, no. 4, pp. 442–450, 2008.

[7] N. L. Johnston and P. J. Riordan, "Tooth follicle extirpation and uvulectomy," *Australian Dental Journal*, vol. 50, no. 4, pp. 267–272, 2005.

[8] G. Holan and E. Mamber, "Extraction of primary canine tooth buds: prevalence and associated dental abnormalities in a group of Ethiopian Jewish children," *International Journal of Paediatric Dentistry*, vol. 4, no. 1, pp. 25–30, 1994.

[9] S. N. Dewhurst and C. Mason, "Traditional tooth bud gouging in a Ugandan family: a report involving three sisters," *International Journal of Pediatric Dentistry*, vol. 11, no. 4, pp. 292–297, 2001.

[10] S. Accorsi, M. Fabiani, N. Ferrarese, R. Iriso, M. Lukwiya, and S. Declich, "The burden of traditional practices, *ebino* and tea-tea, on child health in Northern Uganda," *Social Science & Medicine*, vol. 57, no. 11, pp. 2183–2191, 2003.

31

Chair-Side Direct Microscopy Procedure for Diagnosis of Oral Candidiasis in an Adolescent

Mathieu Lemaitre,[1] **Sarah Cousty,**[2] **and Mathieu Marty**(iD)[3]

[1]Department of Biology, Toulouse Dental School, University of Toulouse III, Toulouse University Hospital, Toulouse, France
[2]Department of Oral Surgery, Toulouse Dental School, University of Toulouse III, Toulouse University Hospital, Toulouse, France
[3]Department of Pediatric Dentistry, Toulouse Dental School, University of Toulouse III, Toulouse University Hospital, Toulouse, France

Correspondence should be addressed to Mathieu Marty; martymat@hotmail.fr

Academic Editor: Jose López-López

Oral candidiasis is caused by fungi of the genus *Candida* and one of the most common opportunistic fungal infections of the human oral cavity. Given the clinical variability of this disease, microbiological techniques are often required for clinical confirmation, as well as establishing a differential diagnosis with other diseases. The aim of this brief technical report is to illustrate a simple chair-side method, which can provide immediate microscopic diagnosis of this disease. We present the case of a 14-year-old boy suffering from a denture-related erythematous stomatitis, diagnosed and followed-up with a simplified direct microscopy technique. It enables an accurate diagnosis with a noninvasive and painless sampling method, linked to laboratory results.

1. Introduction

Oral candidiasis is caused by fungi of the genus *Candida* and one of the most common opportunistic fungal infections of the human oral cavity. One hundred fifty species of this genus have been isolated in the oral cavity, 80% of which correspond to *Candida albicans* [1]. An oral candidiasis infection could either be acute or chronic, and classified as either pseudomembranous or erythematous. Oral candidiasis represents one of the most frequent mucosal diseases as all types of infection can be found [2]. An increased incidence of infection can be linked to various predisposing factors, such as prolonged antibiotic therapy, malnutrition, endocrine disorders, HIV infection, xerostomia, smoking, poor oral hygiene, and the use of prosthetic dentures [3]. Typically, a diagnosis of oral candidiasis is based on clinical symptoms [4] and usually straightforward in cases of acute pseudomembranous candidiasis, especially in infants. However, given the clinical variability of this disease, microbiological techniques are often required for clinical confirmation, as well as establishing a differential diagnosis with other diseases. In addition, cases characterized by resistance to antifungal drugs, particularly in chronic patients, may benefit from an additional microbiological test. Several methods are currently used to isolate and identify *Candida* species, including direct microscopy of smears, stains, cultures, and genetic methods (PCR) [5]. Also new identification methods are tested to provide rapid and accurate detection [6]. A recent literature review demonstrated the advantages of direct microscopy in the diagnosis of oral candidiasis in children and adolescents [7]. The aim of this brief technical report is to illustrate a simple chair-side method which can provide immediate microscopic diagnosis of this disease.

2. Case Report

To illustrate this method, we present the case of a 14-year-old boy suffering from a denture-related erythematous stomatitis (Figure 1). Denture-related stomatitis is defined as an inflammatory process of the oral mucosa underlying a removable dental prosthesis. In young patients, a denture-related

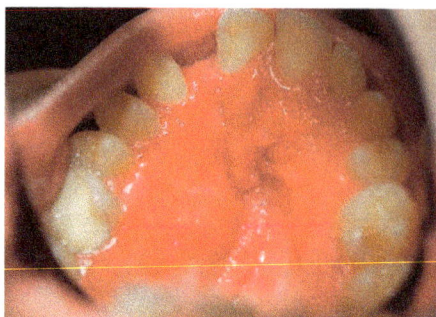

FIGURE 1: Erythematous, denture-related candidiasis in a 14-year-old boy (photography taken in an intraoral mirror).

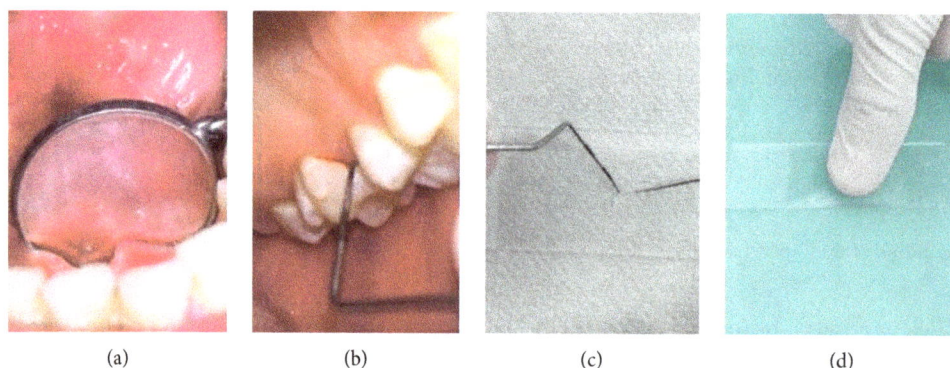

| (a) | (b) | (c) | (d) |

FIGURE 2: Step-by-step procedure for sampling.

stomatitis could be due to a complication of a pediatric prosthetic denture or can occur during long-term orthodontic treatment with a removable material. This pathology has been described among both children and teenagers, and diagnosis methods and treatment have been proposed [8–11]. Here, a removable orthodontic appliance was worn for two years to compensate a dental agenesis.

A classical microscopical procedure typically involves removing a representative sample from the infected site (exfoliative cytology) which is transferred to a microscopic slide and treated with potassium hydroxide (KOH), Gram stain, or periodic acid-Schiff (PAS) stain. A sample collection was performed and sent to laboratory for cultivation and the result was positive for *Candida albicans*.

Then we provided simplified, direct microscopy method as comparison. In this method, the patient's saliva was collected on the floor of the mouth. An intraoral mirror was placed horizontally beneath the tongue, in contact with mucosa. When saliva covers the mirror, it is removed from the mouth and laid on the slide (Figure 2(a)). The sample was subsequently collected with a sterile probe directly placed into the patient's saliva (Figure 2(c)), and a cover slip was mounted. An important point to note is that the sulcus area is the optimal site to collect the sample using this method (Figure 2(b)). The practitioner should press with his or her finger on the slide to spread the sample. The sample was then analyzed under a phase contrast optical microscope (Figure 2(d)). The most interesting magnification is ×1000 as it allows nonpathogenic yeast forms to be differentiated from opportunistic hyphal

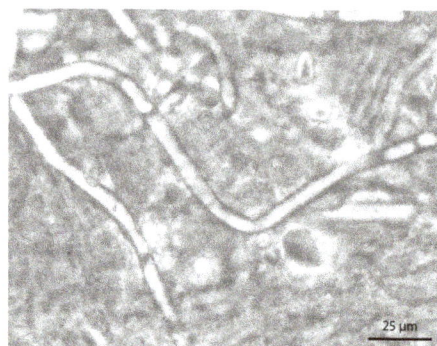

FIGURE 3: Candida hyphae (×1000 in patient's saliva).

forms. In pathological conditions, several hyphae are visible on each screen, mixed with oral bacteria and cells (Figure 3). Importantly, this method is valuable for determining the efficacy of treatment. The treatment consisted in 3 weeks of local treatment using antifungal agent (amphotericin B), and the modification of the prosthetic appliance for a fixed one. Another laboratory analysis by cultivation was negative. At the two years follow-up, the same procedure showed a normalization of oral flora, with absence of hyphae (Figure 4(b)), linked to a clinical improvement (Figure 4(a)).

3. Conclusion

Direct microscopy is widely used in laboratories to diagnose candidiasis. It enables an accurate diagnosis with a noninvasive

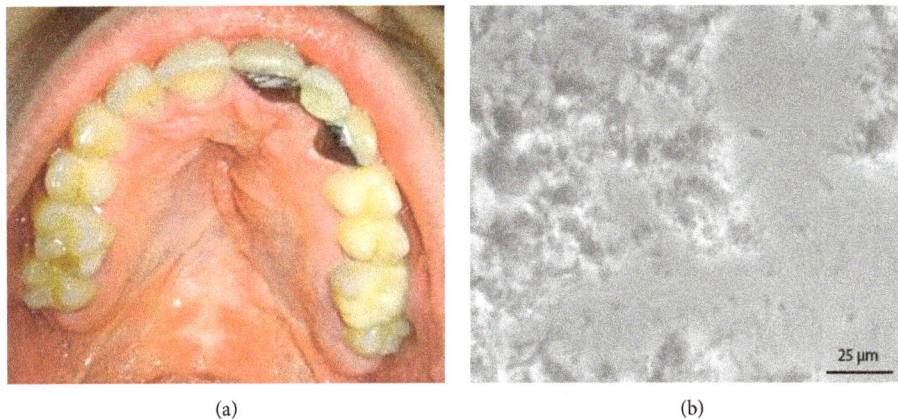

(a)   (b)

FIGURE 4: (a) Clinical improvement at the 2 years follow-up. (b) Normalization of oral flora after treatment (×1000 in patient's saliva).

and painless sampling method, particularly well-suited to young patients. A classical procedure, which involves sample collection and shipment to a laboratory, takes more time and expense. Moreover, the method presented here does not require any fixation or sample treatment. Therefore, it is a cost-effective way to examine a patient's oral microbiota and determine any potential imbalance. Although direct microscopy is not as specific as culture, it appears to be a procedure of choice for a first-line diagnosis. Of course, a complete clinical examination remains absolutely necessary, as well as an extensive medical history, in order to study any associated general disease. Moreover, this approach requires experience in detecting yeast through microscopic observation which is not a transversal competence within clinicians. However the identification is not very difficult, and a simple, short-time formation may be sufficient. In this way, more practitioners will increasingly have access to this method; therefore, further awareness of this simple microscopic analysis will allow clinicians to make an immediate chair-side diagnosis. Furthermore, as it was the case for intraoral cameras, given the progress of microscopic devices, they can be integrated in the concept of person-centered care as an element of education and prevention to understand diagnoses and make informed treatment decisions [12]. Potential development of smartphone-based microscopes will provide easier access for clinicians to microscopy. Smartphone-based microscopes have already been in use to detect parasite [13] or obtain live-cells images [14]. This is a promising approach to perform accurate chair-side diagnosis in the future.

Ethical Approval

All procedures performed in the study involving human participants were in accordance with the ethical standards of Toulouse University and with the 1964 Helsinki declaration and its amendments.

Consent

Informed consent was obtained from all patients and their parents. All the authors gave their consent for publication.

References

[1] L. Coronado-Castellote and Y. Jiménez-Soriano, "Clinical and microbiological diagnosis of oral candidiasis," *Journal of Clinical and Experimental Dentistry*, vol. 5, no. 5, pp. e279–e286, 2013.

[2] P. J. Giannini and K. V. Shetty, "Diagnosis and management of oral candidiasis," *Otolaryngologic Clinics of North America*, vol. 44, no. 1, pp. 231–240, 2011.

[3] N. Aslani, G. Janbabaei, M. Abastabar et al., "Identification of uncommon oral yeasts from cancer patients by MALDI-TOF mass spectrometry," *BMC Infectious Diseases*, vol. 18, no. 1, p. 24, 2018.

[4] P. A. Krishnan, "Fungal infections of the oral mucosa," *Indian Journal of Dental Research*, vol. 23, no. 5, pp. 650–659, 2012.

[5] J. M. Aguirre-Urízar, "Oral Candidiasis," *Revista Iberoamericana de Micología*, vol. 19, pp. 17–21, 2002.

[6] H. Noguchi, T. Iwase, D. Omagari et al., "Rapid detection of *Candida albicans* in oral exfoliative cytology samples by loop-mediated isothermal amplification," *Journal of Oral Science*, vol. 59, no. 4, pp. 541–547, 2017.

[7] M. Marty, E. Bourrat, F. Vaysse, M. Bonner, and I. Bailleul-Forestier, "Direct microscopy: a useful tool to diagnose oral candidiasis in children and adolescents," *Mycopathologia*, vol. 180, no. 5-6, pp. 373–377, 2015.

[8] M. H. Figueiral, A. Azul, E. Pinto, P. A. Fonseca, F. M. Branco, and C. Scully, "Denture-related stomatitis: identification of aetiological and predisposing factors-a large cohort," *Journal of Oral Rehabilitation*, vol. 34, no. 6, pp. 448–455, 2007.

[9] A. M. Iacopino and W. F. Wathen, "Oral candida infection and denture stomatitis: a comprehensive review," *Journal of the American Dental Association*, vol. 123, no. 1, pp. 46–51, 1992.

[10] C. O. Mosca, M. D. Moragues, S. Brena, A. C. Rosa, and J. Pontón, "Isolation of *Candida dubliniensis* in a teenager with denture stomatitis," *Medicina Oral, Patologia Oral Y Cirugia Bucal*, vol. 10, no. 1, pp. 28–31, 2005.

[11] M. H. Figueiral, P. A. Fonseca, M. M. Lopes, E. Pinto, T. Pereira-Leite, and B. Sampaio-Maia, "Effect of denture-related stomatitis fluconazole treatment on oral *Candida albicans* susceptibility profile and genotypic variability," *Open Dentistry Journal*, vol. 9, no. 1, pp. 46–51, 2015.

[12] M. Walji, N. Karimbux, and A. Spielman, "Person-centered care: opportunities and challenges for Academic Dental Institutions and Programs," *Journal of Dental Education*, vol. 81, no. 11, pp. 1265–1272, 2017.

32

Ellis-van Creveld Syndrome: A Rare Clinical Report of Oral Rehabilitation by Interdisciplinary Approach

Talib Amin Naqash [ID],[1] **Ibrahim Alshahrani** [ID],[2] **and Siripan Simasetha**[3]

[1]*Department of Prosthetic Dentistry, King Khalid University College of Dentistry, Abha, Saudi Arabia*
[2]*Department of Pediatric Dentistry and Orthodontic Sciences, King Khalid University College of Dentistry, Abha, Saudi Arabia*
[3]*Dental Department, Bhumibol Adulyadej Hospital, The Royal Thai Air Force, Bangkok, Thailand*

Correspondence should be addressed to Talib Amin Naqash; go4talib@yahoo.com

Academic Editor: Konstantinos Michalakis

Ellis-van Creveld syndrome (EVC) is a very rare genetic disorder that affects various tissues of ectodermal and mesodermal origin; patients with EVC present with typical oral deficiencies. The affected individuals are quite young at the time of oral evaluation. It is, therefore, important that these individuals are diagnosed and receive dental treatment at an early age for their physiologic and psychosocial well-being. Albeit there are numerous articles penned on the EVC, the treatise from an oral perspective is inadequate, covering only oral exhibitions and the preventive treatments. This article reviews the literature and serves as the first disquisition for oral rehabilitation of an EVC patient utilizing surgical, orthodontic, restorative, and prosthodontic management.

1. Introduction

Ellis-van Creveld syndrome (EVC) is a rare autosomal recessive disorder with characteristic clinical manifestations, resulting from a genetic mutation in two genes, *EVC1* and *EVC2*, mapping both in locus 16 on the short arm of chromosome 4 (4p16) in a head-to-head configuration [1, 2]. EVC presents with a distinctive tetrad of disproportionate dwarfism, bilateral postaxial polydactyly, ectodermal dysplasia, and congenital heart malformations [3]. It is also known as chondroectodermal dysplasia and mesoectodermal dysplasia; dysplasia is an abnormality in form or development [4].

Pediatricians Richard W. B. Ellis of Edinburgh and Simon van Creveld of Amsterdam were the first to describe a case of EVC in 1940 [5]. The syndrome had been partially described previously in several reports, but work of Ellis and van Creveld defined it [6, 7]. In literature, detailed description of clinical presentation in finite case series or single reports is found [3–13].

EVC presents with a characteristic tetrad of clinical manifestations [3]:

(1) Chondrodysplasia of the long, tubular bones resulting in disproportionate dwarfism, and an exceptionally long trunk is the most common clinical feature, producing a serious ossification defect [6]. The severity of short limbs increases from the proximal to the distal portions [6].

(2) Bilateral postaxial polydactyly of the hands, with the supernumerary finger, usually being on the ulnar side [6]. Fingers are sausage shaped with wide hands and feet [14].

(3) Hidrotic ectodermal dysplasia with dystrophic, small dysplastic nails, thin sparse hair, and oral manifestations [12].

(4) Congenital heart malformations in 50% to 60% of cases, the most common being a single atrium and a ventricular septal defect [6]. The associated cardiorespiratory problems are described as the primary cause of decreased life expectancy in these patients [15].

According to Winter and Geddes, oral manifestations in EVC are characteristic and remarkable [16]. The most common finding is the fusion of the anterior portion of the upper lip to the maxillary gingival margin, obliterating mucolabial fold, causing the upper lip to present a slightly V-notch in the middle [14, 17]. The anterior portion of the lower alveolar ridge is often jagged [7]. Multiple small accessory labiogingival frenula, serrated incisal edges, diastemas, teeth of abnormal form, enamel hypoplasia, and hypodontia are other features [3, 16]. Varela and Ramos stated that malocclusion is secondary to oral abnormalities and is of no specific type [18].

2. Clinical Report

A 15-year-old female was referred to the Department of Prosthetic Dentistry for evaluation and prosthetic dental treatment of congenitally absent maxillary lateral incisors and mandibular incisors (Figure 1). The patient was attending a regular school but had concerns about her esthetics.

Pregnancy and delivery were uneventful, and no exposure to radiation or drugs had occurred during pregnancy. At birth, however, the patient presented with short limbs, a long trunk, and polydactyly of hands. Medical history revealed that the patient has an atrial septal defect and was being planned for surgical closure. Psychomotor development was within the normal range. Extra oral examination showed that the patient has short limb dwarfism (131 cm), with a long trunk and weighed 37.1 kg. Polydactyly of hands was observed with dysplastic and atrophic finger and toe nails (Figure 2). Hair was thin and sparse.

Intraoral examination showed absence of maxillary lateral incisors, mandibular central and lateral incisors, microdontia of the maxillary left canine, unilateral crossbite on the left side, partial end-to-end occlusal relationship on the right side, and alveolar ridge defect in the anterior mandible (Figure 3).

The examination of soft tissues showed presence of a large maxillary labial frenum attached to alveolar ridge causing obliteration of vestibule and midline diastema. Laterally, there were multiple small accessory labial frenula (Figure 3). The remaining oral mucosa was normal.

A panoramic radiograph confirmed agenesis of the maxillary lateral incisors, mandibular incisors, and all third molars (Figure 4).

Dental procedure that involved manipulation of gingival tissue or perforation of the oral mucosa was performed under proper antibiotic cover, as per revised guidelines from American Heart Association, to prevent infective (bacterial) endocarditis [19].

Treatment started with supragingival periodontal therapy for removal of plaque and calculus, and to improve oral health. It was followed by maxillary labial frenectomy and vestibular deepening, using electrosurgery. Electrocautery procedure offered minimal time consumption, bloodless field during the surgical procedure with no requirement of sutures, and absence of postoperative complications [20].

Following postoperative healing, orthodontic examination revealed that the patient had a unilateral crossbite on the left side. Cervical Vertebrae Maturation Index (CVMI),

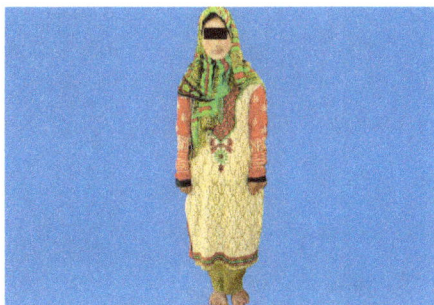

FIGURE 1: Patient with Ellis-van Creveld syndrome.

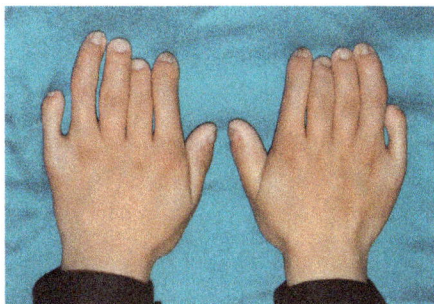

FIGURE 2: Hands showing polydactyly and hypoplastic nails.

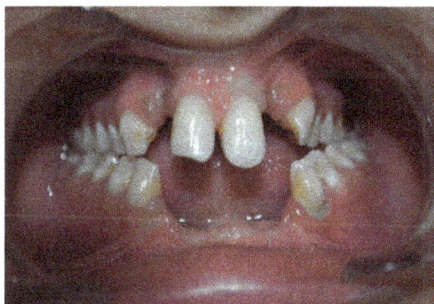

FIGURE 3: Absent maxillary lateral incisors and mandibular incisors, large maxillary labial frenum, multiple accessory labial frenula, midline diastema, mandibular anterior ridge defect, and crossbite.

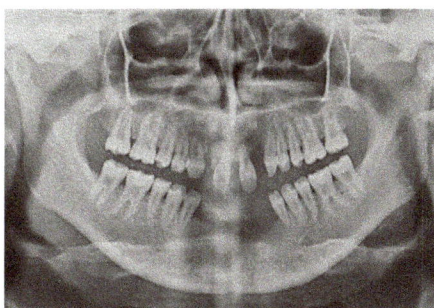

FIGURE 4: Panoramic radiograph showing agenesis of maxillary lateral incisors, mandibular incisors, and all 4 third molars.

using lateral cephalogram (Figure 5), depicted the patient to be in CVMI Stage V [21, 22]. As such, the patient was put on Quad Helix, a slow maxillary expansion appliance, aimed at

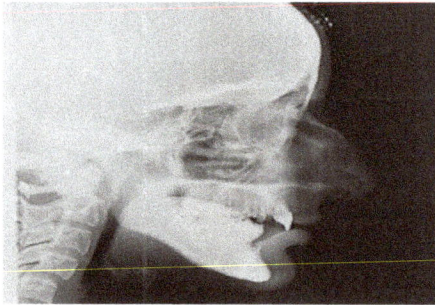

FIGURE 5: Lateral cephalogram.

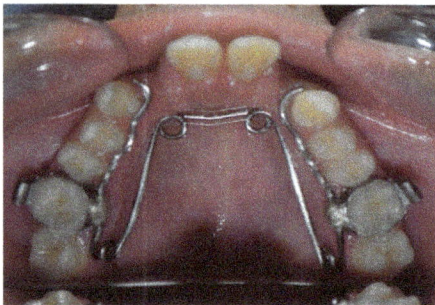

FIGURE 6: Quad helix cemented to maxillary molars.

FIGURE 7: Andrew's removable component with Ceka Preciline attachments.

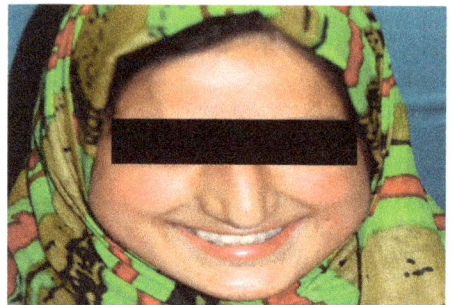

FIGURE 8: Clinical view after oral rehabilitation.

dentoalveolar expansion of the arch on the left side and correction of partial end-to-end occlusion on the right side [23, 24]. The appliance was fabricated from 36 mil stainless steel wire and was soldered with bands. Initial activation of 8 mm was done extraorally, and the bands were cemented with glass ionomer cement (Ketac Cem Glass Ionomer Cement, 3M) on maxillary molars (Figure 6). The patient was seen every four weeks for three months unless the appliance achieved 8 mm intraoral activation. After twelve-week treatment, crossbite was corrected and the appliance was removed. A retention appliance was placed for three months to prevent relapse.

After correction of crossbite, crown build-up, with glass ionomer cement (Vitremer, 3M), was done on the maxillary left canine, to correct microdontia.

Andrew's Bridge System was designed for rehabilitation of mandibular incisors on lower canines, keeping in view Seibert's class III ridge defect in the anterior mandible [25]. Andrew's Bridge System is a fixed removable prosthesis that is indicated in patients with large ridge defects. It provides maximum aesthetics, is hygienic, and has a good fit with minimal trauma to soft tissues or underlying bone at an economic price [26, 27]. Bar and Clip attachments (Preci-Horix, Ceka) were used to secure removable and fixed component (Figure 7).

Dental implants were planned for maxillary lateral incisors, but the patient was reluctant to undergo invasive treatment option, owing to her concerns about the cardiac defect. Therefore, six units metal ceramic fixed dental prosthesis (Ivoclar Vivadent) was fabricated in the maxillary arch, from canine to canine region, with maxillary canines and central incisors as abutments.

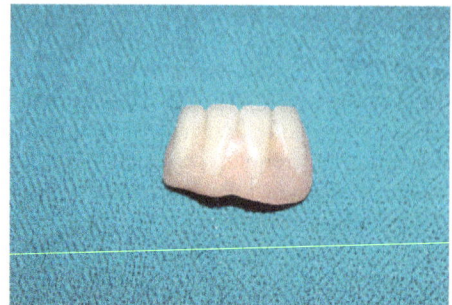

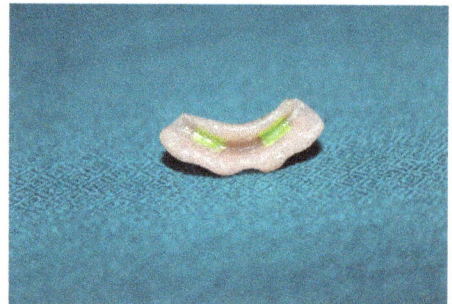

The patient was trained to properly insert and remove the removable prosthesis that was fabricated over the fixed component of Andrew's Bridge System, and proper oral hygiene instructions (including interdental brush) were given to the patient.

Follow-up was done for six months, and no complication after treatment was noted.

3. Discussion

The presentation of medically compromised and syndromic children in the dental office is a great challenge to oral health care providers [28]. Various syndromes are identified earlier in childhood and demand special attention right from the birth [28]. EVC is one of these syndromes with variable phenotype affecting multiple organs [11].

There is no definitive cure for EVC [29]. The management is multidisciplinary which involves several specialists: a cardiologist, a pediatrician, an orthopedician, a prosthodontist, an oral and maxillofacial surgeon, an orthodontist, and a periodontist [13, 30].

The approach to dental management will depend on each particular case [6]. Preventive measures include dietary counseling, plaque control, oral hygiene instructions, fluoride varnish application, or daily fluoride mouth rinses [3, 6, 31].

To maintain space and to improve function, esthetics, and speech, removable or fixed dental prosthesis (considering age) is recommended [28]. Restoration of hypoplastic and decayed teeth is indicated to preserve tooth structure and to improve esthetics; taking into account possible presence of enlarged pulp chambers [6, 30]. For soft tissue anomalies, surgical correction is advised [31]. Parental and child counseling is often required to treat psychological trauma due to compromised oral and medical health [28].

4. Summary

EVC is a rare autosomal recessive disorder with variable expression, diagnosed by its characteristic clinical manifestations. Dental and oral manifestations of EVC are definitive; dentist plays a vital role in its early diagnosis and treatment planning and to establish a differential diagnosis with other clinically similar entities. EVC has high mortality in early life due to cardiac and respiratory problems; those who survive require multidisciplinary treatment planning in terms of preventing oral diseases and providing rehabilitation. Early treatment can help the patient to prevent various problems and undue psychological trauma.

After completion of the treatment, esthetics, function and phonetics improved remarkably. The patient was happy and comfortable with the oral rehabilitation, and the post treatment esthetic outcome helped her to improve her quality of life (Figure 8).

Acknowledgments

The authors acknowledge the support of King Khalid University, Abha, Saudi Arabia, in preparation of this manuscript.

References

[1] M. H. Polymeropoulos, S. E. Ide, M. Wright et al., "The gene for Ellis van Creveld syndrome is located on chromosome 4p16," *Genomics*, vol. 35, no. 1, pp. 1–5, 1996.

[2] M. Galdzicka, S. Patnala, M. G. Hirshman et al., "A new gene, EVC2, is mutated in Ellis van Creveld syndrome," *Molecular Genetics and Metabolism*, vol. 77, no. 4, pp. 291–295, 2002.

[3] F. N. Hattab, O. M. Yassin, and I. S. Sasa, "Oral manifestations of Ellis-van Creveld syndrome. Report of 2 siblings with unusual dental anomalies," *Journal of Clinical Pediatric Dentistry*, vol. 22, pp. 159–165, 1998.

[4] D. Tahririan, A. Eshghi, P. Givehchian, and M. A. Tahririan, "Chondroectodermal dysplasia: a rare syndrome," *Journal of Dentistry*, vol. 11, pp. 361–364, 2014.

[5] R. W. Ellis and S. van Creveld, "A syndrome characterized by ectodermal dysplasia, polydactyly, chondrodysplasia and congenital morbus cordis. Report of 3 cases," *Archives of Disease in Childhood*, vol. 15, no. 82, pp. 65–84, 1940.

[6] A. Cahuana, C. Palma, W. Gonzales, and E. Gean, "Oral manifestations in Ellis-van Creveld syndrome: report of five cases," *Pediatric Dentistry*, vol. 26, no. 3, pp. 277–282, 2004.

[7] M. Atasu and S. Biren, "Ellis-van Creveld syndrome: dental, clinical, genetics and dermatoglyphic findings of a case," *Journal of Clinical Pediatric Dentistry*, vol. 24, pp. 141–145, 2000.

[8] V. A. Mckusick, J. A. Egeland, R. Eldridge, and D. E. Krusen, "Dwarfism in the Amish I. The Ellis van Creveld syndrome," *Bulletin of the Johns Hopkins Hospital*, vol. 115, pp. 306–336, 1964.

[9] M. L. Martinez Frias and A. Sanchez Cascos, "Ellis-van Creveld syndrome," *Revista Clínica Española*, vol. 133, no. 4, pp. 311–318, 1974.

[10] C. Stoll, B. Dott, M. P. Roth, and Y. Alembik, "Birth prevalence rates of skeletal dysplasia," *Clinical Genetics*, vol. 35, no. 2, pp. 88–92, 1989.

[11] G. Baujat and M. Le Merrer, "Ellis-van Creveld syndrome," *Orphanet Journal of Rare Diseases*, vol. 2, no. 1, p. 27, 2007.

[12] K. M. Zangwill, D. K. Boal, R. L. Ladda, J. M. Opitz, and J. F. Reynolds, "Dandy-Walker malformation in Ellis-van Creveld syndrome," *American Journal of Medical Genetics*, vol. 31, no. 1, pp. 123–129, 1998.

[13] J. A. Hanemann, B. C. de Carvalho, and E. C. Franco, "Oral manifestations in Ellis-van Creveld syndrome: report of a case and review of the literature," *Journal of Oral and Maxillofacial Surgery*, vol. 68, no. 2, pp. 456–460, 2010.

[14] C. Sergi, T. Voigtlander, S. Zoubaa et al., "Ellis-van Creveld syndrome: a generalized dysplasia of enchondral ossification," *Pediatric Radiology*, vol. 31, no. 4, pp. 289–293, 2001.

[15] D. Alves-Pereira, L. Berini-Aytes, and C. Gay-Escoda, "Ellis-van Creveld syndrome. Case report and literature review," *Medicina Oral, Patologia Oral y Cirugía Bucal*, vol. 14, no. 7, pp. E340–E343, 2009.

[16] G. B. Winter and M. Geddes, "Oral manifestations of chondroectodermal dysplasia (Ellis-van Creveld syndrome). Report of a case," *British Dental Journal*, vol. 122, pp. 103–107, 1967.

[17] P. Babaji, "Oral abnormalities in the Ellis-van Creveld syndrome," *Indian Journal of Dental Research*, vol. 21, no. 1, pp. 143–145, 2010.

[18] M. Varela and C. Ramos, "Chondroectodermal dysplasia (Ellis-van Creveld syndrome): a case report," *European Journal of Orthodontics*, vol. 18, no. 1, pp. 313–318, 1996.

[19] D. K. Lam, A. Jan, G. K. Sándor, C. M. Clokie, and American Heart Association, "Prevention of infective endocarditis: revised guidelines from the American Heart Association and the implications for dentists," *Journal-Canadian Dental Association*, vol. 74, no. 5, pp. 449–453, 2008.

[20] Devishree, S. K. Gujjari, and P. V. Shubhashini, "Frenectomy: a review with the reports of surgical techniques," *Journal of Clinical and Diagnostic Research*, vol. 6, no. 9, pp. 1587–1592, 2012.

[21] B. Hassel and A. G. Farman, "Skeletal maturation evaluation using cervical vertebrae," *American Journal of Orthodontics and Dentofacial Orthopedics*, vol. 107, no. 1, pp. 58–66, 1995.

[22] R. C. Santiago, L. F. de Miranda Costa, R. W. Vitral, M. R. Fraga, A. M. Bolognese, and L. C. Maia, "Cervical vertebral maturation as a biological indicator of skeletal maturity," *Angle Orthodontist*, vol. 82, no. 6, pp. 1123–1131, 2012.

[23] S. J. Chaconas and J. A. de Alba y Levy, "Orthopedic and orthodontic applications of the quad-helix appliance," *American Journal of Orthodontics*, vol. 72, no. 4, pp. 422–428, 1977.

[24] R. W. Bench, "The quad helix appliance," *Seminars in Orthodontics*, vol. 4, no. 4, pp. 231–237, 1998.

[25] J. S. Seibert, "Reconstruction of deformed partially edentulous ridges using full thickness onlay grafts: part I–technique and wound healing," *Compendium of Continuing Education in Dentistry*, vol. 4, no. 5, pp. 437–453, 1983.

[26] R. J. Everhart and E. Cavazos Jr., "Evaluation of a fixed removable partial denture: Andrews Bridge System," *Journal of Prosthetic Dentistry*, vol. 50, no. 2, pp. 180–184, 1983.

[27] J. A. Andrews and W. F. Biggs, "The Andrews bar-and-sleeve-retained bridge: a clinical report," *Dentistry Today*, vol. 18, no. 4, pp. 94–99, 1999.

[28] R. Kalaskar and A. R. Kalaskar, "Oral manifestations of Ellis-van Creveld syndrome," *Contemporary Clinical Dentistry*, vol. 3, no. 5, pp. S55–S59, 2012.

[29] R. Kamal, P. Dahiya, S. Kaur, R. Bhardwaj, and K. Chaudhary, "Ellis-van Creveld syndrome: a rare clinical entity," *Journal of Oral and Maxillofacial Pathology*, vol. 17, no. 1, pp. 132–135, 2013.

[30] T. Susami, T. Kuroda, H. Yoshimasu, and R. Suzuki, "Ellis-van Creveld syndrome: craniofacial morphology and multidisciplinary treatment," *Cleft Palate-Craniofacial Journal*, vol. 36, no. 4, pp. 345–352, 1999.

[31] M. L. Hunter and G. J. Roberts, "Oral and dental anomalies in Ellis-van Creveld syndrome (Chondroectodermal dysplasia): report of a case," *International Journal of Paediatric Dentistry*, vol. 8, no. 2, pp. 153–157, 1999.

33

Removal of Implant and New Rehabilitation for Better Esthetics

Wilson Matsumoto (ID), **Victor Garone Morelli, Rossana Pereira de Almeida,**
Alexandre Elias Trivellato, Cássio Edvard Sverzut, and Takami Hirono Hotta

Dental School of Ribeirão Preto, Dental Materials and Prosthodontic Department, University of São Paulo, Ribeirão Preto, SP, Brazil

Correspondence should be addressed to Wilson Matsumoto; wmatsumoto@forp.usp.br

Academic Editor: Jamil Awad Shibli

Tooth loss can result in loss of facial esthetics, in addition to its effect on mastication, swallowing, and speech. Adequate planning is required in order for the prosthetic treatment of the teeth and implants to be successful. Here, we present a clinical case demonstrating that improper positioning of an implant can make prosthetic rehabilitation unfeasible, necessitating new surgical and rehabilitation planning to achieve the desired esthetics. The patient had a missing right lateral incisor and cuspid, and a buccally directed implant. The preferred treatment regimen involved the removal of this implant and placement of another one more properly positioned distally and three dimensionally. The repositioning of the implant made rehabilitation treatment with a mesial cantilever possible. Due to esthetic considerations, gingival conditioning in the cantilever region was performed in the temporary prosthesis phase. The changes adopted in planning the surgery and rehabilitation resulted in good esthetics as well as functional outcomes.

1. Introduction

It is known that tooth loss negatively affects swallowing, chewing, phonetics, and mandibular posture, as well as the patient's facial esthetics, all of which may lead to social and emotional discomfort. Consequently, when the treatment option involves the placement of implants, appropriate care must be taken to ensure the accurate three-dimensional placement of the implant [1], and that the implant is in harmony with the opposing and adjacent teeth [2], especially when esthetic areas are involved [3] where there is the necessity to precisely evaluate the existence of bone and soft tissue deficiencies.

The papillae adjacent to the single-unit crown should mimic those of a healthy tooth, in both height and embrasure fill, and the midbuccal gingival margins should harmonize with those of the adjacent teeth [3, 4]; however, the progressive involution of the alveolar bone begins following tooth loss, and it can be accompanied by a marked reduction in both the quality and quantity of hard and soft tissues [5], and the final result may not be acceptable from an esthetic point of view.

As a dental procedure, diagnostic waxing-up can be used to visualize the final result of prosthetic treatment [1], thereby allowing an analysis of the emergency profile and the shape and size of the teeth, as well as the surgical guide to check the correct position of the implant during the placement [6, 7]. The use of techniques, such as computerized guided surgery, stereolithographs, and three-dimensionally printed surgical guides, has made the results of implant prosthesis treatment better and more predictable [8].

However, despite all prior care, the implant can be placed in an improper position, making prosthetic restoration impracticable [9]. In this situation, removal of the implant or its repositioning have been proposed [10], and several types of procedures can be used to solve this problem [9, 11–13]. In this context, the professional should select the option that best suits the specific case, seeking the preservation of soft tissues and the patient's comfort and welfare. Here, we present a case in which the removal of a buccally positioned implant was required, and we demonstrate a new surgical procedure and successful prosthetic treatment.

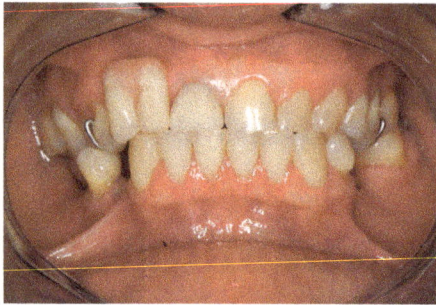

FIGURE 1: Temporary crown on teeth 11 adapted to the removable prosthesis.

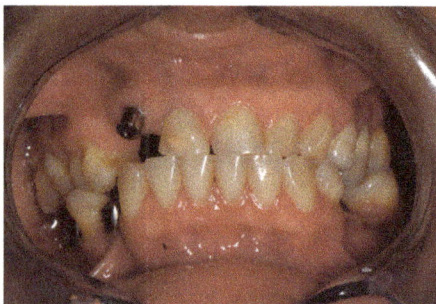

FIGURE 3: Removal of the implant with a retrieval tool.

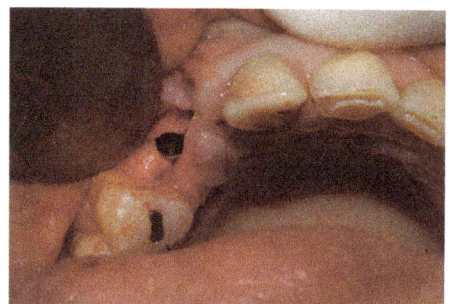

FIGURE 2: Poorly positioned implant.

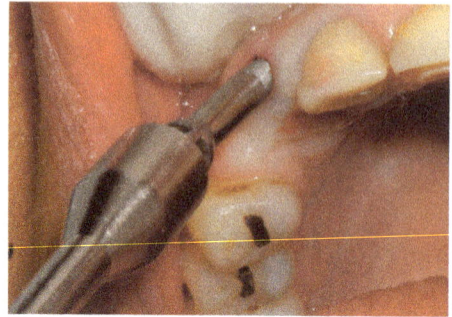

FIGURE 4: Installation of the new implant.

2. Case Report

A 44-year-old female patient reported to the Department of Oral and Maxillofacial Surgery, and Periodontology at the Dental School of Ribeirao Preto, University of São Paulo for a placement of implants. During the initial examination, it was observed that the right upper central incisor had an unsatisfactory temporary Richmond type crown that was changed by a metal core, post, and new temporary crown. The new temporary crown was fitted to the removable partial denture that was used by the patient (Figure 1). Surgical guides were made and the patient was referred for implant placement, in the region of teeth 12, 35, 36, 44, and 46.

After approximately 8 months, it was verified that the implant located in the anterior region was positioned further apical and buccal (Figure 2) making it impossible to fabricate a successful implant crown from an esthetic point of view.

The implant was gradually removed using the implant removal instrument (Implant Retrieval Tool; Nobel Biocare), with antirotational movement (Figure 3). Following this surgical procedure, a new implant was installed (cone morse 3.5 × 11 mm, Conexão, Brazil), with a torque of 30 N, and positioned in the mesiodistal direction. Specifically, the implant was placed closer to tooth 14 in the buccal-palatine direction on the bone ridge (located around 1 mm for the palatal from an imaginary curvature passing through the buccal surfaces of the present teeth and 1 mm infraosseo in the coronoapical direction) (Figure 4).

After the surgery, the removable partial denture was removed. This was followed by the fabrication of a temporary fixed partial prosthesis with retention used during the

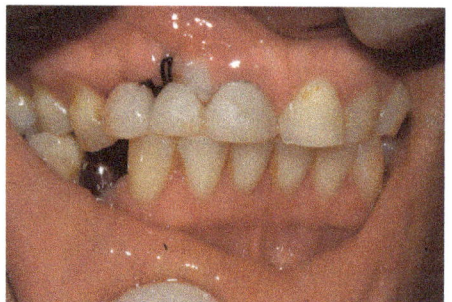

FIGURE 5: Installation of the temporary fixed partial denture.

osseointegration phase on teeth 11 and 14 (Figure 5): this was only for esthetic purpose. This was in addition to the installation of prostheses on the implants in the regions of teeth 35, 36, 44, and 46.

Immediately after the second stage surgery, the temporary fixed partial denture was performed using the healing cap as an abutment and a lateral incisor as a mesial cantilever. Following the rehabilitation procedures, this temporary fixed partial denture was changed to a provisional fixed prosthesis with the mesial cantilever screwed into the implant. During this phase, periodic acrylic resin implements were added to the temporary prosthesis to promote gingival conditioning (Figures 6 and 7) and black triangle closure (Figures 8 and 9) and also to improve gingival esthetics.

At the end of two months, the implant prosthesis with a mesial cantilever was installed (Figure 10). This case report

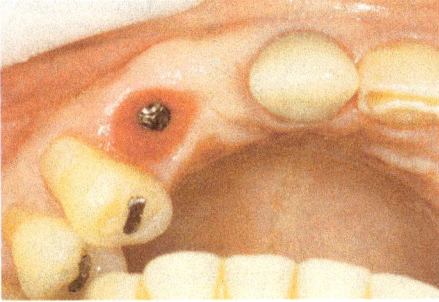

FIGURE 6: Occlusal view of the gingival conditioning.

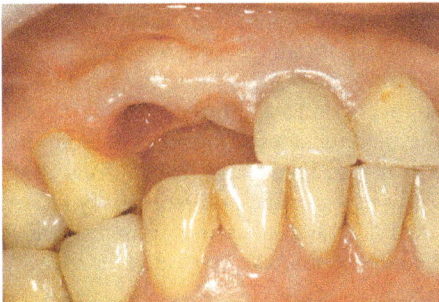

FIGURE 7: Buccal view of the gingival conditioning.

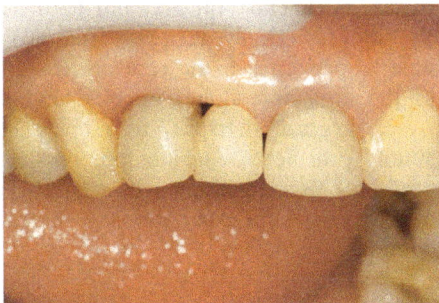

FIGURE 8: Presence of the black triangle before gingival conditioning.

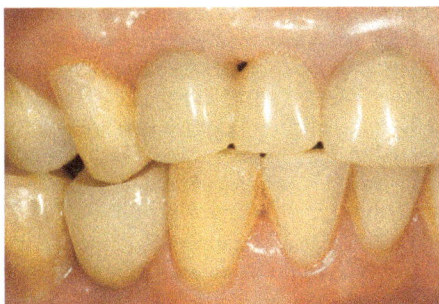

FIGURE 9: Gradual closing of the black triangle.

was approved by the institution's Ethics Committee on Human Research and followed the ethical principles of the Declaration of Helsinki, in addition to complying with specific legislation.

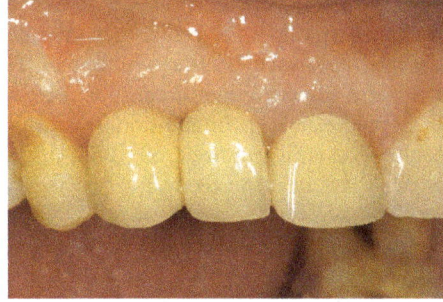

FIGURE 10: Final appearance of the implant prosthesis.

3. Discussion

From an esthetic point of view, a misplaced implant, especially in the anterior region, generally results in an unsatisfactory prosthesis. Since esthetics is a primary requirement of the treatment regimen, this error is prevented through appropriate planning of the surgery for implant placement.

A typical successful course of treatment involves, but is not limited to, clinical exams, mounted casts in the semi-adjustable articulator, a diagnostic waxing-up, radiographic images, surgical guides, and bone and/or soft tissue grafts which are part of a set of procedures that must be strictly followed [14].

The introduction of the cone beam computerized tomography (CBCT) in dentistry has made it possible to perform a precise preoperative evaluation of the implant sites and sophisticated surgical guide in dental implantology [8, 15]. The guided implant protocols have made the clinicians simplify their procedures starting from the diagnostic phase up to the realization of the final prosthetic restoration [7]. However, as these resources are not always available for a large part of the population, even with the best preparation and planning, undesirable occurrences can result into a detriment or can even render the treatment impracticable [10], a development which, without a doubt, will likely generate dissatisfaction, frustration, the necessity of other surgery, and loss of time for the patient.

Until recently, the removal of an implant resulted in a heavy loss of bone tissue and the necessity of bone grafting procedures [16]. However, technological advancements have led to the development of instruments that facilitate implant removal via conservative and easy procedures [13, 17].

Some points are worth making for this report. In this case, despite the careful presurgical planning, complications during the surgery resulted in a case with no prosthetic solution, even if using angled implant abutment due to the buccal positioning of the implant. The angled abutment presented a metallic platform wider than the straight one, thereby negatively affecting esthetics. This condition could have been avoided if the positioning of the implant had been 1 to 2 mm more palatal from an imaginary line passing through the buccal surfaces of the other teeth [1, 6]. This would facilitate prosthetic procedures, preserve facial esthetics, and conserve bone tissue on the buccal surfaces.

The apical placement of the implant is another deficient aspect of the case study, because it created a misalignment in relation to the natural teeth. Ideally, it should have been placed 3 to 4 mm apical to the cementoenamel junction of the adjacent teeth [6] to achieve the esthetic goal. This would have resulted in a smooth gingival contour, without abrupt changes in tissue height [1]. In addition, this implant positioning would necessarily require a very long clinical crown, disproportionate to adjacent teeth and visible during the patient's smile.

Therefore, due to the poor prognosis, the treatment option was to remove the implant and carefully replace it with a new one that was three-dimensionally well positioned, enabling the prosthetic rehabilitation. Among the various possibilities [9, 11, 12], the selected technique allowed the implant to be removed quickly, atraumatically, and without the need for incisions or manipulation of bone tissue. Considering the prosthetic planning, even if the implant had been adequately placed in the apicocoronal and buccopalatal direction, the prosthetic resolution for the implant in the site of tooth 12 would be a distal cantilever of tooth 13. This is a controversial option from a mechanical and biological point of view [18]. Another option could have been a fixed partial denture using the implant abutment in the site of tooth 12 and a tooth abutment on tooth 14, which was also not considered as the first choice [19, 20]. The surgeon was then asked to place the new implant in the mesiodistal direction, closest to tooth 14, in the position of tooth 13, to serve as an abutment for a mesial cantilever prosthesis in the site of tooth 12, avoiding the trauma caused by the placement of another implant [21]. In addition, studies have shown that the lateral incisor had the thinnest alveolar ridge compared to the central incisor and cuspid, probably due to the presence of the lateral fossa which creates the buccal concavity adjacent to the lateral incisor [15].

Regarding the immediate provisionalization, because the temporary prosthesis was retained only by tooth 11, its main objective was the patient's satisfaction with the esthetics during the period of osseointegration [1, 22] despite some benefit in preserving the tissue integrity. It is important to emphasize that this temporary restoration presented no functional characteristic. In other words, occlusal loads were not incident on it, and after second stage surgery, the prosthesis was adjusted and additionally retained on the healing cap.

After the osseointegration period and during the prosthetic treatment, the alignment of the gingival height and adequate conformation of the gingival papilla between the first right upper premolar and the implant were verified. According to Buser et al. [1], the harmony of the gingival margins around the implant and the adjacent tooth requires sufficient height and thickness of the bone, mainly in the buccal side, which was verified in the present case. However, in the cantilever region, there was a need for tissue conditioning by the gradual addition of self-curing resin, giving an oval characteristic to the pontic of the provisional prosthetic restoration to conform to the underlying soft tissue. As bone and connective tissue grafts were not performed, the shape of the interproximal papilla was not completely reestablished. It was necessary to modify the interproximal contact from point to facet of contact with the goal of reducing the

black triangle and improving the esthetics of the region, as suggested by Jivraj and Chee [3].

The maxillary anterior region may be the implant site that requires the most rigorous preoperative assessment [15]. In the present case, the esthetic result was satisfactory, mainly when compared with the initial aspect, even with no bone or soft tissue graft procedures. Two other factors should be considered in a treatment and not only the result of the treatment itself [7]: (1) the economic condition of the patient because of the cost of sophisticated procedures and exams, and (2) the patient satisfaction with the final result of the treatment. Still, according to Stajčić et al. [4], studies have shown that there is no definitive evidence in improving esthetics with the use of bone and soft tissue grafts, justifying the option of the selected treatment. Furthermore, in the present case, the economic condition of the patient was considered as important.

Another important aspect was the position of the new implant, in the mesiodistal direction closest to tooth 14. This allowed the placement of a mesial cantilever that is more favorable to the occlusal loads than a distal cantilever [3], and the screw-type prosthesis is more easily retrievable than the cemented type and, therefore, technical and sometimes biological complications can be treated more easily [23].

4. Conclusion

Regardless of the cause, when an implant is not well positioned, prosthetic rehabilitation may not be mechanically, functionally, and esthetically adequate, and may even be impracticable to perform. In the case presented here, the removal of the implant and new surgical and prosthetic planning were necessary. Despite the esthetic limitations of the resulting prosthetic rehabilitation, considering that no bone and soft tissue grafting has been performed, it was in agreement with the expectations of the patient and the prosthodontist.

References

[1] D. Buser, W. Martin, and U. C. Belser, "Optimizing esthetics for implant restorations in the anterior maxilla: anatomic and surgical considerations," *International Journal of Oral & Maxillofacial Implants*, vol. 19, no. 7, pp. 43–61, 2004.

[2] O. D. Moráguez, F. Vailati, and U. C. Belser, "Malpositioned implants in the anterior maxilla: a novel restorative approach to reestablish peri-implant tissue health and acceptable esthetics. Part II: case report and discussion," *Journal of Esthetic Dentistry*, vol. 10, no. 4, pp. 522–533, 2015.

[3] S. Jivraj and W. Chee, "Treatment planning of implants in the aesthetic zone," *British Dental Journal*, vol. 201, no. 2, pp. 77–89, 2006.

[4] Z. Stajčić, L. J. Stojčev Stajčić, M. Kalanović, A. Đinić, N. Divekar, and M. Rodić, "Removal of dental implants: review of five different techniques," *International Journal of Oral & Maxillofacial Surgery*, vol. 45, no. 5, pp. 641–648, 2016.

[5] Y. Kim, B. Kim, H. Lee, J. Hwang, and P. Yun, "Surgical repositioning of an unrestorable implant using a trephine bur: a

case report," *International Journal of Periodontics & Restorative Dentistry*, vol. 30, no. 2, pp. 181–185, 2010.

[6] S.-R. Jung, J. D. Bashutski, and M. L. Linebaugh, "Application of modified bony lid technique to remove or replace compromised implants: case series," *Implant Dentistry*, vol. 22, no. 3, pp. 206–211, 2013.

[7] J. L. Rumfola, S. Andreana, L. Colucci, and Y. Tsay, "Restoring unfavorably positioned implants in anterior maxilla: case report," *New York State Dental Journal*, vol. 79, no. 5, pp. 40–44, 2013.

[8] C. H. Li and C. T. Chou, "Bone sparing implant removal without trephine via internal separation of the titanium body with a carbide bur," *International Journal of Oral & Maxillofacial Surgery*, vol. 43, no. 2, pp. 248–250, 2014.

[9] W. Chee and S. Jivraj, "Failures in implant dentistry," *British Dental Journal*, vol. 202, no. 3, pp. 123–129, 2007.

[10] F. I. Muroff, "Removal and replacement of a fractured dental implant: case report," *Implant Dentistry*, vol. 12, no. 3, pp. 206–210, 2003.

[11] J.-B. Lee, "Selectable implant removal methods due to mechanical and biological failures," *Case Reports in Dentistry*, vol. 2017, Article ID 9640517, 7 pages, 2017.

[12] G. E. Romanos, B. Gupta, and S. E. Eckert, "Distal cantilevers and implant dentistry," *International Journal of Oral & Maxillofacial Implants*, vol. 27, no. 5, pp. 1131–1136, 2012.

[13] T. L. Schlumberger, J. F. Bowley, and G. I. Maze, "Intrusion phenomenon in combination tooth-implant restorations: a review of the literature," *Journal of Prosthetic Dentistry*, vol. 80, no. 2, pp. 199–203, 1998.

[14] C. M. Becker, D. A. Kaiser, and J. D. Jones, "Guidelines for splinting implants," *Journal of Prosthetic Dentistry*, vol. 84, no. 2, pp. 210–214, 2000.

[15] L. Levin, "Dealing with dental implant failures," *Journal of Applied Oral Science*, vol. 16, no. 3, pp. 171–175, 2008.

[16] G. J. Conte, P. Rhodes, D. Richards, and R. T. Kao, "Considerations for anterior implant esthetics," *Journal of the California Dental Association*, vol. 130, no. 7, pp. 528–534, 2002.

[17] M. Colombo, C. Mangano, E. Mijiritsky, M. Krebs, U. Hauschild, and T. Fortin, "Clinical applications and effectiveness of guided implant surgery: a critical review based on randomized controlled trials," *BMC Oral Health*, vol. 17, no. 1, p. 150, 2017.

[18] T. Testori, T. Weinstein, F. Scutella, H. L. Wang, and G. Zucchelli, "Implant placement in the esthetic area: criteria for positioning single and multiple implants," *Periodontology 2000*, vol. 77, no. 1, pp. 176–196, 2018.

[19] F. G. Mangano, P. Mastrangelo, F. Luongo, A. Blay, S. Tunchel, and C. Mangano, "Aesthetic outcome of immediately restored single implants placed in extraction sockets and healed sites of the anterior maxilla: a retrospective study on 103 patients with 3 years of follow-up," *Clinical Oral Implants Research*, vol. 28, no. 3, pp. 272–282, 2017.

[20] W. Zhang, A. Skrypczak, and R. Weltman, "Anterior maxilla alveolar ridge dimension and morphology measurement by cone beam computerized tomography (CBCT) for immediate implant treatment planning," *BMC Oral Health*, vol. 15, no. 1, p. 65, 2015.

[21] N. Khzam, H. Arora, P. Kim, A. Fisher, N. Mattheos, and S. Ivanovski, "Systematic review of soft tissue alterations and esthetic outcomes following immediate implant placement and restoration of single implants in the anterior maxilla," *Journal of Periodontology*, vol. 86, no. 12, pp. 1321–1330, 2015.

[22] W. G. Van Nimwegen, G. M. Raghoebar, N. Tymstra, A. Vissink, and H. J. A. Meijer, "How to treat two adjacent missing teeth with dental implants. A systematic review on single implant-supported two-unit cantilever FDP's and results of a 5-year prospective comparative study in the aesthetic zone," *Journal of Oral Rehabilitation*, vol. 44, no. 6, pp. 461–471, 2017.

[23] I. Sailer, S. Mühlemann, M. Zwahlen, C. H. F. Hämmerle, and D. Schneider, "Cemented and screw-retained implant reconstructions: a systematic review of the survival and complication rates," *Clinical Oral Implants Research*, vol. 23, no. 6, pp. 163–201, 2012.

34

Partial Mandibulectomy Rehabilitation of Keratocystic Odontogenic Tumour Case in Neutral Zone

Mohamad Syahrizal Halim ⓘ[1] **and Tengku Fazrina Tengku Mohd Ariff**[2]

[1]*Conservative Dentistry Unit, School of Dental Sciences, Universiti Sains Malaysia, Health Campus, 16150 Kota Bharu, Kelantan, Malaysia*
[2]*Centre for Restorative Dentistry Studies, Faculty of Dentistry, Jalan Hospital, Universiti Teknologi MARA, Sungai Buloh Campus, 47000 Sungai Buloh, Selangor Darul Ehsan, Malaysia*

Correspondence should be addressed to Mohamad Syahrizal Halim; drmatchah@yahoo.com

Academic Editor: Luis M. J. Gutierrez

Restoring the patient's missing dentition secondary to partial mandibulectomy of KCOT is important to improve function and aesthetics. The patient presented with a significant loss of alveolar bone which makes the fabrication of rehabilitation prosthesis a significant challenge. A neutral-zone impression technique is helpful in determining the exact space to be restored without compromising aesthetics and it avoids functional muscle displacement that may displace the prosthesis. This article describes the neutral zone impression technique to record a patient's functional muscular movement in guiding the setting of acrylic teeth and denture flange in the neutral zone area. This technique is very useful for postsurgical cases with significant loss of alveolar bone.

1. Introduction

Keratocystic odontogenic tumour (KCOT) is a benign intraosseous neoplasm which can occur in a unicystic or multicystic form and originate from odontogenic tissue [1]. Originally known as an odontogenic keratocyst, WHO has reclassified this lesion into a new name to reflect the aggressive nature of this benign neoplasm. Its aggressive and infiltrative behaviour is due to its propensity to grow inside the jaws, with minimal expansion [2]. These features warrant aggressive surgical removal to prevent recurrence of the lesion.

KCOT surgical treatment may cause the patient to have functional and aesthetic problems. This is due to the aggressive surgical treatment performed by the surgeon which includes at least 2 mm surgical removal from the margin's lesion. This is done to prevent recurrence as the lesion can infiltrate the head and neck bone. The overall rate of occurrences of postsurgical treatment of KCOT are 23.09% [3].

Rehabilitation of patient postsurgical segmental mandibulectomy gives significant challenges to a dentist. The patient may present with a significant loss in vertical and horizontal alveolar bone which will make the fabrication of rehabilitation prosthesis a setback. After a surgical procedure, the patient is left with a space that used to be occupied with teeth and alveolus. This loss in space will allow the tongue and buccal mucosa tissue to occupy the space which will make the neutral zone smaller. A problem may also arise since there is no alveolar ridge to serve as a guide in the placement of the prosthetic teeth during acrylic denture setting. Minute displacement in the functional space will compromise denture stability, disturb patient speech, and interfere with patient masticatory function.

Preferably, the loss in vertical and horizontal bone should be replaced with vascularized bone graft or alloplastic material, which may involve another surgery for the former graft. Most of the patients who have been diagnosed with this neoplasm are reluctant to undergo through the surgical and emotional stress from another surgery. So this method of rehabilitation by removable of a partial denture recorded in the neutral zone is an alternative for patients who refuse such emotional and physical stress. This method will also serve as an interim prosthesis before future implant treatment consideration.

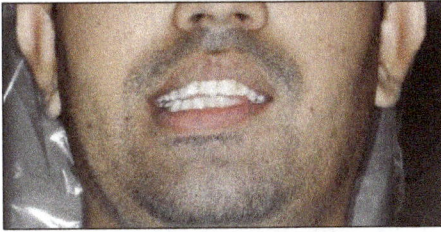

FIGURE 1: Facial profile at initial presentation.

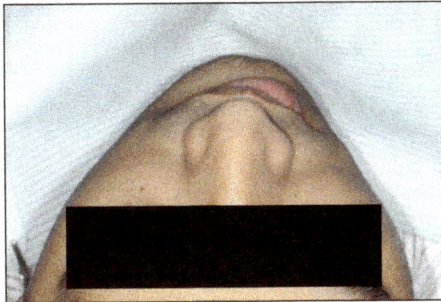

FIGURE 2: Coronal view profile at initial presentation.

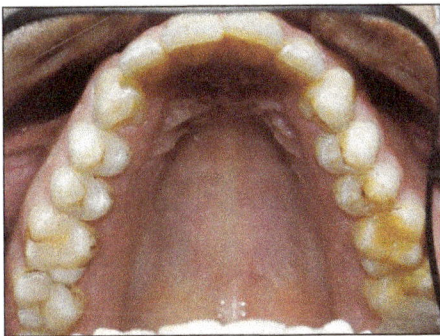

FIGURE 3: Preoperative maxillary occlusal view.

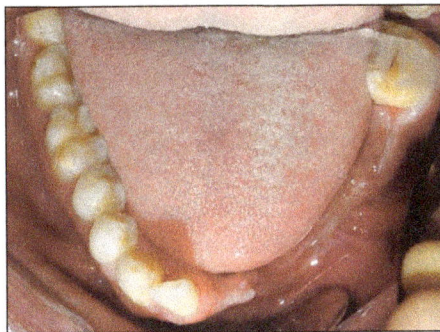

FIGURE 4: Preoperative mandibular occlusal view, note the tongue occupying the edentulous area.

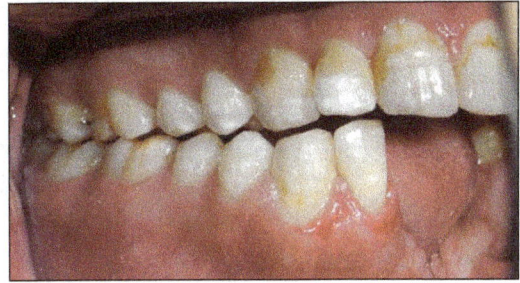

FIGURE 5: Preoperative right buccal view at maximum intercuspation.

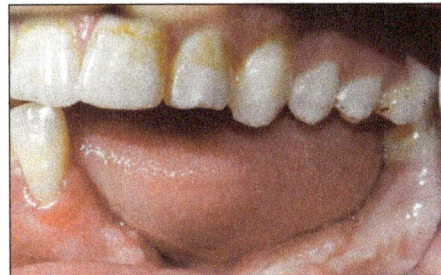

FIGURE 6: Left buccal view at maximum intercuspation. Note the tongue occupying the edentulous space.

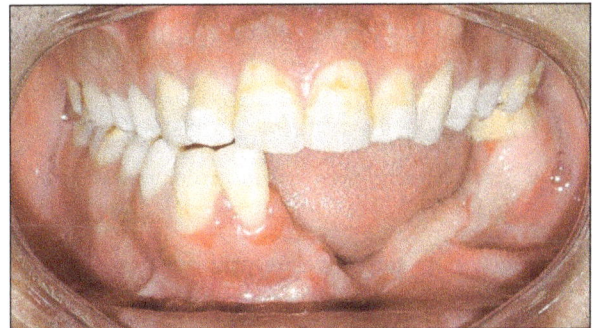

FIGURE 7: Preoperative frontal view with teeth at maximum intercuspation.

The purpose of this paper is to highlight the importance of the neutral zone for a mandibular partial denture in the rehabilitation of partial mandibulectomy of KCOT. This ensures that the polished surface of the denture does not encroach the functional movement on the lingual and buccal musculature and eventually minimizes denture displacement.

1.1. Case. A 29-year-old Pakistani male was referred to the Oral Surgery Department for rehabilitation of the left edentulous mandible secondary to partial mandibulectomy surgery. He had undergone two operations for the left body of a mandible keratocyst odontogenic tumour (KCOT). The patient has been diagnosed with (KCOT) in Pakistan, where he received his first surgical treatment. A second surgical partial mandibulectomy was attempted due to recurrence. He has been reviewed regularly and he requested to have a replacement of his missing teeth on the lower left side due to a difficulty in eating and the effect on his appearance (Figure 1).

Clinical examination reveals an asymmetrical face with a slightly depressed left lower body of the mandible on a class I skeletal pattern (Figures 1 and 2). The patient reported an absence of paraesthesia on the left mandible.

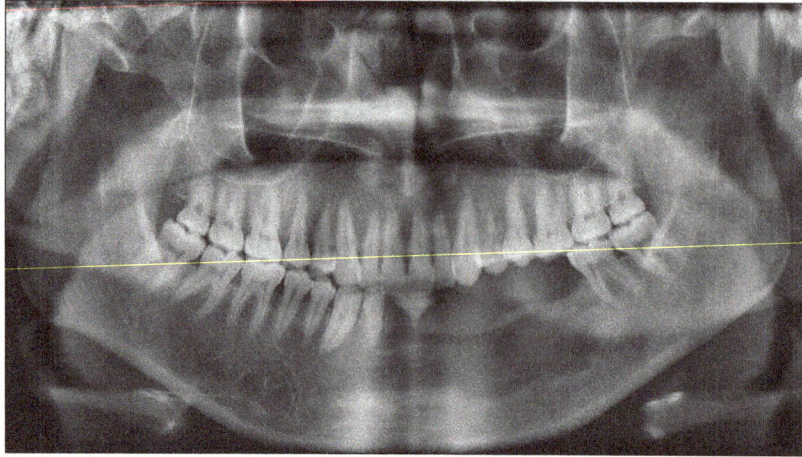

FIGURE 8: Orthopantomogram.

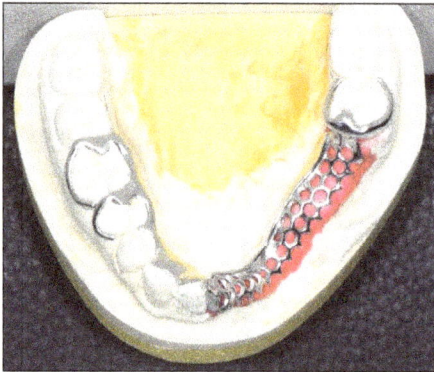

FIGURE 9: Cobalt-chrome frame constructed on the working model.

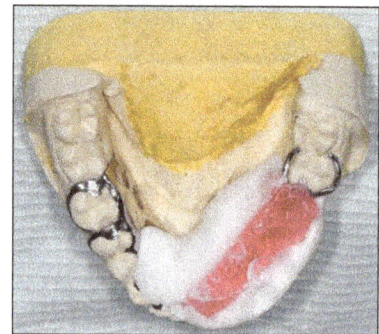

FIGURE 12: The obtained functional impression.

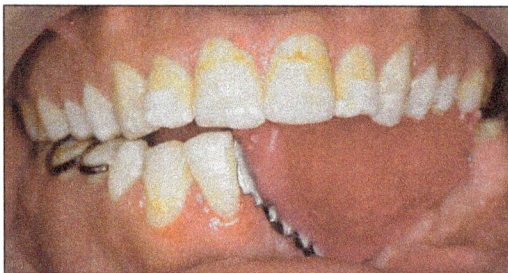

FIGURE 10: Wax bite record.

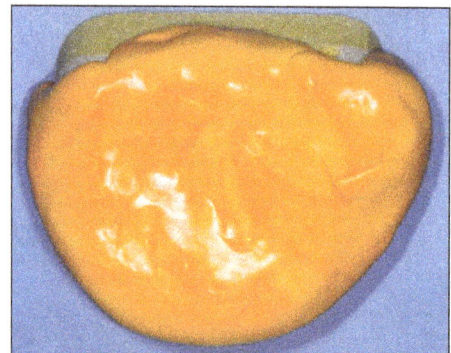

FIGURE 13: Putty index to serve as a guide for the arrangement of acrylic teeth.

The smile line was high exposing the gingiva on the upper maxillary incisors.

Intraorally, the oral hygiene was fair with the presence of mild gingivitis. The dentition on the maxillary arch was unrestored (Figure 3). The left edentulous mandible was irregular basal bone with firm mucosa covering the bone from 41 until 37. There were marked loss of bony structure horizontally and vertically. This has caused the tongue to occupy the space that used to be occupied by

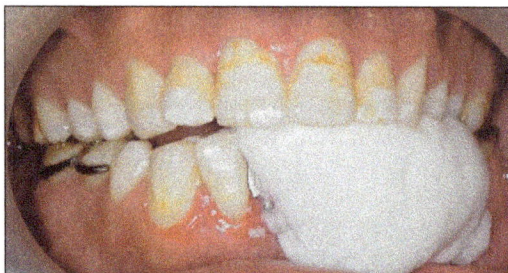

FIGURE 11: Functional impression obtained to record the neutral zone.

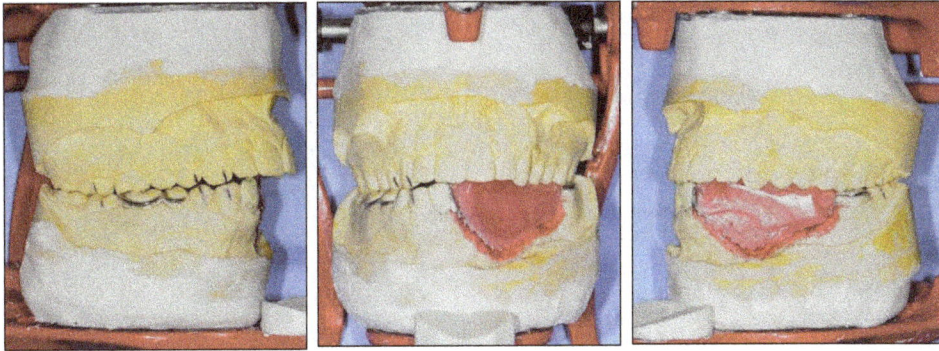

FIGURE 14: Working model with bite registration mounted on an articulator.

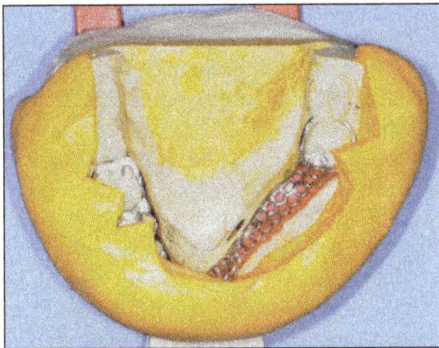

FIGURE 15: The sectioned putty index showing space for teeth arrangement within the neutral zone.

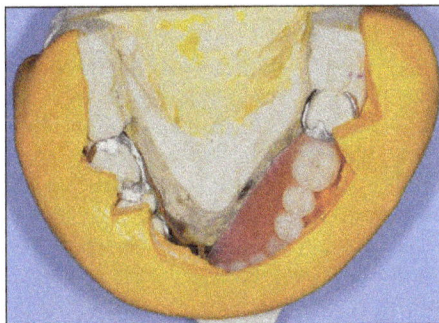

FIGURE 16: Teeth arranged in the neutral zone.

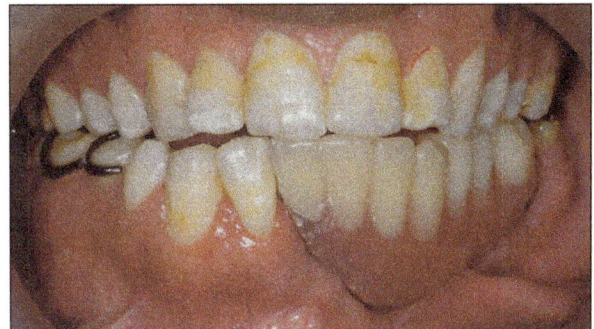

FIGURE 17: Intraoral facial view at ICP.

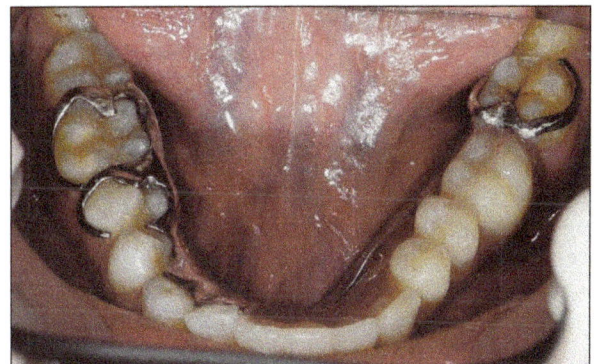

FIGURE 18: Occlusal view of prosthesis intraorally.

teeth and alveolus in the left mandibular segment (Figures 4, 5, and 6). The healing of the operation site was uneventful (Figures 6 and 7).

An orthopantomogram was taken to evaluate the remaining bony structure of the mandible (Figure 8). Radiographically, the operation site (lower left posterior segment) has no abnormalities. The remaining basal bone was adequate in thickness to support the mandible with an irregular margin. There are no radiopaque abnormalities suggestive of new pathology.

1.2. Procedures. Primary impression was made using alginate (Kromopan, Lascod, Illinois, USA) to obtain a set of study cast. A special tray was constructed using a light-cured acrylic resin tray material (plaque photo; W + P Dental,

Hamburg, Germany). After border moulding, a secondary impression was taken with a polyether impression (Impregum Penta Soft, 3M-ESPE, Minnesota, USA) and poured with type IV die stone (Vel-Mix, SDS, Kerr, Orange CA) for the construction of the lower cobalt-chrome partial denture frame (Figure 9).

After the framework try-in procedure, the bite was registered with a block of wax (Figure 10). The borders of the wax rim were adjusted so that the lingual flange was harmonized with the resting and active positions of the floor of the mouth. The buccal width extension was also modified to be a little bit short of the reflection of the cheek. Then, a functional impression procedure was made using a tissue conditioner (F.I.T.T., SDS, Kerr, Orange, CA) to record the neutral zone while the patient was instructed to do basic functional movements in the mouth (Figures 11 and 12).

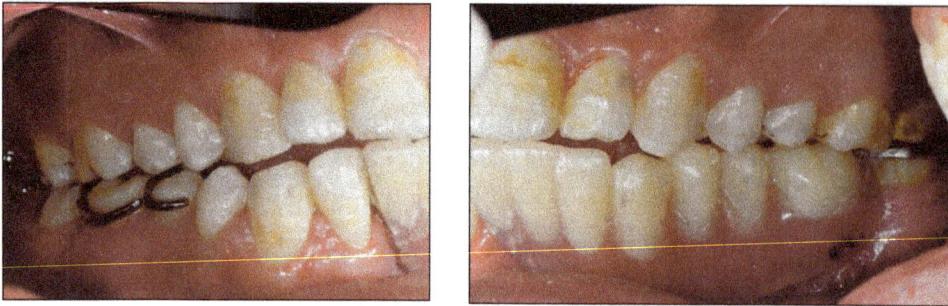

FIGURE 19: Buccal views after prosthesis delivery.

Laboratory putty (Zetaflow Putty, Zhermack SpA, Italy) was then used to record the space obtained from the functional impression (Figure 13). The cast was then mounted (Figure 14) and the putty index was sectioned to visualize the space available for teeth arrangement (Figures 15 and 16). The prosthesis was issued one week after the try-in procedure (Figures 17, 18, and 19).

2. Discussion

The keratocystic odontogenic tumour (KCOT), once known as odontogenic keratocyst (OKC), is a benign unicystic or multicystic odontogenic tumour with an aggressive and infiltrative behavior. It is considered a neoplastic lesion due to its locally destructive behavior, with the basal layer of the KCOT budding through connective tissue [4] and the genetics factor involving the tumour suppressor gene PTCH ("patched") being suppressed [5]. KCOT has also been known to have a high recurrence rate. According to Voorsmit et al. [6] and Irvine and Bowerman [7], the recurrence rate was between 2.5% and 62%. The recurrence rate of KCOT was low when aggressive treatment was done [8]. This happens when the epithelial lining was not completely removed, and this may give rise to new lesion formation. Daughter cells, microcysts, or an epithelial island which may exist in the original walls of the KCOT can contribute to the recurrent lesion [6].

Treatment of KCOT can be divided into conservative and aggressive treatment. Conservative treatment involves enucleation with curettage of marsupialization, which is usually a treatment reserved for a cyst-oriented lesion. Aggressive treatment is usually done using the ostectomy technique and chemical curettage with Carnoy's solution of en bloc resection [9]. The latter technique will result in significant loss of alveolar bone that affects a patient's function as well as aesthetics. In this patient, the alveolar bone loss was vertical as well as horizontal which has left the edentulous site less than ideal for any prosthetic to be emplaced or restorative treatment to be done (Figures 6 and 7).

The patient's left mandibular alveolar bone was completely removed and the basal bone was preserved (Figures 6 and 8). This allows the restorative dentist to have a foundation to start rehabilitation. The basal bone can act as a guide for bone augmentation, and it can also preserve the patient's facial profile. This can minimize the psychological effect due to facial disfigurement after surgical removal of

the lesion and reconstruction. If the left body of the mandible was completely removed, the surgeon needs to reconstruct the defect by an autogenous bone graft from a distant site [10]. Nowadays, a surgeon prefers the use of a vascularized bone graft in mandibular reconstruction since it promises a success rate of up to 90% [11]. The patient was not receiving any bone augmentation since the basal bone was intact.

Several options were given to the patient regarding the rehabilitation of his left mandibular defect. An implant that retained fixed partial dentures is a promising option given its high success rate. Prior to that, the left body of the mandible needs to be augmented to restore the bone height and width to provide a sound platform for placement. This is to ensure that the implant is not subjected to a high-tipping force resulting from an increased coronal : root ratio in implant restoration. Since the recurrence rate of KCOT was high, it is wise to defer the implant treatment and observe for any sign of recurrence. The recurrence of KCOT can take place up to 5–7 years after treatment [9] and prolonged follow-up is crucial. The patient wished to have a long-term provisional replacement for his missing teeth on the left of the mandible and a cobalt-chrome partial denture was suggested. The cobalt-chrome partial denture was chosen due to the rigidity of the framework and superior surface polishability compared to an acrylic partial denture. The partial denture can also serve as a template for bone augmentation and for the placement of future implants. The partial denture can restore the function of the patient and will improve his aesthetics and confidence in dealing with society (Figure 20).

In this patient, a partial denture needs to be constructed in a neutral zone, a space that is free of muscle movement. This space is a result of a balanced interaction between the tongue's outward movement together with buccal mucosa and lip inward movement during this function [12]. By placing the denture teeth and flange in the neutral zone, this can avoid breaching the buccal space occupied by the cheek and lip as well as the lingual space occupied by the tongue, creating a partial denture that exists in muscle balance. Although this practice can usually be done on a full lower denture, in this case since the alveolar bone has a marked loss in the vertical and horizontal direction together with a collapsed left lip and reduced cheek support, the neutral-zone impression serves as a guide for teeth arrangement.

Upon issue of the lower partial denture, the patient was very satisfied with the result. He was happy to have his lower

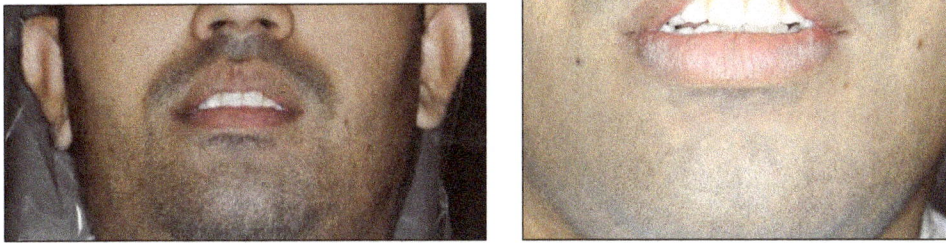

FIGURE 20: Postoperative photograph. Note that the collapse of the buccal cheek has been restored symmetrically.

lip and cheek restored to the original contour and was satis-fied with his smile (Figure 20). He was able to eat comfortably with the partial denture. His speech was improved after the prosthesis was issued. The patient was given instructions to maintain good oral hygiene and to observe the left edentu-lous site for any sign of recurrence or to report any sign and symptom immediately for further management. He was given a follow-up review every six months.

3. Conclusions

In the present case, we demonstrate the construction of a removable partial denture recorded at a neutral zone result-ing in an adequate restoration of a patient's aesthetics and function with minimal displacement from the normal soft tissue movement. The neutral-zone impression technique also allows a dental technician to arrange the acrylic teeth in an area with minimal deviation. The marked loss of alveolar bone secondary to surgical removal can give diffi-culty to the technician to arrange acrylic teeth in the actual position, which can later cause discomfort to the patient and may result in partial denture instability.

References

[1] H. Philipsen, D. Gardner, K. Heikinheimo et al., "Pathology and genetics of head and neck tumours," *World Health Orga-nization Classfication of Tumours*, vol. 9, pp. 296–300, 2005.

[2] S. C. White and M. J. Pharoah, "Oral radiology—e-book: principles and interpretation," in *Elsevier Health Sciences*, pp. 351–355, Elsevier, 2014.

[3] T. Kaczmarzyk, I. Mojsa, and J. Stypulkowska, "A systematic review of the recurrence rate for keratocystic odontogenic tumour in relation to treatment modalities," *International Journal of Oral & Maxillofacial Surgery*, vol. 41, no. 6, pp. 756–767, 2012.

[4] E. Ahlfors, Å. Larsson, and S. Sjögren, "The odontogenic keratocyst: a benign cystic tumor?," *Journal of Oral and Maxillofacial Surgery*, vol. 42, no. 1, pp. 10–19, 1984.

[5] M. Michael Cohen Jr., "Nevoid basal cell carcinoma syndrome: molecular biology and new hypotheses," *International Journal of oral and Maxillofacial Surgery*, vol. 28, no. 3, pp. 216–223, 1999.

[6] R. A. C. A. Voorsmit, P. J. W. Stoelinga, and U. J. G. M. van Haelst, "The management of keratocysts," *Journal of Maxillo-facial Surgery*, vol. 9, no. 4, pp. 228–236, 1981.

[7] G. H. Irvine and J. E. Bowerman, "Mandibular keratocysts: surgical management," *British Journal of Oral and Maxillofa-cial Surgery*, vol. 23, no. 3, pp. 204–209, 1985.

[8] J. Madras and H. Lapointe, "Keratocystic odontogenic tumour: reclassification of the odontogenic keratocyst from cyst to tumour," *Texas Dental Journal*, vol. 125, no. 5, pp. 446–454, 2008.

[9] T. A. Morgan, C. C. Burton, and F. Qian, "A retrospective review of treatment of the odontogenic keratocyst," *Journal of Oral and Maxillofacial Surgery*, vol. 63, no. 5, pp. 635–639, 2005.

[10] R. Marx, "Philosophy and particulars of autogenous bone grafting," *Oral and Maxillofacial Surgery Clinics of North America*, vol. 5, pp. 599–612, 1993.

[11] D. A. Hidalgo and A. L. Pusic, "Free-flap mandibular reconstruction: a 10-year follow-up study," *Evaluation*, vol. 21, no. 639, 1999.

[12] A. G. Wee, R. B. Cwynar, and A. C. Cheng, "Utilization of the neutral zone technique for a maxillofacial patient," *Journal of Prosthodontics*, vol. 9, no. 1, pp. 2–7, 2000.

35

Clinical and Radiographic Success of Selective Caries Removal to Firm Dentin in Primary Teeth: 18-Month Follow-Up

Tássia Carina Stafuzza,[1] Luciana Lourenço Ribeiro Vitor (iD),[1] Daniela Rios (iD),[1] Thiago Cruvinel Silva (iD),[1] Maria Aparecida Andrade Moreira Machado (iD),[1,2] and Thais Marchini Oliveira (iD)[1,2]

[1]Department of Pediatric Dentistry, Orthodontics, Public Health, Bauru School of Dentistry, University of São Paulo, Bauru, SP, Brazil
[2]Hospital for the Rehabilitation of Craniofacial Anomalies, University of São Paulo, Bauru, SP, Brazil

Correspondence should be addressed to Thais Marchini Oliveira; marchini@usp.br

Academic Editor: Ali I. Abdalla

The selective caries removal is increasingly spreading in daily clinical practice because this minimally invasive technique treats deep carious lesion and decreases the risk of pulp exposure. This case report was aimed at describing the selective removal to firm dentin on the primary mandibular left first molar of a girl aged 7 years and 6 months. The Mineral Trioxide Aggregate (MTA Angelus™) was used as liner, and the tooth was definitively restored with resin-modified glass ionomer cement (Vitremer™). The clinical and radiographic following-up was performed at 6, 12, and 18 months after treatment. The treatment showed satisfactory results after 18-month following-up, suggesting that this minimally invasive approach for carious lesion removal can replace the total removal, when properly indicated. Notwithstanding, further randomized clinical trials with longer following-up periods are still necessary.

1. Introduction

Currently the literature reports many studies on selective caries removal [1–6]. The selective removal to firm dentin [7] enables the change in the carious lesion microenvironment, decreases the number and bacterial diversity which stops the carious lesion progression, reduces the risk of pulp exposure [8], and preserves pulp vitality [6]. Although growing evidences indicate that minimally invasive approaches are effective to treat carious lesions [9], selective caries removal success may depend on the appropriate use of liners and restorative materials.

Many bacteriostatic, bactericidal, and remineralizing materials can be applied to the remaining dentin after selective caries removal [1, 10], but no consensus exist on which liner would be the most suitable for teeth undergoing selective caries removal [5, 10]. Randomized clinical trials and systematic reviews are necessary to clarify the persistent doubts.

Faced with this reality, caries tissue management techniques have been widely discussed [5, 9, 11]. Thus, this case report describes the selective removal to firm dentin in the primary mandibular left first molar of a girl aged 7 years and 6 months using the Mineral Trioxide Aggregate (MTA Angelus) as a pulp protective material.

2. Case Report

A girl aged 7 years and 6 months searched treatment at the Pediatric Dentistry Clinic of the Bauru School of Dentistry, University of São Paulo. During the anamnesis, the mother reported no spontaneous pain in the primary mandibular left first molar what was confirmed by the girl during the clinical examination. In the clinical and radiographic examination, the presence of deep occlusal carious lesion close to the pulp was observed (Figures 1(a) and 1(b)).

First, topical anesthesia was performed with benzocaine (Benzotop DFL) applied to the previously dried mucosa with

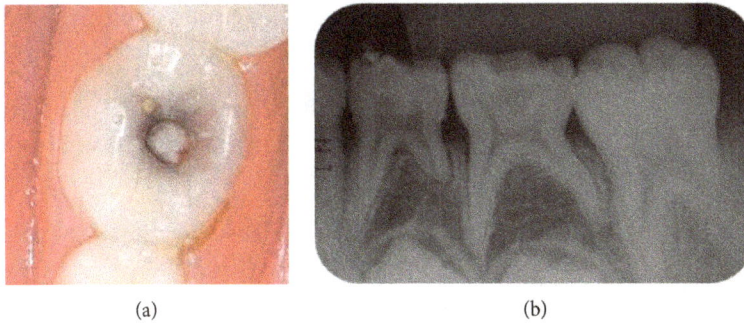

FIGURE 1: (a) Initial clinical aspect of the primary mandibular left first molar. (b) Initial periapical radiograph of the primary mandibular left first molar. Note the proximity of the carious lesion to the pulp.

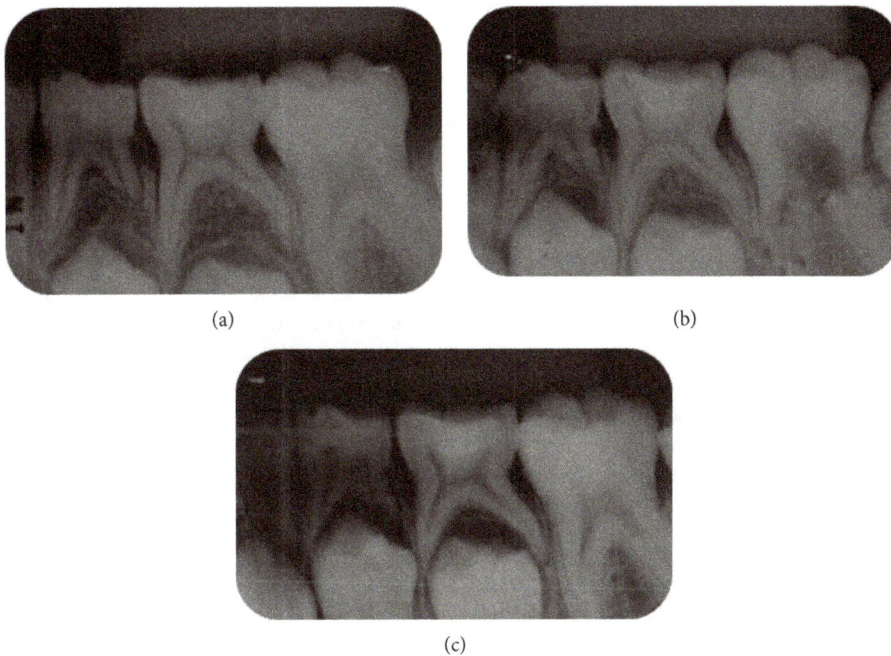

FIGURE 2: Radiographic following-up: (a) 6 months, (b) 12 months, and (c) 18 months.

the aid of a cotton pellet. Local infiltrative anesthesia of inferior alveolar nerve was performed with articaine 4% and epinephrine 1 : 100.000 [12–15]. After rubber dam isolation, the total caries removal was performed on the lateral walls of the cavity with low-speed round burs (sizes 4, 5, and 6, KG Sorensen, São Paulo, Brazil). Selective caries removal was executed on pulpal wall with hand excavators until firm dentin, and it was possible to observe that the remaining dentin had a darker color and leathery consistency. Before applying the protective material, the cavity was cleaned and dried with sterile cotton pellet. The MTA (Angelus, Londrina, PR, Brazil) was mixed according to the manufacturer's in-structions on a sterile glass plate and directly placed on the pulpal wall reaching a thickness of 2 mm. The resin-modified glass ionomer cement (RMGIC) (Vitremer, 3M/ESPE, Min-nesota, USA) was mixed at 1 : 1 powder/liquid ratio and applied to the cavity with a Centrix syringe (Centrix™, Nova DFL, Taquara, Rio de Janeiro, RJ, Brazil). At the end, the patient's occlusion was checked.

During the 18-month following-up period, no pain, mo-bility, sensitivity to percussion, abscess/fistula, restoration failure (such as partial fracture or loss of restoration), internal/external resorption, signs of furcal impairment, and advanced rhizolysis stage were observed (Figures 2(a)–Figures 2(c) and 3).

3. Discussion

With the diagnosis of deep caries lesion without pulp in-volvement, there were two possible treatment options: total or selective caries removal. Total caries removal could lead to pulp exposure. In addition, the removal of all carious dentin from the cavity is no longer necessary to manage the carious lesion [9]. So, for this case, we choose the selective caries removal to avoid greater damage to the tooth [1–3, 9] and to minimize the potential complications of complete excava-tion of carious dentin close to the pulp by avoiding pul-potomy and a breach in the pulp [1–3].

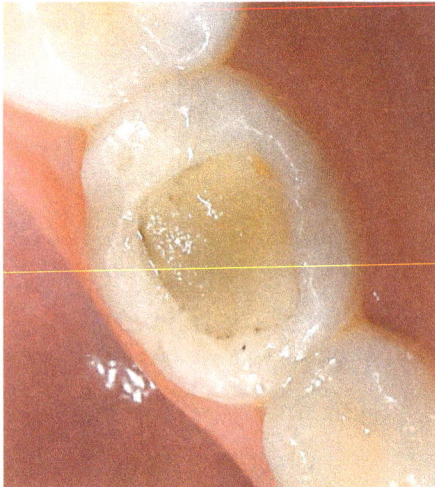

FIGURE 3: Clinical aspect at 18 months of follow-up.

Another advantage of the proposed treatment is the permanence of the primary teeth in the oral cavity until its natural exfoliation period [16], a fact that should be highlighted in the dental treatment of children. In this case report, the patient was seven and a half years old, which suggests that the primary molar will remain for at least 3-4 years in her mouth. With all this preexfoliation time, it has become imperative to perform a minimally invasive treatment that preserves the prognosis of dental longevity.

Scientific evidence reported significant chemical and morphological differences between dentin in permanent and primary teeth. The diameter of the dentinal tubules is larger in the primary teeth. This structural feature suggests that primary teeth may be more susceptible to sensitivity and transmission of harmful substances to pulp [17]. Thus, to ensure a correct indication of the therapy, the first primary molar treated in this case report did not present painful symptomatology, periapical lesion, fistula, or abscess, keys to success in minimally invasive dentistry.

The carious dentin is divided into two parts: the outermost part, infected dentin, which must be removed, and the innermost part, affected dentin, which should be preserved because it can be remineralized [18]. The main difficulty of selective removal to firm dentin is the subjective criteria to evaluate the amount of carious tissue to be removed [3]. To overcome this problem, the literature has determined that the best guide to be given is the operator's tactile feel [7]. In this case report, the dentin was removed until a harder tissue with leather consistency was found based on tactile perception of the operator [3, 7]. No caries detector dye was used.

The ideal liner to be placed on the remaining dentin after selective caries removal is still a subject that raises many doubts. Good results were obtained in studies that used calcium hydroxide as liner material [19–22], but the histological evaluation demonstrated that a lower inflammation and hyperemia of pulp and a thicker dentin bridge with formation of odontoblastic layer are more frequent with the use of MTA [23]. It can maintain the vitality of the remaining pulp, allowing it to continue to exhibit normal physiological functions [24, 25]. Thus, current clinical trials should evaluate the combined effect of carious tissue removal strategies with restorative procedures, including the use of liners [5]. MTA is a biocompatible material with satisfactory physical and chemical properties [24], and it has been constantly used in indirect pulp treatments of permanent and primary teeth [1, 26, 27, 28].

Currently, the literature lacks scientific evidence on the suitable restorative material for selective removal to firm dentin. Thus, ionomeric cements were chosen because they are less sensitive to the technique and can be placed in the cavity in only one increment [29]. Furthermore, RMGIC enables repair in case of failures in the restorations, assuring the minimally invasive approach [29].

In this case report, we applied a methodology standardized by the literature to evaluate the dentin-pulp complex response [1, 4]. Clinical and radiographic follow-up was performed at 6, 12, and 18 months [15]; however, other studies have follow-up times with longer evaluation periods [2, 3, 6]. In this way, the follow-up of this clinical case will continue to be performed.

The satisfactory outcomes of this case report agree with those reported by the literature evidencing that the sealed dentin is capable of remineralizing due to changes in the microenvironment [2] caused by the lack of substrates for the bacteria [3, 30]. Thus, new strategies for the management of the carious tissue may target alternative approaches in the treatment of the most advanced stages of the carious lesion, especially with benefits for the children.

Consent

Informed consent was obtained from all individual participants included in the study.

References

[1] M. A. Petrou, F. A. Alhamoui, A. Welk, M. B. Altarabulsi, M. H. Alkilzy, and C. Splieth, "A randomized clinical trial on the use of medical Portland cement, MTA and calcium hydroxide in indirect pulp treatment," *Clinical Oral Investigations*, vol. 18, no. 5, pp. 1383–1389, 2013.

[2] D. M. Dalpian, T. M. Ardenghi, F. F. Demarco, F. Garcia-Godoy, F. B. de Araujo, and L. Casagrande, "Clinical and radiographic outcomes of partial caries removal restorations performed in primary teeth," *American Journal of Dentistry*, vol. 27, no. 2, pp. 68–72, 2014.

[3] R. Franzon, L. F. Guimaraes, C. E. Magalhaes, A. N. Haas, and F. B. Araujo, "Outcomes of one-step incomplete and complete excavation in primary teeth: a 24-month randomized controlled trial," *Caries Research*, vol. 48, no. 5, pp. 376–383, 2014.

[4] F. Schwendicke, H. Schweigel, M. A. Petrou et al., "Selective or stepwise removal of deep caries in deciduous molars: study protocol for a randomized controlled trial," *Trials*, vol. 16, no. 1, p. 10, 2015.

[5] F. Schwendicke, J. E. Frencken, L. Bjørndal et al., "Managing carious lesions: consensus recommendations on carious tissue

removal," *Advances in Dental Research*, vol. 28, no. 2, pp. 58–67, 2016.

[6] R. Brignardello-Petersen, "Stepwise and partial caries removal probably have high success rates up to 3 years after treatment of deep carious lesions, but partial caries removal is more likely to preserve tooth vitality," *Journal of the American Dental Association*, vol. 148, no. 4, p. e38, 2017.

[7] N. P. Innes, J. E. Frencken, L. Bjørndal et al., "Managing carious lesions: consensus recommendations on terminology," *Advances in Dental Research*, vol. 28, no. 2, pp. 49–57, 2016.

[8] D. Ricketts, T. Lamont, N. P. T. Innes, E. Kidd, and J. E. Clarkson, "Operative caries management in adults and children," *Cochrane Database of Systematic Reviews*, vol. 28, no. 3, p. CD003808, 2013.

[9] F. Schwendicke, "Contemporary concepts in carious tissue removal: a review," *Journal of Esthetic and Restorative Dentistry*, vol. 29, no. 6, pp. 404–408, 2017.

[10] M. A. Pereira, R. B. D. Santos-Júnior, J. A. Tavares et al., "No additional benefit of using a calcium hydroxide liner during stepwise caries removal: a randomized clinical trial," *Journal of the American Dental Association*, vol. 148, no. 6, pp. 369–376, 2017.

[11] J. E. Frencken, N. P. Innes, and F. Schwendicke, "Managing carious lesions: why do we need consensus on terminology and clinical recommendations on carious tissue removal?," *Advances in Dental Research*, vol. 28, no. 2, pp. 46–48, 2016.

[12] A. P. Fernandes, N. Lourenço Neto, N. C. Teixeira Marques et al., "Clinical and radiographic outcomes of the use of Low-Level Laser Therapy in vital pulp of primary teeth," *International Journal of Paediatric Dentistry*, vol. 25, no. 2, pp. 144–150, 2015.

[13] N. Lourenço Neto, N. C. Marques, A. P. Fernandes et al., "Clinical and radiographic evaluation of Portland cement added to radiopacifying agents in primary molar pulpotomies," *European Archives of Paediatric Dentistry*, vol. 16, no. 5, pp. 377–382, 2015.

[14] N. C. Marques, N. L. Neto, C. de Oliveira Rodini et al., "Low-level laser therapy as an alternative for pulpotomy in human primary teeth," *Lasers in Medical Science*, vol. 30, no. 7, pp. 1815–1822, 2015.

[15] B. Z. Mello, T. C. Stafuzza, L. L. Vitor, D. Rios, M. A. Machado, and T. M. Oliveira, "Alternative approach for carious tissue removal in primary teeth," *European Archives of Paediatric Dentistry*, vol. 17, no. 5, pp. 413–417, 2016.

[16] N. P. Innes and D. J. Evans, "Modern approaches to caries management of the primary dentition," *British Dental Journal*, vol. 214, no. 11, pp. 559–566, 2013.

[17] D. A. Sumikawa, G. W. Marshall, L. Gee, and S. J. Marshall, "Microstructure of primary tooth dentin," *Pediatric Dentistry*, vol. 21, no. 7, pp. 439–444, 1999.

[18] T. Fusayama, "Two layers of carious dentin; diagnosis and treatment," *Operative Dentistry*, vol. 4, no. 2, pp. 63–70, 1979.

[19] A. E. Bressani, A. A. Mariath, A. N. Haas, F. Garcia-Godoy, and F. B. de Araujo, "Incomplete caries removal and indirect pulp capping in primary molars: a randomized controlled trial," *American Journal of Dentistry*, vol. 26, no. 4, pp. 196–200, 2013.

[20] M. Hayashi, M. Fujitani, C. Yamaki, and Y. Momoi, "Ways of enhancing pulp preservation by stepwise excavation–a systematic review," *Journal of Dentistry*, vol. 39, no. 2, pp. 95–107, 2011.

[21] A. S. Pinto, F. B. De Araujo, R. Franzon et al., "Clinical and microbiological effect of calcium hydroxide protection in indirect pulp capping in primary teeth," *American Journal of Dentistry*, vol. 19, no. 6, pp. 382–386, 2006.

[22] M. J. Tuculina, M. Raescu, I. T. Dascalu et al., "Indirect pulp capping in young patients: immunohistological study of pulp-dentin complex," *Romanian Journal of Morphology and Embryology*, vol. 54, no. 4, pp. 1081–1086, 2013.

[23] M. Aeinehchi, B. Eslami, M. Ghanbariha, and A. S. Saffar, "Mineral trioxide aggregate (MTA) and calcium hydroxide as pulp-capping agents in human teeth: a preliminary report," *International Endodontic Journal*, vol. 36, no. 3, pp. 225–231, 2003.

[24] T. M. Oliveira, A. B. Moretti, V. T. Sakai et al., "Clinical, radiographic and histologic analysis of the effects of pulp capping materials used in pulpotomies of human primary teeth," *European Archives of Paediatric Dentistry*, vol. 14, no. 2, pp. 65–71, 2013.

[25] N. Lourenço Neto, N. C. Marques, A. P. Fernandes et al., "Immunolocalization of dentin matrix protein-1 in human primary teeth treated with different pulp capping materials," *Journal of Biomedical Materials Research Part B: Applied Biomaterials*, vol. 104, no. 1, pp. 165–169, 2016.

[26] F. Leye Benoist, F. Gaye Ndiaye, A. W. Kane, H. M. Benoist, and P. Farge, "Evaluation of mineral trioxide aggregate (MTA) versus calcium hydroxide cement (Dycal(®)) in the formation of a dentine bridge: a randomised controlled trial," *International Dental Journal*, vol. 62, no. 1, pp. 33–39, 2012.

[27] V. George, S. K. Janardhanan, B. Varma, P. Kumaran, and A. M. Xavier, "Clinical and radiographic evaluation of indirect pulp treatment with MTA and calcium hydroxide in primary teeth (in-vivo study)," *Journal of Indian Society of Pedodontics and Preventive Dentistry*, vol. 33, no. 2, pp. 104–110, 2015.

[28] N. P. Menon, B. R. Varma, S. Janardhanan, P. Kumaran, A. M. Xavier, and B. S. Govinda, "Clinical and radiographic comparison of indirect pulp treatment using light-cured calcium silicate and mineral trioxide aggregate in primary molars: a randomized clinical trial," *Contemporary Clinical Dentistry*, vol. 7, no. 4, pp. 475–480, 2016.

[29] R. Franzon, N. J. Opdam, L. F. Guimaraes et al., "Randomized controlled clinical trial of the 24-months survival of composite resin restorations after one-step incomplete and complete excavation on primary teeth," *Journal of Dentistry*, vol. 43, no. 10, pp. 1235–1241, 2015.

[30] M. Maltz, L. S. Alves, J. J. Jardim, S. Moura MdoS, and E. F. de Oliveira, "Incomplete caries removal in deep lesions: a 10-year prospective study," *American Journal of Dentistry*, vol. 24, no. 4, pp. 211–214, 2011.

36

Glanzmann's Thrombastenia: The Role of Tranexamic Acid in Oral Surgery

Rocco Franco ⓘD,[1] Michele Miranda ⓘD,[2] Laura Di Renzo ⓘD,[1] Antonino De Lorenzo ⓘD,[1] Alberta Barlattani,[3] and Patrizio Bollero[2]

[1]Section of Clinical Nutrition and Nutrigenomic, Department of Biomedicine and Prevention, School of Applied Medical-Surgical Sciences, University of Rome Tor Vergata, Via Montpellier 1, 00133 Rome, Italy
[2]Department of Systems Medicine, Medical School, University of Rome Tor Vergata, Rome, Italy
[3]Department of Clinical Sciences and Translational Medicine, University of Rome Tor Vergata, Rome, Italy

Correspondence should be addressed to Rocco Franco; roccofr91@gmail.com

Academic Editor: Wasiu L. Adeyemo

Glanzmann's thrombastenia (GT) is the most frequent inherited condition. GT is a genetic autosomal recessive disease caused by the alteration of the genes ITGA2B and ITGB3, located on the chromosome 17. The incidence of GT is calculated in 1 on 1000000. The patients, during their life, show episodes of mucocutaneous bleeding, epistaxis, and gingival bleeding. Some subjects required continuous bleeding transfusion. The aim of this case report is to demonstrate that oral assumption of tranexamic acid is a gold standard to prevent excessive bleeding. The patient GM of 36 years old with GT type 1 needs dental extractions of the teeth 4.7 and 4.8 at the "Tor Vergata" University Hospital in Rome. The specialist suggests that 3 days before surgery, the patient must take 6 vials every day of tranexamic acid that is used in obstetrics and gynecology. The teeth were extracted and applied suture. The patient is observed and is recommended mouth rinse with tranexamic acid. No bleeding complications were observed.

1. Introduction

Platelets are an important component in the hemostasis process. The damage of endothelium releases some proteins (i.e., collagen and thromboplastin) that avoid the aggregation of the platelet. The surface of the platelet permits the aggregation of procoagulant factor that activates the coagulation pathway. The platelet acquired disorders are more frequent in the clinical practice and are the result from the induction of the use of medications. The inherited conditions are very rare. The most frequent inherited condition is the Glanzmann's thrombastenia (GT). GT is a genetic autosomal recessive disease caused by the alteration of the genes ITGA2B and ITGB3, located on the chromosome 17. The gene codes for a platelet surface receptor GPIIb/GPIIIa, now known as ITG $\alpha IIb\beta 3$, that is, a large heterodimeric cell transmembrane receptor, comprised of a larger αIIb and a smaller $\beta 3$ subunits. It is expressed in a large quantity on the surface of the platelet, up to 100000 copies. When a platelet is active, the integrin changes conformation and are exposed areas that bind fibrinogen and other soluble adhesive proteins such as Von Willenbrand factor. These proteins mediate the aggregation between a platelet in a Ca++ dependent manner [1]. The receptor also transmits signals into the platelet, mediates interactions with the cytoskeleton, and assures the transport of fibrinogen to alfa granules. The incidence of GT is calculated in 1/1000000. It is more common in some ethnic groups that have a high incidence of consanguinity such as Iraqui Jews and French Gypsies. Purpura is the initial manifestation of GT. The patients, during their life, showed episodes of mucocutaneous bleeding, epistaxis, and gingival bleeding. The subject, during invasive surgical acts or after accidental injuring, required bleeding transfusion. The gravity of bleeding is linked to the type of mutation. GT is classified into three subclasses (type 1, type 2, and other variant) characterized by the ability of platelets to retract a

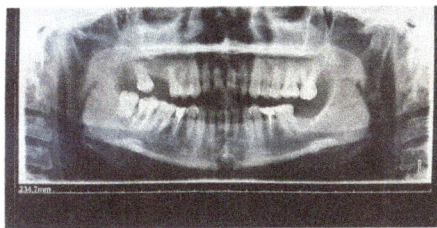

FIGURE 1: Initial radiography.

fibrin clot and store fibrinogen. Patients with type I have platelets with no ability to retract a fibrin clot and lack internal stores of fibrinogen; patients with type II have platelets with a reduced ability to retract a fibrin clot and low levels of platelet fibrinogen, while for other variant, the platelets have a differential ability to retract a fibrin clot and contain appreciable levels of platelet fibrinogen. The different types of GT have different quantities of integrin receptor: type I has <5% GPIIb±IIIa, type II $10 \pm 25\%$, and other variant can have 100% of the normal receptor. Patients with GT need not take therapy daily but will always require treatment during surgical procedures, controlling bleeding after injury, and during spontaneous bleeding episodes. In general, the bleeding tendency in GT decreases with age. Local bleeding can be treated by local measures, such as fibrin sealants [2]. Regular dental care is essential to prevent gingival bleeding. Bleeding following trauma or surgical procedures could be severe, and transfusions are often given by precaution. For teeth extractions or for hemorrhage accompanying the loss of deciduous teeth, hemostasis can be significantly improved by the application of individually prepared plastic splints that provide physical support for hemostasis [3]. The correct management during dental surgery is very complex. The effectivity of transfusion is very discussed for negative effects. The administration of antifibrinolytic agents blocks the formation of fibrin and is a high-grade alternative [4]. Oral tranexamic acid is a method used in obstetrics and gynecology to treat menorrhagia. Oral surgery usually makes use of intravenous infusion or mouth rinse. The importance of the tranexamic acid use is discussed in a multitude of clinical studies. Tranexamic acid is an antifibrinolytic agent and inhibits the degradation of thrombus and consequently blocks bleeding. In dentistry, only the utilization of tranexamic acid mouth rinse is based on a significant literature [5]. Moreover, tranexamic acid does not require a period of hospitalization and consequently a great economic saving. The oral assumption is a new method utilized in oral surgery; only in obstetrics and gynecology, its assumption is based on important scientific literature. The aim of this case report is to describe the safety and practicality of oral tranexamic acid in dentistry and the total absence of adverse effects with respect to platelet concentrate.

2. Case Presentation

The patient GM of 36 years old with GT type 1 needs extractions of the dental teeth 4.7 and 4.8 for an endoperio lesion, diagnosed by ortopanthomography, at the "Tor Vergata" University Hospital in Rome (Figure 1).

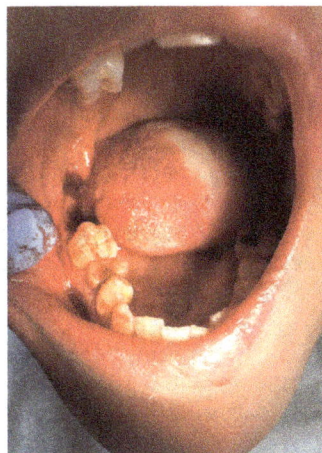

FIGURE 2: Postsurgery.

Past laboratory tests revealed normal platelet counts and morphology, prolonged bleeding times, clotting time of 4.15 minutes, decreased clot retraction (20%), and abnormal platelet aggregation responses to physiologic stimuli such as adenosine diphosphate and epinephrine used during the aggregometer study. They have no family history of any bleeding disorder. The diagnosis occurred prematurely for the presence of frequent epistaxis, and the diagnosis was ascertained by light transmission aggregometry (LTA). The LTA evaluates shape change, lag phase, percent of aggregation, slope of aggregation, and deaggregation before and after the addition of an agonist (ADP, collagen, epinephrine, arachidonic acid, ristocetin, thrombin receptor-activating peptide, and thromboxane A2 mimetic). There was no history of consanguineous marriages in the family. The patient is looked after at the hematological center of Rome "Tor Vergata". Preoperative examination was conducted by anesthesiologists. A hematological consult was requested. Oral surgery is classified as simple surgery because risk of bleeding is low. The hematology has advised against performing blood transfusions. The specialist suggests that 3 days before surgery, the patient must take by mouth 6 vials every day of tranexamic acid because the half-life of this drug is 2 hours [6]. The patient shows loss of multiple teeth and had executed other dental extraction with the same methods with no adverse events. A prophylactic assumption of amoxicillina and clavulanic acid has been started one day at the dose of 2 g daily before the surgery and continued for another 4 days.

A peripheral block of the inferior alveolar nerve with bupivacaine without adrenaline and paraperiosteal anesthesia with articain and adrenaline in concentration 1/100000 was also performed. The surgery was conducted with atraumatic technique without osteotomies and mucoperiosteal flaps. The syndesmotomy of the elements 4.7 and 4.8 was performed; they were dislocated through a straight lever and extracted through an appropriate clamp (Figure 2). The socket was courted, washed with saline solution. At the end, oxidized regenerated cellulose was inserted in the socket, and the mucous membrane was sutured with silk 3-0.

Postoperative indications of oral surgery were given to the patient; she was monitored for about 4 hours postintervention. During the postoperatory time, an intravenous paracetamol infusion was performed because it does not interfere with the platelet aggregation. Mouth rinse with tranexamic acid was recommended to the patient. During the hospitalization, no major episode of bleeding was observed. The patient did not present any problems of any kind, and after 7 days, the sutures were removed. A maximum dose of 4 g daily of paracetamol is prescribed. Other nonsteroidal anti-inflammatory drugs are dissuaded because they stop the platelet aggregation. The patient did not present excessive and uncontrolled bleeding during the postoperative period and during the days following the operation.

3. Discussion

GT is a rare pathology that complicates surgical treatment for possible uncontrolled bleeding. A correct management of oral surgery in literature is the employment of endovenous tranexamic acid or platelet transfusion. Tranexamic acid, as shown in literature, works by slowing the breakdown of blood clots, which helps to prevent prolonged bleeding. It belongs to antifibrinolytic drugs. This drug is used to prevent excessive bleeding during menstrual period. Tranexamic acid is well tolerated; nausea and diarrhea are the most common adverse events. Increased risk of thrombosis with the drug has not been demonstrated in all clinical trials.

The blood or platelet transfusion in a GT patient has a high risk of alloimmunization (cross-reaction) against platelet glycoprotein IIb and/or IIIa. Specifically, the patient produce auto-antibodies against the glycoprotein. The occurrence of such alloantibodies is usually due to repeated blood transfusion and greatly complicates the treatment of these patients since they prevent effective platelet transfusion and might, theoretically, cause posttransfusion purpura [7].

Other rare reaction against transfusion observed in all patients are acute hemolytic reaction, allergic reaction, anaphylactic reaction, coagulation problems in massive transfusion, febrile nonhemolytic reaction, metabolic derangements, mistransfusion (transfusion of the incorrect product to the incorrect recipient), septic or bacterial contamination, transfusion-associated circulatory overload, transfusion-related acute lung injury, urticarial reaction, delayed hemolytic reaction, posttransfusion purpura, transfusion-associated graft-versus-host disease, transfusion-related immunomodulation, and infectious complications [8]. These complications are very rare, and the medical guidelines have greatly reduced these complications. In literature, only 16 studies treat the correct management during oral surgery of GT. Eight studies recommended platelet transfusion before oral surgery together with the use of endovenous tranexamic acid [9–16], four studies, in alternative to transfusion, recommended the use of recombinant-activated factor VII [17–20], one study recommended the use of plasma rich in platelet [21], and another the use of acrylic splint [22]. Two studies recommended the intravenous infusion of an antifibrinolytic agent [9, 23].

Oral surgery is classified as surgery with low risk of bleeding and are influenced by local factors such as inflammation and the grade of complexity. In this case report, we use the oral assumption of tranexamic acid for the presence of low adverse effects (nausea and diarrhea) compared to transfusion and practicality of employment. The patient had no adverse events and no excessive bleeding. The patient did not need blood transfusion. No cases in literature describe a similar method. This new method is more comfortable because the patient starts therapy domiciliary, and the oral surgery must carry out without the use of the platelet transfusion. The platelet transfusion required a period of hospitalization to observe possible adverse effects, and this is not an ambulatory procedure. Also, the transfusion has a higher economic cost. For this reason, the procedure with tranexamic acid can be performed in ambulatory. Only in obstetrics and gynecology, during menorrhagia, its assumption is based on important scientific literature. In gynecology, the recommended dose is 2–4.5 g/day. This drug is not influenced by food and has a half-life of 2 hours [24]. It is used also in orthopedic surgery [25]. The oral assumption of tranexamic acid shows a gold standard to prevent bleeding in patients affected by GT. New future studies must confirm our results with a major number of patients.

References

[1] T. Solh, A. Botsford, and M. Solh, "Glanzmann's thrombasthenia: pathogenesis, diagnosis, and current and emerging treatment options," Journal of Blood Medicine, vol. 6, pp. 219–227, 2015.

[2] A. T. Nurden, M. Fiore, P. Nurden, and X. Pillois, "Glanzmann thrombasthenia: a review of ITGA2B and ITGB3 defects with emphasis on variants, phenotypic variability, and mouse models," Blood, vol. 118, no. 23, pp. 5996–6005, 2011.

[3] A. T. Nurden, X. Pillois, and D. A. Wilcox, "Glanzmann thrombasthenia: state of the art and future directions," Seminars in Thrombosis and Hemostasis, vol. 39, no. 6, pp. 642–655, 2013.

[4] C. Sebastiano, M. Bromberg, K. Breen, and M. T. Hurford, "Glanzmann's thrombasthenia: report of a case and review of the literature," International Journal of Clinical and Experimental Pathology, vol. 3, no. 4, pp. 443–447, 2010.

[5] B. S. Coller and S. J. Shattil, "The GPIIb/IIIa (integrin $\alpha IIb\beta 3$) odyssey: a technology-driven saga of a receptor with twists, turns, and even a bend," Blood, vol. 112, no. 8, pp. 3011–3025, 2008.

[6] H. Leminen and R. Hurskainen, "Tranexamic acid for the treatment of heavy menstrual bleeding: efficacy and safety," International Journal of Women's Health, vol. 4, pp. 413–421, 2012.

[7] P. Bierling, P. Fromont, A. Elbez, N. Duedari, and N. Kieffer, "Early immunization against platelet glycoprotein IIIa in a newborn Glanzmann type I patient," Vox Sanguinis, vol. 55, no. 2, pp. 109–113, 1988.

[8] S. Sharma, P. Sharma, and L. N. Tyler, "Transfusion of blood and blood products: indications and complications," American Family Physician, vol. 83, no. 6, pp. 719–724, 2011.

[9] E. Segna, A. Artoni, R. Sacco, and A. B. Giannì, "Oral surgery

in patients with Glanzmann thrombasthenia: a case series," *Journal of Oral and Maxillofacial Surgery*, vol. 75, no. 2, pp. 256–259, 2017.

[10] I. Varkey, K. Rai, A. M. Hegde, M. S. Vijaya, and V. I. Oommen, "Clinical management of Glanzmann's thrombasthenia: a case report," *Journal of Dentistry*, vol. 11, no. 2, pp. 242–247, 2014.

[11] A. Gopalakrishnan, R. Veeraraghavan, and P. Panicker, "Hematological and surgical management in Glanzmann's thrombasthenia: a case report," *Journal of the Indian Society of Pedodontics and Preventive Dentistry*, vol. 32, no. 2, pp. 181–184, 2014.

[12] A. Ranjith and K. Nandakumar, "Glanzmann thrombasthenia: a rare hematological disorder with oral manifestations: a case report," *The Journal of Contemporary Dental Practice*, vol. 9, no. 5, pp. 107–113, 2008.

[13] R. Conte, D. Cirillo, F. Ricci, C. Tassi, and P. L. Tazzari, "Platelet transfusion in a patient affected by Glanzmann's thrombasthenia with antibodies against GPIIb-IIIa," *Haematologica*, vol. 82, no. 1, pp. 73-74, 1997.

[14] A. W. Sugar, "The management of dental extractions in cases of thrombasthenia complicated by the development of isoantibodies to donor platelets," *Oral Surgery, Oral Medicine, Oral Pathology*, vol. 48, no. 2, pp. 116–119, 1979.

[15] R. F. Perkin, G. C. White, and W. P. Webster, "Glanzmann's thrombasthenia: report of two oral surgical cases using a new microfibrillar collagen preparation and EACA for hemostasis," *Oral Surgery, Oral Medicine, Oral Pathology*, vol. 47, no. 1, pp. 36–39, 1979.

[16] M. Sugimura, A. Yoshioka, M. Morishita et al., "Tooth extraction in a patient with Glanzmann's thrombasthenia," *International Journal of Oral Surgery*, vol. 4, no. 3, pp. 130–135, 1975.

[17] M. C. Valera, P. Kemoun, S. Cousty, P. Sie, and B. Payrastre, "Inherited platelet disorders and oral health," *Journal of Oral Pathology & Medicine*, vol. 42, no. 2, pp. 115–124, 2013.

[18] V. T. Lombardo and G. Sottilotta, "Recombinant activated factor VII combined with desmopressin in preventing bleeding from dental extraction in a patient with Glanzmann's thrombasthenia," *Clinical and Applied Thrombosis/Hemostasis*, vol. 12, no. 1, pp. 115-116, 2006.

[19] U. Hennewig, H. J. Laws, S. Eisert, and U. Göbel, "Bleeding and surgery in children with Glanzmann thrombasthenia with and without the use of recombinant factor VII a," *Klinische Pädiatrie*, vol. 217, no. 6, pp. 365–370, 2005.

[20] A. Chuansumrit, M. Suwannuraks, N. Sri-Udomporn, B. Pongtanakul, and S. Worapongpaiboon, "Recombinant activated factor VII combined with local measures in preventing bleeding from invasive dental procedures in patients with Glanzmann thrombasthenia," *Blood Coagulation & Fibrinolysis*, vol. 14, no. 2, pp. 187–190, 2003.

[21] M. Fernandes Gomes, R. M. de Melo, G. Plens, E. M. Pontes, M. M. Silva, and J. C. da Rocha, "Surgical and clinical management of a patient with Glanzmann thrombasthenia: a case report," *Quintessence International*, vol. 35, no. 8, pp. 617–620, 2004.

[22] D. N. Mehta and R. Bhatia, "Dental considerations in the management of Glanzmann's thrombasthenia," *International Journal of Clinical Pediatric Dentistry*, vol. 3, no. 1, pp. 51–56, 2010.

[23] F. C. Bisch, K. J. Bowen, B. S. Hanson, V. L. Kudryk, and M. A. Billman, "Dental considerations for a Glanzmann's thrombasthenia patient: case report," *Journal of Periodontology*, vol. 67, no. 5, pp. 536–540, 1996.

[24] K. Wellington and A. J. Wagstaff, "Tranexamic acid: a review of its use in the management of menorrhagia," *Drugs*, vol. 63, no. 13, pp. 1417–1433, 2003.

[25] E. Kayupov, Y. A. Fillingham, K. Okroj et al., "Oral and intravenous tranexamic acid are equivalent at reducing blood loss following total hip arthroplasty: a randomized controlled trial," *The Journal of Bone and Joint Surgery*, vol. 99, no. 5, pp. 373–378, 2017.

37

Sectional Fixed Orthodontic Extrusion Technique in Management of Teeth with Complicated Crown-Root Fractures: Report of Two Cases

S. Nagarajan M. P. Sockalingam (iD), **Katherine Kong Loh Seu, Halimah Mohamed Noor, and Ahmad Shuhud Irfani Zakaria**

Department of Operative Dentistry, Faculty of Dentistry, National University Malaysia (UKM), Jalan Raja Muda Abdul Aziz, 50300 Kuala Lumpur, Malaysia

Correspondence should be addressed to S. Nagarajan M. P. Sockalingam; drnaga67@gmail.com

Academic Editor: H. Cem Güngör

Complicated crown-root fractures account for a small percentage of traumatic dental injuries seen in children; however, management of these injuries can be very challenging to clinicians. Factors such as complexity of the injury, patient's age and dentition stage, patient's cooperation, and parental demands may have some bearing on the type of treatment undertaken and its outcomes. In some children, these injuries may have significant impact on their quality of life. The purpose of this article is to describe two cases of complicated crown-root fracture which were successfully managed through orthodontic extrusion using a sectional fixed orthodontic technique. The basis for the treatment technique and its favourable outcomes were highlighted with its advantages and drawbacks.

1. Introduction

Dentoalveolar trauma accounts for 76% of cases seen among children with maxillofacial injuries [1]. In the context of dental injuries alone, the prevalence has been reported to be between 15 and 20% in the permanent dentition of children and adolescents [2, 3]. A large proportion of the dental injuries was due to accidental fall and sport-related activities [4].

Of the different types of dental injuries, the crown fracture which accounts for a third of the injuries is the commonest type reported. In contrast, crown-root fracture only represents 0.3–5% of the injuries stated [5]. Crown-root fracture involves the fracture of enamel, dentin, and cementum with or without the involvement of the pulp [6]. Both the upper central and lateral incisors are the commonest teeth affected by dental injuries [3, 7].

Crown-root fracture especially the complicated type with pulp involvement is one of the most difficult types of dental injury to treat. Factors such as the complexity and direction of fracture, size and mobility of the fractured tooth fragment, subgingival extension of the fracture line, stage root development, alveolar fracture, soft tissue injuries, and the pulp status of the affected tooth at the time of presentation may contribute toward the outcomes of the treatment [8]. Besides these tooth-related factors, additional considerations such parental demand and attitude, patient's cooperation and medical condition, oral condition, and teeth alignment may dictate the possible treatment options to be considered.

This case report highlighted two clinical cases of complicated crown-root fracture of permanent central incisors in growing children with complex fracture lines. The challenges and possible treatment options with the basis of treatment selection were discussed. In addition, the preparation of the affected teeth prior to the root canal treatment and the use of sectional fixed orthodontic extrusion technique were also explained.

2. Case Report 1

An eight-year-old girl was referred by her general dental practitioner (GDP) to the National University of Malaysia (UKM) Paediatric Dental Clinic for management of an upper anterior tooth with a complicated crown-root fracture. The tooth fractured two days earlier due to a fall at a poolside. The patient was medical fit and healthy.

Clinical examination revealed an oblique fracture from the labial surface of the upper left permanent central incisor (tooth 21) extending palatally 3.5 mm beneath the gingival margin (Figures 1 and 2). The upper coronal two-thirds of the crown structure was mobile, and the tooth did not response to sensibility testing. A periapical radiograph showed evidence of a crown-root fracture of the tooth 21, and the tooth has an immature apex (Figure 3).

The fractured crown was pushed into its original position with gentle pressure with digits and held in position by composite resin during the initial stages to allow commencement of the root canal treatment. This allowed minimal interference of the palatal gum tissue and therefore reduced the risk of contamination. An access cavity was made through the crown (Figure 4). The canal was chemomechanically prepared, dried, and filled with nonsetting calcium hydroxide (Figure 5). A week later, apexification was carried out, where the canal was filled with 4 mm of a bioceramic material (EndoSequence®, BC RRM Fast Set Putty™, Brasseler, USA) plug. The following week, the canal was obturated with thermoplasticised GP, and the access cavity was restored with the self-cured GIC (Figure 6).

Subsequently, in order to allow adequate exertion of the orthodontic forces to the root portion, the coronal crown fragment had to be removed and kept in a container of normal saline for hydration. The missing palatal aspect of the crown was filled with self-cured glass ionomer cement from the base of the fracture to above the gingival margin to prevent gingival ingrowth. Following that, four brackets were placed on the labial surfaces of the upper incisors. Extrusion of the fractured tooth was initiated with a sectional fixed orthodontic technique using a 0.014 × 0.025 rectangular nickel-titanium (NiTi) archwire (Figure 7). The patient was reviewed every month. After 4 months, the palatal fracture margin of the tooth was raised to the gum level. At this stage, the brackets were removed and a periapical radiograph was taken to assess the root filling and the root status. The periapical radiograph did not show any remarkable changes (Figure 8). The stored coronal fragment was reattached to the extruded tooth with composite resin (Figure 9). A supracrestal fibrotomy was performed around the extruded tooth with a surgical scalpel blade, and the tooth was splinted on its palatal aspect with the adjacent teeth using a composite-wire splint for 6 months. Post-op reviews at 3, 6, and 12 months of the tooth did not reveal any unremarkable clinical changes.

3. Case Report 2

A ten-year-old was brought to the to the National University of Malaysia (UKM) Paediatric Dental Clinic

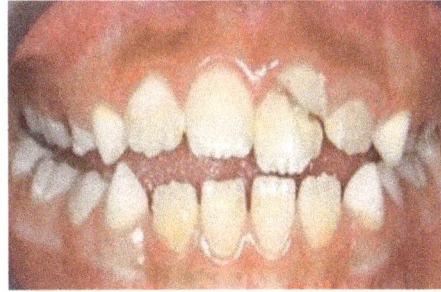

FIGURE 1: Pretreatment photograph of tooth 21 with crown-root fracture (frontal view).

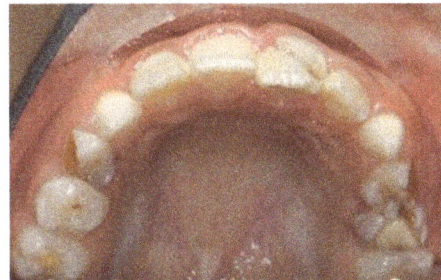

FIGURE 2: Pretreatment photograph of tooth 21 with crown-root fracture (palatal view).

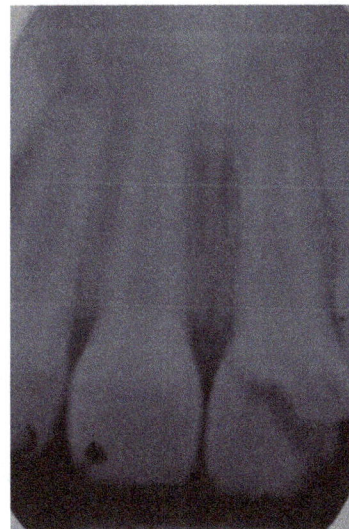

FIGURE 3: Periapical radiograph of tooth 21 showing the extent of the crown-root fracture.

a month after an alleged fall at school by his mother. The patient had some discomfort during eating and felt there is something loose behind his front tooth. He was medically fit and well.

Clinical examination showed a crown-root fracture of the upper right permanent central incisor (tooth 11) (Figure 10). The oblique fracture line extended in a labiopalatal direction with the palatal margin extending 3.5 mm subgingivally (Figure 11). Cone Beam Computer Tomography

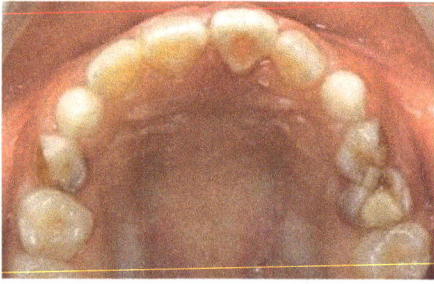

Figure 4: Location of the root canal treatment access on the palatal of the fractured tooth 21 after repositioning of the fractured fragments.

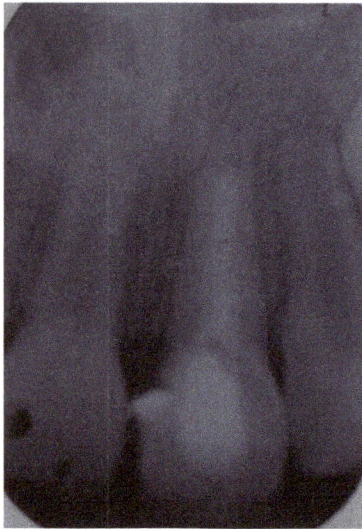

Figure 7: Sectional fixed orthodontic appliance in place for extrusion of fractured tooth 21.

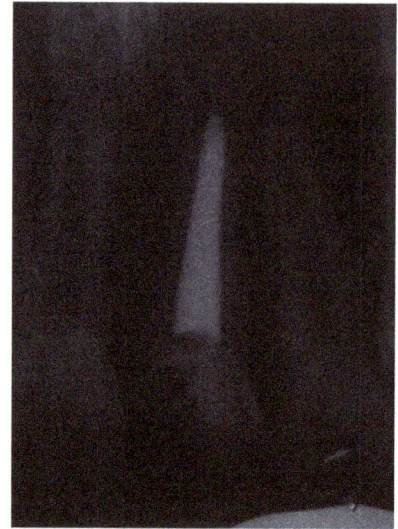

Figure 5: Root canal of tooth 21 filled with nonsetting calcium hydroxide.

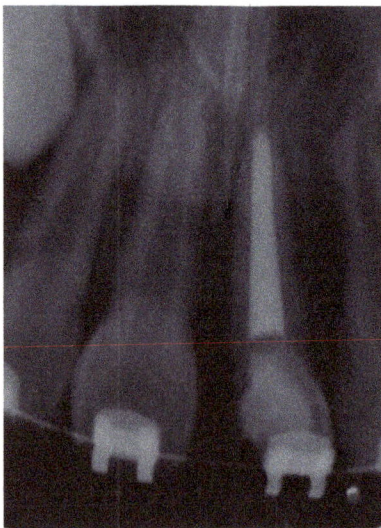

Figure 8: Periapical radiograph of tooth 21 following extrusion prior to reattachment of the fractured fragment of the tooth.

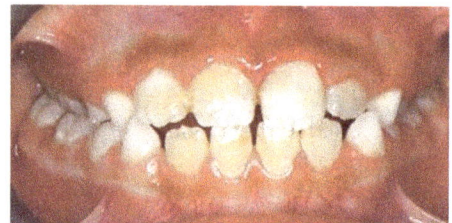

Figure 6: Obturation of the root canal of tooth 21 with bioceramics and gutta-percha.

(CBCT) images of the tooth showed a complicated crown-root fracture, and the tooth has an almost matured root apex (Figure 12). Sensibility test was negative.

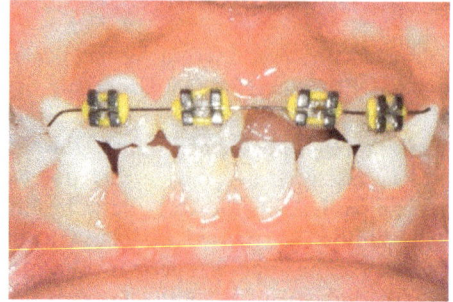

Figure 9: Final restoration of tooth 21 using the patient's own fractured fragment of the tooth.

The palatal mobile tooth fragment was removed under local anaesthesia, and palatal fracture margin was identified. After haemostasis control, self-cured GIC was placed on the palatal aspect of the tooth similar to that in Case 1. A week later, a root canal treatment was initiated with chemo-mechanically preparation. Thereafter, the canal was filled with 4 mm of a bioceramic material (EndoSequence®, BC RRM Fast Set Putty™, Brasseler, USA) plug. The following week, the canal was obturated with thermoplasticised GP, and four orthodontic brackets were placed on the labial surfaces of tooth 12 to tooth 22 (Figure 13). A short span

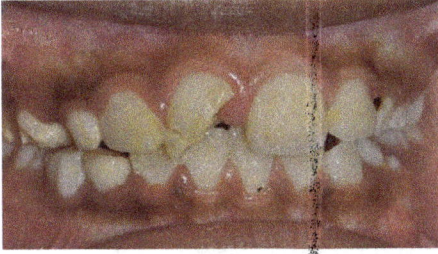

FIGURE 10: Pretreatment photograph of tooth 11 with crown-root fracture (frontal view).

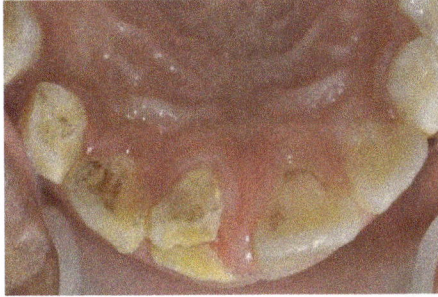

FIGURE 11: Pretreatment photograph of tooth 11 with crown-root fracture (palatal view).

0.014×0.025 rectangular nickel-titanium (NiTi) archwire was used to extrude the tooth fractured palatal margin further gingivally (Figure 14). The patient was reviewed monthly. Five months later, sufficient amount of the palatal margin of the fractured tooth was clinically visible for composite build-up (Figure 15). A palatal wire-composite splint was placed for 6 months following a supracrestal fibrotomy around the tooth. The tooth was successfully reviewed at 3-, 6- (Figure 16), and 12-month intervals without any evidence of pathosis.

4. Discussion

Two important questions that are often thought of by clinicians pertaining dental injuries are, Is it possible to save the injured tooth? Is it desirable to save the injured tooth? A multitude of problems such tooth, patient, and parental related factors may dictate the decision process to either save the tooth or extract it [8]. Another concern in a growing child, losing a tooth at such a tender age may have a significant effect on the child's quality of life. Studies have shown that traumatic dental injuries can bring about a strong and prolong impact on the emotion and social well-being on the affected children [9, 10]. Parents also often hope in desperation that clinicians can do something to salvage the traumatised tooth.

There are few treatment options available to manage teeth with complicated crown-root fractures [11, 12]:

(i) Removal of the fractured coronal fragment and restoration of the tooth if the fracture line has not encroached into the biologic width.

(ii) Removal of the coronal fragment and supplement with gingivectomy or/and osteotomy to expose the fracture line in order to establish biologic width prior to restoration.

(iii) Removal of the coronal fragment and initiation of endodontic treatment and restoration of tooth with a postcrown.

(iv) Removal of the coronal fragment and initiation of endodontic treatment and followed by either orthodontic or surgical extrusion of the apical fragment prior to restoration with a postcrown.

(v) In severe crown-root fracture, the tooth may have to be extracted and replaced with a removal or fixed prosthesis.

If a decision to save the tooth is taken, one should ensure the restorability of the remaining tooth structure after the removal of the mobile coronal fragment and availability of adequate root length. Generally, teeth with crown-root fractures require a multidisciplinary intervention especially if the teeth need to be saved. Three main issues need to be considered prior to treatment:

(i) If the tooth needs RCT, how to prevent contamination of the canal form the subgingival tissue?

(ii) How to bring the subgingival fracture margin to equigingival or supragingival level?

(iii) How to provide a lasting and aesthetic restoration that not only provides good coronal seal but also has self-cleansing margins?

In the cases presented, both the teeth had complicated crown-root fracture and required RCT. One of the main challenges in carrying out RCT on crown-root fractured teeth is bleeding and crevicular fluid contamination from the gums which usually occurs after removal of the mobile coronal fragment. Two different approaches were undertaken to minimise the degree of contamination: in Case 1, the fractured crown was repositioned and held together in the reduced position with composite resin. The RCT was carried through the fractured crown. In Case 2, the coronal fragment was too loose for reattachment and had to be removed. GIC was placed on the palatal defect up to the supragingival level after control of gum bleeding. The GIC forms a continues rim with the tooth and allowed the gums to heal without any ingrowth into the defective area prior to the commencement of the RCT. Conventional GIC was used because it has better biocompatibility to gingivae than resin-modified GIC [13]. Since both the traumatised teeth had near completion of the root apices and large pulp canals, apexification was carried out. In both cases, apexification was carried out with a bioceramic material (EndoSequence®, BC RRM Fast Set Putty™, Brasseler, USA) after chemo-mechanical debridement of the canals. The Endo Sequence Root Repair Material is a calcium silicate-based cement which exhibits high biocompatibility and has antibacterial and osteogenic properties. It can be used as an alternative to mineral trioxide aggregate [14, 15].

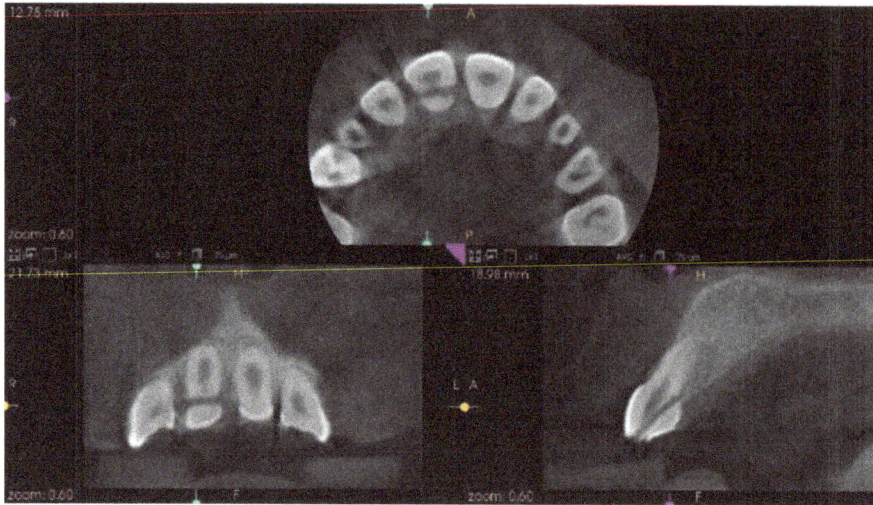

Figure 12: Cone beam computed tomographic view of tooth 11 in various planes showing the extent of the fracture.

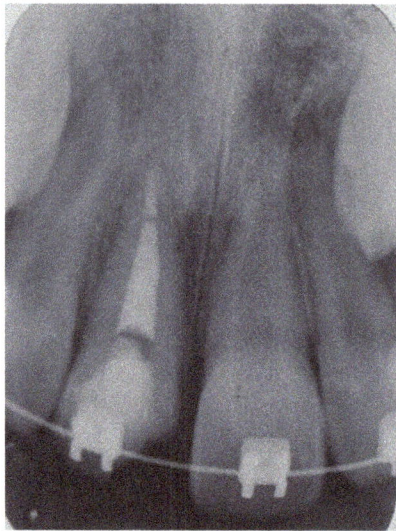

Figure 13: Obturation of the root canal of tooth 11 with bioceramics and gutta-percha.

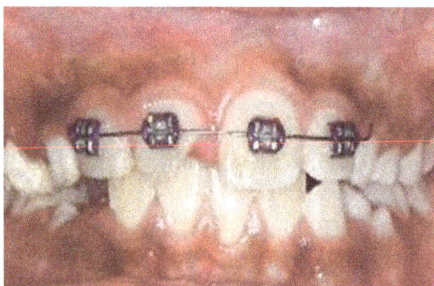

Figure 14: Sectional fixed orthodontic appliance in place for extrusion of tooth 11.

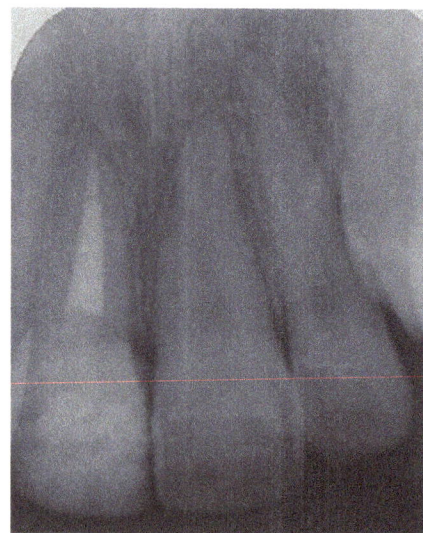

Figure 15: Composite restoration of the fractured tooth 11 after orthodontic extrusion.

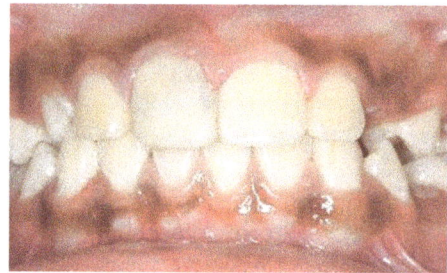

Figure 16: Postoperative periapical radiograph of the fractured tooth 11 at 12 months after extrusion.

Another treatment issue that required much attention was the subgingival fracture margins. In order to provide good and self-cleansing restoration, the restorative margin should be either equigingival or supragingival. As both the traumatic teeth had fractures extending subgingivally and had encroached into the biologic width, extrusion of the apical portion of the teeth was decided to bring the fractured margins close to the desired gum level. In order to achieve this, two options were considered, either the use of orthodontic extrusion or surgical extrusion. Although both methods have proven clinical successes to extrude teeth with minimal complications [16–18], orthodontic extrusion with light forces was used in the current cases due to the patients' age. A sectional fixed orthodontic technique was used for extrusion with four brackets and a short NiTi (0.014 × 0.025) rectangular wire. Use of this technique offers many advantages such good patient compliance, easy access, and less number of teeth involved in bracket placement, easy cleaning, and able to deliver the desired result. Nevertheless, orthodontic extrusion is a much slower process than surgical extrusion, and supracrestal fibrotomy with a retention period of 6 months may be necessary to allow periodontal fibres reattachment and healing [19]. Otherwise, relapse can happen over time.

With regard to restoration of teeth with crown-root facture, factors such as the extent of the fracture, availability of tooth structure, presence of the tooth fragment, occlusion, aesthetic, and patient's age and cooperation may dictate the type of restoration needed. If the fractured coronal fragment is large and available, it could be reused to restore the tooth as demonstrated in Case 1. Another option is to do a composite build-up or composite crown with or without a postcore. Often in a growing child, a ceramic extracoronal crown is not considered as the restorative margins become visible with growth. On the other hand, composite-based restorations allow easy repair and adjustment.

5. Conclusion

The current cases demonstrated the application of multidisciplinary approach in the management of teeth with crown-root fractures. The management displayed three main areas of expertise: the endodontics, orthodontics, and restorative. Each tooth with complicated crown-root fracture has its uniqueness and challenges that need to be taken into consideration during the treatment planning stage. The sectional fixed orthodontics used produced a favourable extrusion of the crown-root fractured teeth and may offer a better alternative to be used than other forms of modified removal appliances.

References

[1] R. Gassner, T. Tuli, O. Hächl, R. Moreira, and H. Ulmer, "Craniomaxillofacial trauma in children: a review of 3,385 cases with 6,060 injuries in 10 years," *Journal of Oral and Maxillofacial Surgery*, vol. 62, no. 4, pp. 399–407, 2004.

[2] L. Andersson, "Epidemiology of traumatic dental injuries," *Journal of Endodontics*, vol. 39, no. 3, pp. S2–S5, 2013.

[3] R. Lam, "Epidemiology and outcomes of traumatic dental injuries: a review of the literature," *Australian Dental Journal* vol. 61, no. 1, pp. 4–20, 2016.

[4] S. Azami-Aghdash, F. E. Azar, F. P. Azar et al., "Prevalence, etiology and type of dental trauma in children and adolescents: systematic review and meta-analysis," *Medical Journal Islamic Republic of Iran*, vol. 29, no. 4, p. 234, 2015.

[5] S. Olsburgh, T. Jacoby, and I. Krejci, "Crown fractures in the permanent dentition: pulpal and restorative considerations," *Dental Traumatology*, vol. 18, no. 3, pp. 103–115, 2002.

[6] J. O. Andreasen and F. M. Andreasen, "Classification, aetiology and epidemiology," in *Textbook and Colour Atlas of Traumatic Injuries to the Teeth*, pp. 218-219, Blackwell Munksgaard, Copenhagen, Denmark, 4th edition, 2011.

[7] U. Glendor, "Epidemiology of traumatic dental injuries—a 12-year review of the literature," *Dental Traumatology*, vol. 24, no. 6, pp. 603–611, 2008.

[8] V. K. Kulkarni, D. S. Sharma, N. R. Banda, M. Solanki, V. Khandelwal, and P. Airen, "Clinical management of a complicated crown-root fracture using autogenous tooth fragment: a biological restorative approach," *Contemporary Clinical Dentistry*, vol. 4, no. 1, pp. 84–87, 2013.

[9] T. D. Berger, D. J. Kenny, M. J. Casas, E. J. Barrett, and H. P. Lawrence, "Effects of severe dentoalveolar trauma on the quality-of-life of children and parents," *Dental Traumatology*, vol. 25, no. 5, pp. 462–469, 2009.

[10] F. B. Freire-Maia, S. M. Auad, M. H. Abreu et al., "Oral health-related quality of life and traumatic dental injuries in young permanent incisors in Brazilian schoolchildren: a multilevel approach," *PLoS One*, vol. 10, no. 8, article e0135369, 2015.

[11] G. J. Brown and R. R. Welbury, "Root extrusion, a practical solution in complicated crown-root incisor fractures," *British Dental Journal*, vol. 189, no. 9, pp. 477-478, 2000.

[12] L. F. Fariniuk, E. L. Ferreira, G. C. Soresini, A. E. Cavali, and F. Baratto Filho, "Intentional replantation with 180-degree rotation of a crown–root fracture: a case report," *Dental Traumatology*, vol. 19, no. 6, pp. 321–325, 2003.

[13] I. A. Rodriguez, C. A. Ferrara, F. Campos-Sanchez, M. Alaminos, J. U. Echevarria, and A. Campos, "An in-vitro biocompatibility study of conventional and resin-modified glass ionomer cements," *Journal of Adhesive Dentistry*, vol. 15, no. 6, pp. 541–546, 2013.

[14] M. Tanomaru, R. Viapiana, and J. Guerreiro, "From MTA to new biomaterials based on calcium silicate," *Odovtos International Journal of Dental Science*, vol. 18, no. 1, pp. 18–22, 2016.

[15] S. Utneja, R. R. Nawal, S. Talwar, and M. Verma, "Current perspectives of bio-ceramic technology in endodontics: calcium enriched mixture cement—review of its composition, properties and applications," *Restorative Dentistry and Endodontics*, vol. 40, no. 1, pp. 1–13, 2015.

[16] N. Bach, J. F. Baylard, and R. Voyer, "Orthodontic extrusion: periodontal considerations and applications," *Journal of Canadian Dental Association*, vol. 70, no. 11, pp. 775–780, 2004.

[17] S. R. Fidel, R. A. Fidel-Junior, L. M. Sassone, C. F. Murad, and R. A. Fidel, "Clinical management of complicated crown root fracture; a case report," *Brazilian Dental Journal*, vol. 22, no. 3, pp. 258–262, 2011.

[18] A. Elkhadem, S. Mickan, and D. Richards, "Adverse events of surgical extrusion in treatment for crown-root and cervical root fractures: a systematic review of case series/reports," *Dental Traumatology*, vol. 30, no. 1, pp. 1–14, 2014.

[19] O. Malmgren, B. Malmgren, and A. Frykholm, "Rapid orthodontic extrusion of crown root and cervical root fractured teeth," *Dental Traumatology*, vol. 7, no. 2, pp. 49–54, 1991.

Permissions

The contributors of this book come from diverse backgrounds, making this book a truly international effort. This book will bring forth new frontiers with its revolutionizing research information and detailed analysis of the nascent developments around the world.

We would like to thank all the contributing authors for lending their expertise to make the book truly unique. They have played a crucial role in the development of this book. Without their invaluable contributions this book wouldn't have been possible. They have made vital efforts to compile up to date information on the varied aspects of this subject to make this book a valuable addition to the collection of many professionals and students.

This book was conceptualized with the vision of imparting up-to-date information and advanced data in this field. To ensure the same, a matchless editorial board was set up. Every individual on the board went through rigorous rounds of assessment to prove their worth. After which they invested a large part of their time researching and compiling the most relevant data for our readers.

The editorial board has been involved in producing this book since its inception. They have spent rigorous hours researching and exploring the diverse topics which have resulted in the successful publishing of this book. They have passed on their knowledge of decades through this book. To expedite this challenging task, the publisher supported the team at every step. A small team of assistant editors was also appointed to further simplify the editing procedure and attain best results for the readers.

Apart from the editorial board, the designing team has also invested a significant amount of their time in understanding the subject and creating the most relevant covers. They scrutinized every image to scout for the most suitable representation of the subject and create an appropriate cover for the book.

The publishing team has been an ardent support to the editorial, designing and production team. Their endless efforts to recruit the best for this project, has resulted in the accomplishment of this book. They are a veteran in the field of academics and their pool of knowledge is as vast as their experience in printing. Their expertise and guidance has proved useful at every step. Their uncompromising quality standards have made this book an exceptional effort. Their encouragement from time to time has been an inspiration for everyone.

The publisher and the editorial board hope that this book will prove to be a valuable piece of knowledge for researchers, students, practitioners and scholars across the globe.

List of Contributors

Kazuhiro Murakami, Kazuhiko Yamamoto, Tsutomu Sugiura and Tadaaki Kirita
Department of Oral and Maxillofacial Surgery, Nara Medical University, Kashihara, Nara, Japan

Stefan Ihde
Dental Implants Faculty, International Implant Foundation, 116 Leopold Street, 80802 Munich, Germany

Łukasz Pałka
Reg-Med Dental Clinic, Rzeszowska 2, 68-200 Żary, Poland

Maciej Janeczek
Department of Biostructure and Animal Physiology, Wroclaw University of Environmental and Life Sciences, Kożuchowska 1,51-631 Wroclaw, Poland

Piotr Kosior
Department of Conservative Dentistry and Pedodontics, Wroclaw Medical University, Krakowska 26, 50-425 Wroclaw, Poland

Maciej Dobrzyński
Department of Conservative Dentistry and Pedodontics, Wroclaw Medical University, Krakowska 26, 50-425 Wroclaw, Poland

Jan Kiryk
Private Dental Clinic Maciej Kozłowski, Spokojna 23, 56-400 Oleśnica, Poland

Farah Asa'ad, Gionata Bellucci, Luca Ferrantino and Davide Trisciuoglio
Department of Biomedical, Surgical and Dental Sciences, Foundation IRCCS Ca' Granda Polyclinic, University of Milan, Milan, Italy

Silvio Taschieri and Massimo Del Fabbro
Department of Biomedical, Surgical and Dental Sciences, IRCCS Galeazzi Orthopaedic Institute, University of Milan, Milan, Italy

Ayako Taira and Kenichi Sasaguri
Department of Dentistry, Oral and Maxillofacial Surgery, Jichi Medical University, 3311-1 Yakushiji, Shimotsuke, Tochigi 329-0498, Japan

Shiho Odawara
Division of Orthodontics, Department of Oral Science, Kanagawa Dental University, 82 Inaoka-cho, Yokosuka,Kanagawa 238-8580, Japan

Shuntaro Sugihara
Division of Periodontology, Department of Oral Function and Restoration, Kanagawa Dental University,82 Inaoka-cho, Yokosuka, Kanagawa 238-8580, Japan

S. Nagarajan M. P. Sockalingam, Khairil Aznan Mohamed Khan and Elavarasi Kuppusamy
Centre for Family Oral Health, Faculty of Dentistry, e National University of Malaysia (UKM), Bangi, Malaysia

Mônica Fernandes Gomes, Luigi Giovanni Bernardo Sichi, Lilian Chrystiane Giannasi, José Benedito Oliveira Amorim, João Carlos da Rocha, Cristiane Yumi Koga-Ito and Miguel Angel Castillo Salgado
Center of Biosciences Applied to Patients with Special Health Care Needs (CEPAPE), Institute of Science and Technology, São Jose dos Campos Campus, São Paulo State University–UNESP, São Paulo, SP, Brazil

E. I. Ogbureke and C. D. Johnson
Department of General Practice and Dental Public Health, School of Dentistry, The University of Texas Health Science Center at Houston, Houston, TX, USA

M. A. Couey
Department of Oral and Maxillofacial Surgery, School of Dentistry, The University of Texas Health Science Center at Houston, Houston, TX, USA

N. Vigneswaran
Department of Diagnostic and Biomedical Science, School of Dentistry, The University of Texas Health Science Center at Houston,Houston, TX, USA

Ines Kallel, Eya Moussaoui and Nabiha Douki
Department of Dental Medicine, Faculty of Dentistry, Hospital Sahloul, Sousse, Tunisia
Laboratory of Research in Oral Healh and Maxillo Facial Rehabilitation (LR12ES11), Monastir, Tunisia

Faculty of Dental Medicine, University of Monastir, Monastir, Tunisia

Eya Moussaoui
Faculty of Dental Medicine, University of Monastir, Monastir, Tunisia

Dirceu Tavares Formiga Nery
School of Dentistry, Catholic University of Brasília (UCB), Brasília, DF, Brazil

José Ranali
Department of Pharmacology, Anesthesiology and Therapeutics, School of Dentistry, University of Campinas (UNICAMP),Piracicaba, SP, Brazil

Darceny Zanetta Barbosa
Department of Oral and Maxillofacial Surgery and Traumatology, School of Dentistry, Federal University of Uberlandia (UFU),Uberlândia, MG, Brazil

**Helvécio Marangon Júnior, Rafael Martins Afonso Pereira and Patrícia Cristine
de Oliveira Afonso Pereira**
School of Dentistry, University Center of Patos de Minas (UNIPAM), Patos de Minas, MG, Brazil

Davide Augusti and Gabriele Augusti
DDS, Private Dental Practice, Cosmetic and Restorative Dentistry, Via Papa Giovanni XXIII 37, 20091 Bresso Milan, Italy

**Polianne Alves Mendes, Isabela Moreira Neiva, Claudia Borges Brasileiro and
Leandro Napier Souza**
Department of Oral and Maxillofacial Surgery, School of Dentistry, Universidade Federal de Minas Gerais, Belo Horizonte, MG, Brazil

Ana Cristina Rodrigues Antunes Souza
Department of Dentistry, Centro Universit´ario Newton Paiva, Belo Horizonte, MG, Brazil

Qingan Xu
School of Nursing and Medical Technology, Jianghan University, Wuhan, China
Wuhan First Stomatology Hospital, Wuhan, China

Zhou Li
Department of Pediatric Dentistry, Stomatology Hospital of Guangzhou Medical University, Guanghzou, China

Lilies Anggarwati Astuti and Ressy Dwiyanti
Post-Graduate Program of Medical Sciences, Faculty of Medicine, University of Hasanuddin, Makassar, Indonesia

Mochammad Hatta
Molecular Biology and Immunology Laboratory, Faculty of Medicine, University of Hasanuddin, Makassar, Indonesia

Sri Oktawati
Department of Periodontology, Faculty of Dentistry, University of Hasanuddin, Makassar, Indonesia

Rosdiana Natzir
Department of Biochemistry, Faculty of Medicine, University of Hasanuddin, Makassar, Indonesia

Ressy Dwiyanti
Department of Medical Microbiology, Faculty of Medicine, Tadulako University, Palu, Indonesia

Daniel Amaral Alves Marlière
Division of Oral and Maxillofacial Surgery, Piracicaba Dental School, State University of Campinas, 13414-903 Piracicaba,SP, Brazil

Tony Eduardo Costa
Division of Dentistry, Faculty of Medical Science and Health – SUPREMA, 36033-003 Juiz de Fora, MG, Brazil

Saulo de Matos Barbosa
Division of Dentistry, Faculty São Leolpoldo Mandic – SLM, 13045-755 Campinas, SP, Brazil

Rodrigo Alvitos Pereira
Department of Oral and Maxillofacial Surgery, Pedro Ernesto University Hospital, State University of Rio de Janeiro,20551-030 Rio de Janeiro, RJ, Brazil

Henrique Duque de Miranda Chaves Netto
Department of Clinical Dentistry, Juiz de Fora Dental School, Federal University of Juiz de Fora, 36036-300 Juiz de Fora, MG, Brazil

H. Sevilay Bahadır, Gökhan Karadağ and Yusuf Bayraktar
Kırıkkale University Faculty of Dentistry, Department of Restorative Dentistry, Turkey

Saturnino Marco Lupi, Arianna Rodriguez y Baena, Claudia Todaro and Ruggero Rodriguez y Baena
Department of Clinical Surgical, Diagnostic and Pediatric Sciences, University of Pavia, Pavia, Italy

Gabriele Ceccarelli
Department of Public Health, Experimental Medicine and Forensic, Human Anatomy Unit, University of Pavia, Pavia, Italy

Fatme Mouchref Hamasni, Fady El Hajj and Rima Abdallah
Department of Periodontology, Faculty of Dental Medicine, Lebanese University, Hadath, Lebanon

Suraj Arora
Department of Restorative Dentistry, College of Dentistry, King Khalid University, Abha, Asir Province, Saudi Arabia

Gurdeep Singh Gill and Priyanka Setia
Department of Conservative Dentistry and Endodontics, JCD Dental College, Sirsa, Haryana, India

Anshad Mohamed Abdulla
Department of Pediatric Dentistry and Orthodontic Sciences, College of Dentistry, King Khalid University, Abha,Asir Province, Saudi Arabia

Ganapathy Sivadas
Department of Pedodontics and Preventive Dentistry, Faculty of Dentistry, Asian Institute of Medicine, Science and Technology (AIMST) University, Kedah, Malaysia

Vaishnavi Vedam
Department of Oral Pathology, Faculty of Dentistry, Asian Institute of Medicine, Science and Technology (AIMST) University,Kedah, Malaysia

George Borja de Freitas, Evelyne Pedroza de Andrade and Victor Ângelo Montalli
Department of Oral Pathology, São Leopoldo Mandic Institute and Research Center, Campinas, SP, Brazil

Riedel Frota Sá Nogueira Neves, Stefanny Torres dos Santos and Daniella Cristina da Costa Araújo
Department Maxillofacial Surgery, Hospital Getúlio Vargas, Recife, PE, Brazil

M. Ayhan, Sabri Cemil İşler and C. Kasapoglu
Faculty of Dentistry, Department of Oral and Maxillofacial Surgery, Istanbul University, Istanbul, Turkey

Rakshit Vijay Khandeparker and Purva Vijay Khandeparker
Department of Oral and Maxillofacial Surgery, Goa Dental College and Hospital, Bambolim, Goa, India

Anirudha Virginkar
ICU Horizon Hospital, Margao, Goa, India

Kiran Savant
Rejoice Aesthetic Centre, Bangalore, Karnataka, India

S. Nagarajan M. P. Sockalingam, Mohd Safwani Affan Alli Awang Talip and Ahmad Shuhud Irfani Zakaria
Centre for Family Oral Health, Faculty of Dentistry, The National University of Malaysia (UKM), Kuala Lumpur, Malaysia

Layal Ghandour and Samar Bou-Assi
Department of Orthodontics and Dentofacial Orthopedics, Faculty of Dentistry, Lebanese University, Hadath, Lebanon

Hisham F. Bahmad
Department of Anatomy, Cell Biology, and Physiological Sciences, Faculty of Medicine, American University of Beirut,Beirut, Lebanon

Samar Bou-Assi
Division of Orthodontics and Dentofacial Orthopedics, Department of Otolaryngology-Head and Neck Surgery, Faculty of Medicine,American University of Beirut Medical Center, Beirut, Lebanon

Sara Dhoum, Kaoutar Laslami, Fatimazahraa Rouggani, Amal El Ouazzani and Mouna Jabri
Department of Conservative Dentistry and Endodontics, School of Dentistry of Casablanca, Casablanca, Morocco

Turker Yucesoy, Erdem Kilic and Alper Alkan
Oral and Maxillofacial Surgery Department, Dentistry Faculty, Bezmialem Vakif University, Istanbul, Turkey

Fatma Dogruel
Oral and Maxillofacial Surgery Department, Dentistry Faculty, Erciyes University, Kayseri, Turkey

Fahri Bayram
Endocrinology Department, Medicine Faculty, Erciyes University, Kayseri, Turkey

Alper Celal Akcan
General Surgery Department, Medicine Faculty, Erciyes University, Kayseri, Turkey

Figen Ozturk
Pathology Department, Medicine Faculty, Erciyes University, Kayseri, Turkey

Nour Mellouli, Raouaa Belkacem Chebil, Marwa Darej and Lamia Oualha
Oral Medicine and Oral Surgery, Dental Department, University Hospital Sahloul, Sousse, Tunisia
Oral Health and Oro-Facial Rehabilitation Laboratory Research (LR12ES11), Faculty of Dental Medicine, University of Monastir, Avenue Avicenne, 5019 Monastir, Tunisia

Yosra Hasni
Endocrinology Department, University Hospital Farhat Hached, Sousse, Tunisia

Nabiha Douki
Oral Health and Oro-Facial Rehabilitation Laboratory Research (LR12ES11), Faculty of Dental Medicine, University of Monastir, Avenue Avicenne, 5019 Monastir, Tunisia
Endodontics, Dental Department, University Hospital Sahloul, Sousse, Tunisia

Stuardo Valenzuela, José M. Olivares and Nicolás Weiss
Postgraduate Implant Dentistry Department, School of Dentistry, Universidad Andres Bello, Santiago, Chile

Dafna Benadof
School of Dentistry, Universidad Andres Bello, Santiago, Chile

Chithra Aramanadka, Abhay Taranath Kamath and Adarsh Kudva
Department of Oral and Maxillofacial Surgery, Manipal College of Dental Sciences, Manipal, Karnataka, India

Guilherme da Gama Ramos, Danilo Lazzari Ciotti, Raquel Adriano Dantas and Marina Nottingham Guerreiro
São Leopoldo Mandic Institute and Research Center, R. José Rocha Junqueira 13, 13045-755 Campinas, SP, Brazil

Samuel Rehder Wimmers Ferreira and Maide Rehder Wimmers Ferreira Margarido
Paulista Association of Dental Surgeons, Rua José Nardon 177, 13419-000 Piracicaba, SP, Brazil

Tengku Aszraf Tengku Shaeran and A. R. Samsudin
Oral and Maxillofacial Surgery Unit, School of Dental Sciences, University of Science Malaysia (USM), 16150 Kubang Kerian,Kelantan, Malaysia

A. R. Samsudin
Sharjah Institute for Medical Research (SIMR), University of Sharjah, Sharjah, UAE

Emily A. Pope
University of North Carolina School of Dentistry, Chapel Hill, NC, USA

Michael W. Roberts
Department of Pediatric Dentistry, University of North Carolina School of Dentistry, Chapel Hill, NC, USA

E. LaRee Johnson
Department of Pediatric Dentistry, Private Practice of Pediatric Dentistry, Raleigh, NC, USA

Clark L. Morris
Private Practice of Pediatric Dentistry, Raleigh, NC, USA

Mathieu Lemaitre
Department of Biology, Toulouse Dental School, University of Toulouse III, Toulouse University Hospital, Toulouse, France

Sarah Cousty
Department of Oral Surgery, Toulouse Dental School, University of Toulouse III, Toulouse University Hospital, Toulouse, France

Mathieu Marty
Department of Pediatric Dentistry, Toulouse Dental School, University of Toulouse III, Toulouse University Hospital,Toulouse, France

Talib Amin Naqash
Department of Prosthetic Dentistry, King Khalid University College of Dentistry, Abha, Saudi Arabia

Ibrahim Alshahrani
Department of Pediatric Dentistry and Orthodontic Sciences, King Khalid University College of Dentistry, Abha, Saudi Arabia

Siripan Simasetha
Dental Department, Bhumibol Adulyadej Hospital, The Royal Thai Air Force, Bangkok, Thailand

Wilson Matsumoto, Victor Garone Morelli, Rossana Pereira de Almeida, Alexandre Elias Trivellato, Cássio Edvard Sverzut and Takami Hirono Hotta
Dental School of Ribeirão Preto, Dental Materials and Prosthodontic Department, University of São Paulo, Ribeirão Preto, SP, Brazil

Mohamad Syahrizal Halim
Conservative Dentistry Unit, School of Dental Sciences, Universiti Sains Malaysia, Health Campus, 16150 Kota Bharu,Kelantan, Malaysia

Tengku Fazrina Tengku Mohd Ariff
Centre for Restorative Dentistry Studies, Faculty of Dentistry, Jalan Hospital, Universiti Teknologi MARA, Sungai Buloh Campus,47000 Sungai Buloh, Selangor Darul Ehsan, Malaysia

Tássia Carina Stafuzza, Luciana Lourenço Ribeiro Vitor, Daniela Rios, Thiago Cruvinel Silva, Maria Aparecida Andrade Moreira Machado and Thais Marchini Oliveira
Department of Pediatric Dentistry, Orthodontics, Public Health, Bauru School of Dentistry, University of São Paulo,Bauru, SP, Brazil

Maria Aparecida Andrade Moreira Machado and and Thais Marchini Oliveira
Hospital for the Rehabilitation of Craniofacial Anomalies, University of São Paulo, Bauru, SP, Brazil

Rocco Franco, Laura Di Renzo and Antonino De Lorenzo
Section of Clinical Nutrition and Nutrigenomic, Department of Biomedicine and Prevention, School of Applied Medical-Surgical Sciences, University of Rome Tor Vergata, Via Montpellier 1, 00133 Rome, Italy

Michele Miranda and Patrizio Bollero
Department of Systems Medicine, Medical School, University of Rome Tor Vergata, Rome, Italy

Alberta Barlattani
Department of Clinical Sciences and Translational Medicine, University of Rome Tor Vergata, Rome, Italy

S. Nagarajan M. P. Sockalingam, Katherine Kong Loh Seu, Halimah Mohamed Noor and Ahmad Shuhud Irfani Zakaria
Department of Operative Dentistry, Faculty of Dentistry, National University Malaysia (UKM), Jalan Raja Muda Abdul Aziz, 50300 Kuala Lumpur, Malaysia

Index